KU-481-893

Design of Studies for Medical Research

DAVID MACHIN

Division of Clinical Trials and Epidemiological Sciences,
National Cancer Centre, Singapore,
Children's Cancer and Leukaemia Group, University of Leicester, UK
Institute of General Practice and Primary Care, School of Health and Related Sciences,
University of Sheffield, UK

and

MICHAEL J. CAMPBELL

Medical Statistics Group, Institute of General Practice and Primary Care, School of Health and
Related Sciences, University of Sheffield, UK

John Wiley & Sons, Ltd

A 070647

W 20.5

Copyright © 2005   John Wiley & Sons Ltd, The Atrium, Southern Gate, Chichester,
West Sussex PO19 8SQ, England

Telephone   (+44) 1243 779777

Email (for orders and customer service enquiries): cs-books@wiley.co.uk

Reprinted with corrections February 2007
Reprinted March 2007

All Rights Reserved. No part of this publication may be reproduced, stored in a retrieval system or
transmitted in any form or by any means, electronic, mechanical, photocopying, recording, scanning or
otherwise, except under the terms of the Copyright, Designs and Patents Act 1988 or under the terms of a
licence issued by the Copyright Licensing Agency Ltd, 90 Tottenham Court Road, London W1T 4LP, UK,
without the permission in writing of the Publisher. Requests to the Publisher should be addressed to the
Permissions Department, John Wiley & Sons Ltd, The Atrium, Southern Gate, Chichester, West Sussex
PO19 8SQ, England, or emailed to permreq@wiley.co.uk, or faxed to (+44) 1243 770620.

Designations used by companies to distinguish their products are often claimed as trademarks. All brand
names and product names used in this book are trade names, service marks, trademarks or registered
trademarks of their respective owners. The Publisher is not associated with any product or vendor mentioned
in this book.

This publication is designed to provide accurate and authoritative information in regard to the subject matter
covered. It is sold on the understanding that the Publisher is not engaged in rendering professional services. If
professional advice or other expert assistance is required, the services of a competent professional should be
sought.

Other Wiley Editorial Offices

John Wiley & Sons Inc., 111 River Street, Hoboken, NJ 07030, USA

Jossey-Bass, 989 Market Street, San Francisco, CA 94103-1741, USA

Wiley-VCH Verlag GmbH, Boschstr. 12, D-69469 Weinheim, Germany

John Wiley & Sons Australia Ltd, 33 Park Road, Milton, Queensland 4064, Australia

John Wiley & Sons (Asia) Pte Ltd, 2 Clementi Loop #02-01, Jin Xing Distripark, Singapore 129809

John Wiley & Sons Canada Ltd, 22 Worcester Road, Etobicoke, Ontario, Canada M9W 1L1

Wiley also publishes its books in a variety of electronic formats. Some content that appears in print may not
be available in electronic books.

Library of Congress Cataloging-in-Publication Data

Machin, David.
  Design of studies for medical research / David Machin, Michael J. Campbell.
    p. cm.
  Includes bibliographical references and index.
  ISBN 0-470-84495-7 (alk. paper)
    1. Medicine–Research–Methodology.   I. Campbell, Michael J. II. Title.

  R850.M23 2005
  610′.72–dc22

                                                          2004065408

British Library Cataloguing in Publication Data

A catalogue record for this book is available from the British Library

ISBN 978-0-470-84495-3 (P/B)

Typeset by Dobbie Typesetting Ltd, Tavistock, Devon
Printed and bound in Great Britain by Antony Rowe Ltd, Chippenham, Wilts
This book is printed on acid-free paper responsibly manufactured from sustainable forestry
in which at least two trees are planted for each one used for paper production.

To
Christine Machin
and
Jacinta Campbell

THE LIBRARY
KENT & SUSSEX HOSPITAL
TUNBRIDGE WELLS
KENT TN4 8AT

Contents

Preface

There are many textbooks on medical statistics, but the majority concentrate on statistical analysis. However, unless care is taken as to how the data were collected in the first place, no amount of sophisticated analysis can save the experimenter from possibly making misleading conclusions. A poorly designed study is like a house built on sand, easily washed away when the design flaws are pointed out. It appears to us that few textbooks place sufficient emphasis on design of studies and so the purpose of this book is an attempt to fill this gap.

In general design books concentrate on the design of experiments. We have broadened this to include chapters on the design of surveys, epidemiological studies and studies concerned with diagnosis and of prognostic factors. Emphasis is also placed on estimating an appropriate study size and how to choose subjects for inclusion in a study. Much data are captured on forms or questionnaires and since we feel this area to be somewhat neglected by statisticians, we have included a chapter covering it. Although it may not appear to be of immediate relevance to good design, we also cover the essential care to be taken when describing the study design in any eventual publication.

Our plan with this book is to emphasise the importance of good design, whether in preclinical or clinical studies, clinical trials or epidemiological research. We concentrate on research of all types involving human subjects, although many of the designs considered are applicable to laboratory bench and animal studies. We have purposely avoided giving details of statistical analysis, although some of these are unavoidable.

We hope this book will prove useful to investigators with the design of their studies, when completing a research proposal or ethics form, and also for those doing a research methods course.

We would like to thank colleagues in Leicester, Sheffield and Southampton, UK, in Singapore and in Skövde, Sweden, for encouragement and advice. We would also like to thank colleagues, and students for bringing their design problems to us.

David Machin
Michael J. Campbell

Southover, Dorset and Sheffield

July 2004

1 What is Evidence?

Summary

This chapter introduces the ideas associated with evidence-based health care and contrasts this approach with earlier approaches in clinical medicine which had largely relied on describing pathophysiological processes. We consider the nature of proof using evidence and describe the Bradford-Hill criteria which are useful in determining how reliably causation has been established in a study. We define broad areas that distinguish laboratory and animal experiments from studies and clinical trials in humans. Experimental design can be appropriate to research in preclinical, clinical and epidemiological studies. Statistical models are at the heart of the design of studies and the purpose of a good design is to estimate the parameters of a model as efficiently as possible.

We also emphasise the need to check local regulations with respect to ethical clearance of studies and informed consent from the study participants. It is important to develop a formal protocol for any study and describe in general terms the contents of such a protocol. Published guidelines and standards for reporting the results of studies are useful pointers for consideration by the study design teams.

1.1 INTRODUCTION

This is the era of 'evidence-based medicine' (EBM) or more comprehensively 'evidence-based health care' (EBHC). EBM requires that we should consider critically all evidence about whether, for example, a treatment works, an agent causes a disease, or a drug is toxic. This requires a systematic assembly of all available evidence followed by a critical appraisal of this evidence. Before this paradigm had been formulated, biomedical investigators considered it sufficient to understand the pathophysiological process of a disorder. As a consequence the physician would prescribe to patients with relevant symptoms drugs, or other treatments, that had been shown to interrupt this process. Thus the practice of medicine had been based on history taking and clinical examination followed by treatment of symptoms, all based on the accepted pathophysiology of the condition diagnosed at the relevant time.

Design of Studies for Medical Research. D. Machin and M. J. Campbell
© 2005 John Wiley & Sons Ltd. ISBN 0 470 84495 7

Example *– removing the cause – ventricular ectopic beats*

Sackett, Richardson, Rosenberg and Haynes (1997) give an example of a finding that patients who displayed ventricular ectopic beats after a myocardial infarction had occurred were at high risk of sudden death. Following this observation drugs were then widely prescribed to suppress these ectopic beats, on the assumption that removing the cause would reduce the effect. However, subsequent randomised controlled trials which examined clinical outcomes, and not the physiological process alone, showed that use of these drugs actually *increased* death rates rather than decreased them. The use of these drugs is now contra-indicated.

Example *– reducing the risk – premature babies*

Gilman, Cheng, Winter and Scragg (1995) describe a study related to concerns of neonatologists who had always kept premature babies lying on their fronts. One tacit assumption was that, should the premature baby vomit, the baby would be less likely to inhale the vomit. This practice was extended to all babies. However, subsequent epidemiological studies showed that babies who were habitually put on their fronts were exposed to a higher risk of sudden infant death. A 'back-to-sleep' campaign was initiated and the sudden infant deaths in England and Wales dropped from some 2000 to less than 600 per year as a direct consequence. The argument for putting babies to rest on their fronts, albeit reasonable in nature, was not *evidence-based*.

Systematic reviews combine the evidence from individual studies to give a more powerful analysis of any effect. It is important to realise that they can only be as good as their component parts. Thus if the studies being reviewed are of poor quality then inferences drawn from an overview will have to be made with extreme caution. In contrast, if the basic information is of high quality then their collective and systematic review and synthesis clearly adds substantially to the evidence base for clinical medicine.

1.2   EVIDENCE AND PROOF

Any discussion of EBM gives rise to the question, what is evidence? The first concern is with the problem of *proof* and philosophers have long argued over this. In mathematics, the ancient Greeks demonstrated rigorous proofs of many *theorems* (literally God-like things), especially in algebra and geometry, and they thought of these as general laws.

Thus, we know for certain that Pythagoras' Theorem is true. The question arises as to whether one can have similar certainty in other areas of human enquiry.

In the natural sciences, Francis Bacon (1561–1626) described the work of scientists as collecting information and adducing natural laws. However, David Hume (1711–1776) concluded that no number of singular observations, however large, could logically entail an unrestricted general statement. Just because event A follows event B on one occasion, it does not follow that event B will be observed the next time we see A. Thus it does not logically follow, in the manner that a mathematical theorem is true, that A will always follow B whether we observe A and B together on two, twenty or two thousand occasions. The point here is that simply *observing* an association is not proof that an association actually exists.

There may, however, be real reasons why two events are associated, and in general one would hope to discover these. Thus, although we observe that 20 consecutive bed-ridden patients develop pressure sores, this does not logically imply that the 21st patient will do so. However, it does suggest a pattern that would be foolish to ignore when considering appropriate care for patient 21.

'Hume's problem' troubled philosophers as it seemed to discourage endeavours to make sense of nature. It was not until the last century that Karl Popper (1902–1994) proposed the idea of falsifiability. Falsifiability states that laws cannot be shown to be either true or false but that they can only be held *provisionally* true. He pointed out that observations cannot be used to prove laws, but can falsify them. Hume's famous example is the universal law 'all swans are white'. This cannot be proven, no matter how many swans one sees that are white, but it would take only a single black swan to refute the law. This has direct bearing on statistical inference, where, as part of the study design, one sets up a null hypothesis and then tries to refute it with the experimental observations. Failure to reject the null hypothesis does not logically imply that one should accept it, rather it implies that we do not have enough evidence to reject it.

Clinical trials which compare treatments are designed with a null hypothesis in mind, namely that the treatments have no differential effect on patient outcome. We try and disprove this null hypothesis using patient data. However, we can *never* prove a null effect.

The basis of EBM is that any guidance arising from any review of evidence is only *provisional*, albeit based on the best evidence available at the time. We can collect more evidence and, if this concurs with the existing evidence, it may give us greater confidence in our guidelines, but still cannot prove them. However, later evidence may contradict the existing theories (and hence disprove them), however well founded the past evidence is.

This approach may seem rather negative, but in fact it is liberating. What Popper's philosophy gives scientists is the freedom of 'trying their best'. With this they avoid claiming omnipotence, such as would be implied if their statements were assumed true for all time. It gives scientists a model whereby criticism of existing models is actively encouraged. It enables us to differentiate the good scientific theories from the poor. For good ones, one can devise experiments to attempt to falsify the hypotheses arising from the theories. However, all theories are not equally valid. Thus theories that have withstood attempts to disprove them are to be preferred over those that have not been so tested. It is worth pointing out, however, that often the choice of *which* experiments

Table 1.1 The Bradford-Hill criteria to assess causality (after
Hill, 1965; reproduced by permission of the Royal Society of
Medicine)

1.	Temporality
2.	Consistency
3.	Coherence
4.	Strength of association
5.	Biological gradient
6.	Specificity
7.	Plausibility
8.	Freedom from, or control of, confounding and bias
9.	Analogous results found elsewhere

to conduct are financial, social or political decisions. Thus lack of supporting evidence
for a theory may not necessarily be a deficiency of the theory itself, but rather the lack
of will to *test* the theory.

Outside of the realm of mathematics, and in the less predictable fields of the
biomedical and clinical sciences, the nature of human variability has meant that
universal laws are rare. There are some obvious laws, such as if a person is deprived of
oxygen they soon die; but such laws are the exception. Thus if we give a person a large
dose of arsenic, they do not inevitably die. Rather than with establishing universal laws,
biomedical science is concerned with a number of basic questions such as: Does
exposure to substance *A* increase the risk of disease *B*? Does treatment *C* cure more
people with disease *D* than other therapies?

More than a century ago Robert Koch (1843–1910) devised a number of questions
the answers to which could be used to try and decide whether a specific bacterium
caused a particular disease. These were modified by Bradford Hill (Hill, 1965) to a
general examination of whether an event, such as an environmental exposure or
smoking, would increase the risk of disease or prescribing a medical treatment improves
the chance of cure. The Bradford-Hill criteria are summarised in Table 1.1.

In the Bradford-Hill criteria temporality means that the effect follows the cause and
not vice versa. Thus a fall in lung cancer deaths in UK men succeeded a drop in the
numbers of male smokers with a lag in time of some 30 years. This lag lends weight to a
causal link between smoking and lung cancer. Consistency implies that the same fall in
lung cancer deaths has been observed in women, or in other countries where smoking
prevalence has fallen. Coherence means that different study types, such as case–control
and cohort studies addressing the same issue, lead to similar conclusions. Strength of
the association suggests that the stronger the effect the more plausible the causality. For
example, smokers have 10 times the risk of lung cancer compared with non-smokers.
The idea concerning the biological gradient is that if heavy smokers are found to be at
greater risk of lung cancer than light smokers, then the case for causality is
strengthened.

Specificity suggests that if the link were causal, the smokers would be mainly at risk
from respiratory disease mortality, and not from other unrelated types of mortality
such as those arising from road accidents. The relationship appears plausible as
cigarette smoke is inhaled into the lungs and autopsy evidence from smokers and non-
smokers documents clear differences between their respective lungs. A confounding

variable is one that is related to both the exposure and the outcome, but not through a causal pathway. For smoking, genetics has been argued as a confounder on the basis that the impulse to smoke may be genetic – certainly if parents smoke then children are more likely to smoke. Also genes may control the risk of lung cancer. If the genes for smoking and lung cancer were linked then it would appear that smoking and lung cancer were causally related. However, if the genetic theory were true, it would have a hard time to explain away the other causal evidence such as that provided by temporality. Bias could occur in a study or survey because people with lung cancer may be more likely to recall details of their smoking history than people without lung cancer.

Just as in philosophy we cannot prove a universal law, so in medicine we cannot prove absolutely a causal effect. Satisfying the Bradford-Hill criteria increases the likelihood that a causal effect is present, but cannot give an absolute proof of it. Hill (1965) himself admitted: 'none of my nine viewpoints can bring indisputable evidence for or against the cause-and-effect hypothesis and none can be regarded as a sine qua non'.

As one example, this philosophy has considerable implications when epidemiologists try to show that the measles, mumps and rubella (MMR) vaccine does not cause autism. We can never prove the null that that there is no association between the MMR vaccine and autism. All we can do is demonstrate that, if there is a risk, then the risk is very low. It is up to those who advise on public health issues to decide whether the risk of autism is lower and/or less damaging than the competing risks associated with a child having measles. In this respect, temporality was a major issue as in the UK increases in the diagnosis of autism had been linked to the introduction of MMR. However, this increase has not been observed in other countries, none of the other Bradford-Hill criteria are satisfied and there is no clear biological theory linking vaccines to autism.

1.3   COLLECTING THE EVIDENCE

In certain circumstances, evidence for a particular theory may be built up by a series of well-conducted experiments under very controlled (perhaps laboratory) conditions. In contrast, other information may only be obtained incidentally, such as long-term information collected from survivors of the nuclear bombs exploded in the 1940s or by the radiation leakage from Chernobyl nuclear reactors in the 1980s. Thus, it is convenient to distinguish studies in which the investigator conducting *experiments* has total control over the structure of the study and the variables to be some of the observed, and *observational* studies in which the investigator cannot manipulate the values of the variables but merely observe their value.

Control of the 'experiment' is clearly a desirable feature – perhaps easy to attain in the chemistry laboratory but not so easy with living material, particularly if they are animal or human. However, the additional difficulties imposed on the design of studies in human subjects imply that special care should be taken in the design of the studies planned. A good study should answer the questions posed as efficiently as possible. In round terms, this implies with as few subjects as is reasonably possible for a reliable answer to be obtained.

Although 'good science' may lead to an optimal choice of design, the exigencies of 'real life' may cause these ideals to be modified. Nevertheless we can still have some

Table 1.2 Characteristics of laboratory, laboratory animal and human experimental studies

Design feature	Laboratory	Animal	Human
Method of assessments	No restriction	If invasive, may not be acceptable	If invasive, may not be acceptable
Treatment or intervention	No restriction on choice of treatments – other than scientific judgement	Some procedures may bring unacceptable suffering	Implicit that treatments should do some good – thus an innocuous or placebo treatment may not be acceptable
Subject safety issues	None	Minor	Paramount – overriding principle is the safety of the subjects
Protocol review	Scientific only	Scientific and ethical	Scientific and ethical
Consent	None	None	Fully informed consent mandatory
Recruitment	Experiment can be conducted at one calendar time point	Experiment can be conducted at one calendar time point	Usually, subjects recruited one-by-one over calendar time
Time scale	May be relatively short – hours, days or weeks	May be relatively short – days, weeks or months	May be relatively long – weeks, months or years
Study size	All observations planned are made	All observations planned are made	Subjects may refuse to continue in the study at any stage
Observations	Assessed at one calendar time point	Assessed at one calendar time point	Usually, subjects assessed one-by-one over calendar time
Design changes	Immediate	Possibly ethical constraints	Almost certainly requires new ethical approval
Data protection	None	None	Confidentiality and often National Guidelines for storage
Reporting	No formal rules – journal editor's prerogative	No formal rules – journal editor's prerogative	CONSORT for Phase III trials (Begg et al., 1996)

hierarchy in the choice of designs, but where we can enter this hierarchy will depend on circumstance. Thus we do not aim for the 'best' design only the 'best realisable' design in our context.

Table 1.2 illustrates some aspects of the differences that need to be considered when comparing (bench) laboratory-based (non-animal or -human) studies with clinical studies. In some sense the laboratory provides, at least in theory, the greatest flexibility in terms of the experimental design and studies in human subjects should be designed (whenever possible) to be as close to these standards as possible. In general it can be seen that the requirements for human studies are more restrictive. For example safety, in terms of the welfare of the experimental units concerned, is of overriding concern in clinical studies, possibly of little relevance in animal studies and of no relevance to laboratory studies. As a further example, no consent procedures are required for laboratory or animal studies whereas this is a very important consideration in all human experimentation, even in a clinical trial with therapeutic intent.

1.4 TYPES OF STUDY AND HIERARCHY OF DESIGNS

For the purposes of this book we consider three broad areas of medical research. 'Preclinical' studies that are essentially laboratory-based studies and may involve human specimens or directly the humans themselves. These tend to be relatively small and afford a high degree of control for the experimenter. Examples might be studies of changes in brain image after a mental calculation or the elicitation of symptoms in a healthy person by inducing a drop in their blood glucose levels. On the other hand, 'clinical' studies are ones that involve actively intervening in the management of patients in some way, such as in a trial of a new drug. Finally 'epidemiological' studies, including surveys, broadly speaking, do not involve active intervention, but rather observe outcomes to evaluate, for example, a potential risk. Table 1.3 describes a broad

Table 1.3 The relative strength of evidence obtained from alternative designs for preclinical, clinical and epidemiological studies

	Evidence level	Type of study
Preclinical	Strongest	Blinded randomised comparative study
		Non-randomised comparative study
		Before-and-after design
	Weakest	Case-series
Clinical	Strongest	Double-blind randomised controlled trial (RCT)
		Single-blind RCT
		Community intervention study: cluster design
		Non-blinded RCT
		Non-randomised prospective study
		Non-randomised retrospective study
		Before-and-after design (historical control)
	Weakest	Case-series
Epidemiological	Strongest	Cohort study
		Case–control study
		Cross-sectional survey
	Weakest	Case-series

'hierarchy' of designs that give an increasing weight to evidence obtained from these three different types of clinical study.

PRECLINICAL

The design that can provide the strongest evidence is the randomised comparative study in which the experimental units are allocated to an intervention by some form of random mechanism as is described in Chapter 4. In a comparison between two interventions, or an intervention and a control, it is sometimes possible to give the experimental unit both interventions. In that case it is important to randomise the *order* of the interventions. A further refinement is to blind (or mask) the experimenter as to which intervention has been given to which unit. In practice, this can only be done when there are several investigators involved each with different roles in the experimental process, as another desirable feature is that the investigator doing the evaluations is also blind to the intervention received. The measures used for evaluation should also be as objective as is possible in the circumstance. Such a design is termed a *double-blind* (or double-masked) randomised controlled study. There are clearly extensions to this since one could also blind the data analyst. The purpose of the 'blinding' is to make all aspects of the study conduct to be as objective as possible and hence as free as possible from bias.

The weakest level of evidence is provided by a *case-series* that, at one extreme, may be an observation from a single unit.

CLINICAL

In parallel with preclinical studies, the design that provides the strongest type of evidence is again the *double-blind randomised controlled trial* (RCT). In this, the patients are allocated to treatment at random. In this way we can ensure that *in the long run* patients, before treatment commences, will be comparable in the intervention and control groups. Clearly, if one knew which were the important prognostic factors, one could match the patients in the intervention and control groups by other means. However, the advantage that randomisation retains is that it provides for *unknown* as well as the *known* prognostic factors, which could not be achieved by matching. Thus the reason for the intellectual attraction of the double-blind RCT is that it is the *only* design that can give us an absolute certainty that there is no bias in favour of one group compared to another at the start of the trial.

When testing new therapies, we might try a 'before-and-after' design in which outcomes before and after the introduction of the new therapy are compared. This is a very plausible scenario. After all, Alexander Fleming (1881–1955) did not need a clinical trial to demonstrate the efficacy of penicillin. Before penicillin became available most people with certain bacterial infections died, afterwards they survived. The main disadvantage of 'before-and-after' designs is that we have no idea whether the patients in the 'before' group and those in the 'after' group are comparable. Whilst it is hard to imagine the natural history of a disease would change when a new therapy is introduced, it is plausible that the way the disease is diagnosed and patients are recruited for treatment do.

An extension of a 'before-and-after' design is the use of what are known as historical controls. In this case an investigator may have a group of patients on a test therapy, and chooses a comparable group of patients with the same disease treated in the past by a different (comparator or control) treatment.

A case-series may report that a particular compression bandage in patients with venous leg ulcers has been tried and has achieved excellent results. There are many criticisms of this design. Firstly, we do not know how the patients have been selected; the clinical team may have an unerring eye for selecting those patients to be given the bandage who are likely to recover anyway. Secondly, without further evidence of the natural history of the disease, we do not know whether the patients may have recovered naturally, without intervention. Thirdly we do not know whether this type of compression bandage is better or worse than any other.

A rather stronger design is a prospective one called a *quasi-experimental* design. In this patients from one clinic (say) are given the compression bandage and patients in another clinic act as a control group and get standard therapy. The difficulty here is that again patients in the different clinics may not be comparable.

A design that is often used in Health Services Research is a *community intervention* design. This is an extension of a quasi-experimental design. For example, the cure rates for chronic ulcers are observed in two clinics. A new intervention is introduced in one clinic, and after a period of time the cure rates are again measured. An important point is that the subjects at each time point are *different*. Also the allocation of the intervention to the clinic/community is done for pragmatic reasons, such as convenience.

EPIDEMIOLOGICAL

Suppose we wish to investigate the link between chronic cough and smoking. The strongest design would be to choose a group of people, initially free of cough, some of whom were smokers and follow them up for a number of years and see how many develop a cough. This design will conform to the first Bradford-Hill criterion, in that it can test temporality. A weaker design would be a case–control study, which would identify groups of people with and without chronic cough and ask them about their smoking history. Another design would be to simply survey a group of people and ask them whether they have a chronic cough and about their smoking history. The problem with the case–control and survey designs is that they cannot properly test temporality – coughers might choose to smoke to soothe their throats! The weakest design would be a case-series whereby an investigator, say, notes that a series of people who consult about the cough appear to have a high likelihood of being smokers.

1.5   BIOLOGICAL VARIABILITY

Measurements made on human subjects rarely give exactly the same results from one occasion to the next. Even in adults our height varies a little during the course of the day. If one measures blood sugar levels of an individual on one particular day and then again the following day, under exactly the same conditions, greater variation in this than that of height would be expected. Hence were such a subject to receive an intervention (perhaps to lower the blood sugar levels) before the next measure then any lowering observed could not necessarily be ascribed to the intervention itself. The levels of inherent variability may be very high so that, perhaps in the circumstances where a subject has an illness, the oscillations in these may disguise, at least in the early stages of treatment, the beneficial effect of the treatment given to improve the condition.

With such variability it follows that, in any comparison made in a biomedical context, differences between subjects or groups of subjects frequently occur. These differences may be due to real effects, random variation or both. It is the job of the experimenter to decide how this variation should be taken note of in the design of the ensuing study, the purpose being that once at the analysis stage, the variation can be partitioned suitably into that due to any real effect of the intervention or real difference between groups, from the random or chance component.

1.6   STATISTICAL CONSIDERATIONS

STATISTICAL MODELS

Whatever the type of study, it is usually convenient to think of the underlying structure of the design in terms of a statistical model. Once the model is specified the object of the corresponding study is then to estimate the parameters of this model as precisely as is reasonable.

Suppose in a particular experiment, we believed that an outcome y is related to the input x by means of the linear equation

$$y = \beta_0 + \beta_1 x + \varepsilon. \tag{1.1}$$

In equation (1.1), β_0 and β_1 are constants and are termed the parameters of the model. In contrast, ε represents the noise (or error) and this is assumed to be random and have a mean value of 0 across all subjects studied, and variance σ^2. The object of a study would be to estimate β_0 and β_1 in this relationship although often β_1 is the main concern. We write these estimates as b_0 and b_1 to distinguish them from the corresponding parameters.

In a laboratory experiment x might be the amount of an allergen injected under the skin and y the area of the wheal that develops. If the allergen injected results in a wheal in all subjects, but the amount injected does not influence its size, then $\beta_1 = 0$ in equation (1.1). In a clinical trial, x might take values 0 and 1 corresponding to the control and test treatments under study. In this case the null hypothesis of $\beta_1 = 0$ corresponds to no difference in efficacy between the two treatments. For an observational study y might be the diastolic blood pressure (DBP) of the individuals concerned and x their corresponding salt intake in the year before the DBP was measured. In this case, $\beta_1 = 0$ implies that the salt intake does not influence the subsequent DBP.

On the basis of this model, the two fundamental issues in an experiment to consider are:

(1) What levels of the independent variable x to choose?
(2) How many experimental units to observe?

DESIGN EFFECT

The aim of a study is to obtain as good an estimate of β_1 as possible. This implies that, for the design values $x_1, x_2, \ldots, x_N$ under experimental control, we choose their values so that the associated variance of b_1, $\mathrm{Var}(b_1)$, or equivalently its standard error, $SE(b_1)$, is as small as is reasonably possible. The variance of b_1 is expected to be

$$\mathrm{Var}(b_1) = \frac{\sigma^2}{S}, \qquad (1.2)$$

where

$$S = \sum_{i=1}^{N} (x_i - \bar{x})^2$$

and N is the number of experimental units in the particular study. A measure of the efficiency of a particular design

$$E = 1/\mathrm{Var}(b_1). \qquad (1.3)$$

Thus the smaller $\mathrm{Var}(b_1)$ the larger E and so if the values of x are under our control, we might choose them when planning the study to minimise $\mathrm{Var}(b_1)$. This choice is equivalent to choosing them in such a way as to maximise S.

In a design with values of x constrained to be within two limits (say) x_{Min} and x_{Max}, then to minimise $\mathrm{Var}(b_1)$, we would choose half the x's to have the value x_{Min} and half to have x_{Max}. This implies that

$$S = N(x_{\mathrm{Max}} - x_{\mathrm{Min}})^2/4, \qquad (1.4)$$

and so

$$E = \frac{N(x_{\mathrm{Max}} - x_{\mathrm{Min}})^2}{4\sigma^2}. \qquad (1.5)$$

Thus E, the efficiency, gets larger, as $(x_{\mathrm{Max}} - x_{\mathrm{Min}})$ increases.

For a given resource, one can get the most from a study by choice of a good design. The relative efficiency of two designs, I and II, addressing the same question is expressed by the ratio of their efficiencies, and is termed the design effect (DE), that is

$$DE = \frac{E_{II}}{E_I} = \frac{1/\mathrm{Var}(b_{II})}{1/\mathrm{Var}(b_I)} = \frac{\mathrm{Var}(b_I)}{\mathrm{Var}(b_{II})} \qquad (1.6)$$

Suppose we were conducting a trial of a new drug at dose d, and plan to compare this with a placebo (zero dose). In this situation, $x_{\mathrm{Min}}=0$ and $x_{\mathrm{Max}}=d$, then from equation (1.5) $E_I=Nd^2/4\sigma^2$. Alternatively we may choose a lower dose, say $d/2$, for comparison with placebo from which $E_{II}=(Nd^2/4)/4\sigma^2 = Nd^2/16\sigma^2$. Now comparing the two designs, equation (1.6) gives

$$DE = E_{II}/E_I = \frac{Nd^2}{16\sigma^2} \left/ \frac{Nd^2}{4\sigma^2} \right. = \frac{1}{4}.$$

This suggests that the second design is less efficient than the first, even though it is using the same number of experimental units, N.

PREDICTED VALUE

Another way to choose a design is to consider how precisely the predicted value of y at a particular value of x is estimated. That is, once the experiment is complete and we have $y = b_0 + b_1 x$ as our estimate of equation (1.1), the object is to estimate (or predict) the value of y for a given $x = x_0$ say. This gives the estimate as $y_0 = b_0 + b_1 x_0$ and this has variance

$$\text{Var}(y_0) = \sigma^2 \left[\frac{1}{N} + \frac{(x_0 - \bar{x})^2}{S} \right]. \tag{1.7}$$

It can be shown that the 'best' design, that is the one with the minimum variance, again puts half the observations at x_{Min} and half at x_{Max}. This variance is further reduced if the value of x_0 is set equal to $\bar{x}$, which in this case is midway between x_{Min} and x_{Max}. In this situation, equation (1.7) gives $\text{Var}(y_0) = \sigma^2/N$. In contrast, even if the design keeps half the values at x_{Min} and x_{Max}, but x_0 is then set as either x_{Min} or x_{Max} then equation (1.7) is maximised as $\text{Var}(y_0) = 2\sigma^2/N$ or twice the minimum possible value.

Amongst designs that choose different values of x, ones that set the values of x to give the minimal possible variance of an estimate are described as *optimal*.

VERIFYING THE MODEL

A crucial assumption in the above design process is that the supposed linear relationship between y and x of model (1.1) is the true one (or at least close to it). If we are uncertain about this, and this will often be the case, then it would be sensible to plan for observations in the middle of the range of x as well. Thus if we wished to try and test the linearity of the relationship a good design would be to choose equal numbers, $m = N/3$, of experimental units at x_{Min}, $x_{\text{Mean}} [= (x_{\text{Max}} + x_{\text{Min}})/2]$ and x_{Max}.

***Example** – dose response – hepatocellular carcinoma*

In a randomised trial of the use of tamoxifen in patients with inoperable hepatocellular carcinoma, Chow, Tai, Tan *et al.* (2002) randomised patients to $x = 0$, 60 or 120 mg daily in the ratio of 2:1:2. At the design stage of the trial, it was anticipated that the highest tolerable dose of tamoxifen would bring the greatest therapeutic gain. However, there was also concern that additional activity might be slight above a threshold dose level and, should near-therapeutic benefit be demonstrated with a lower dose, this would be desirable – both in cost terms and potential side-effects. This is why the intermediate dose of 60 mg daily was added to the design. In the event, tamoxifen brought no survival advantage for these patients. Indeed there was evidence for declining survival with increasing dose.

In practice, optimal designs, such as these, are not commonly chosen except in clinical trials because experimenters have numerous, sometimes unstated, aims, and so choose designs that try and compromise between them. Thus a design that allocates equal numbers of subjects to a wider set of x's may not be the most efficient in terms of getting the smallest Var(b) but enables the investigator to explore the responses y over a range of x values. However, in a clinical trial, the theory of optimal design suggests that if we believe in a dose–response relationship between a drug and a response, but the main concern is to show that the drug works, then one should choose a two-arm trial. This trial would compare a zero-dose control group, and an intervention group with the maximum tolerable dose.

For an observational study, it may not be possible to manipulate the x values directly, but one can often *choose* subjects who are likely to have a wide variety of these values. Thus, if we were interested in looking at the relationship between salt intake and DBP, we might choose to investigate subjects likely to have a low salt intake and compare these with subjects likely to have a high salt intake, perhaps chosen from geographical areas whose use of salt is known to differ. Within each intake group (say, low and high) there would be similar but not identical intake values.

STUDY SIZE

Although the DE may lead one to choose one design as opposed to another, it is still necessary to decide how large the study should be. This may be done by choosing the number of observations, N, to get the variance within desirable limits which have to be set by the investigating team. This implies that we may choose N to provide a specific value for the $SE(b)$ or equivalently the width of the associated 95% confidence interval (CI) for β. In Chapter 3 we describe in general terms details of how study size may be determined and for specific designs in other relevant chapters.

1.7 INFORMED CONSENT AND ETHICAL APPROVAL

It goes without saying that, before any study can take place, individual subjects have to be identified, and formal processes for their consent will have to be instituted. Clearly, the precise details will depend on the type of study contemplated, for example, whether it involves an invasive procedure, involves completing an epidemiologically based questionnaire received through the post or has therapeutic intent.

It is also usually a requirement, although again details will vary, that all studies of whatever type involving human subjects require ethical approval before they can be carried out. In certain circumstances, these considerations may have major impact on the study design. Thus a preclinical study considering the same question in man, as one that has been asked in animals, may not have the same design. For example, in a dose-finding study the dose range for man may have to avoid low doses (as they would bring no prospect of therapeutic benefit) and high doses (as they may be potentially life-threatening). The measure of drug activity is also likely to be different.

In some countries such as the UK, studies may also be subject to research governance. This means that the studies must be scientifically valid, and have mechanisms in place to ensure that they are properly carried out, written up and

Table 1.4 Major components of a clinical protocol (based on Collins, 2001; reproduced by permission of John Wiley & Sons Ltd)

	Abstract	
1.	Background	
2.	Purpose	
3.	Methods	
		Hypotheses
		Subjects
		Interventions/Comparisons
		Design
		Number of subjects
		Analysis
4.	Recruitment	
5.	Ethics	
6.	Organisation	
7.	Study forms	

disseminated. Investigators are advised to make themselves aware of the local regulations in all of these respects at the planning stage of their study.

1.8   THE STUDY PROTOCOL

For any clinical study, the main features of the study from design to analysis will have been discussed in detail at the planning stage. It is advisable to put a summary of these into a protocol which can then provide a record and reminder of the principal features of the study. Indeed Lassere and Johnson (2002) argue that a formal mechanism for making (trial) protocols, and any amendments thereof, routinely available for examination. Although details will change from study to study, there are common items for most protocols and these are listed in Table 1.4.

The Background provides an in-depth summary with references to relevant published work. Essentially this would contain the information necessary for the Introduction that will be needed for the future paper describing the study results. The purpose of the current study and its importance would be described. The Methods section should address the (major) hypotheses under test, the statistical design, the precise types and numbers of subjects who will be investigated, the interventions they will receive or the comparisons to be made and an indication of the form(s) of statistical analysis. Again, these sections should be at least detailed enough for the subsequent journal submission. This section should also include practical details of how, and from where, the potential subjects are to be identified and screened for entry and the consent procedures.

If the study is multi-centre in nature it will usually be important to describe the relevant responsibilities with details perhaps of how subjects are registered and their progress (through the study) monitored. This section may include such routine details as contact telephone numbers and email addresses. Since recording the information is so important, inclusion of the study forms into the protocol itself is desirable, even if they are quite simple in structure. Finally the protocol should be dated, bound in book form and any subsequent amendments carefully documented. For clinical trials 'Good Clinical Practice' as described by EMEA (2002) will dictate in full the items that are mandatory for such a protocol.

1.9   REPORTING

GUIDELINES

Although we are concerned with aspects of design over a wide range of studies extending from preclinical to large-scale randomised trials and epidemiological studies, it is clear that these studies have to be analysed and interpreted and the conclusions reported. The research is not complete without this final step. Several guidelines, and associated checklists, have been published to assist authors in preparing their work for publication. These guidelines outline the essential features of such reports; in particular they clarify how aspects pertinent to their (statistical) design should be described. Just as an investigator may have a target journal in mind even in the early stages of planning a study, and thereby take note of any journal requirements concerned with aspects of their potential study, it is prudent for the investigating team to cross-check the intended design against these requirements. Anything overlooked at the design stage can then be taken account of in a design modification *before* embarking on the study. In contrast, it is too late to discover such an omission at the time of analysis and reporting.

Guidelines for reporting also give hints on what seemingly extraneous detail information needs to be collected during the experimental process. This may include the details of the consent procedures, or of outcomes in subjects who do not fully comply with the experimental process.

For those studies that do not fit into specific guidelines, it is nevertheless useful to cross-check aspects of design with available guidelines. In these circumstances, it may be useful for an investigator to compile their own checklists that can be updated by their own experience once the study is complete. Such a personal checklist will be a useful guide for the next study.

For certain types of study, including those used in the development stages of a new drug, there may be mandatory guidelines imposed by the regulatory authorities. These may set minimum standards or very specific requirements. Any investigating team ignoring such advice would need to provide cogent reasons for departure. Such departures may be entirely appropriate as new information and new situations are always arising. Should these occur then cross-checking with the regulatory bodies at the design stage is clearly prudent. For non-regulatory situations, teams may be free to have a more flexible approach. However, although flexibility is desirable, care should be taken to ensure this does not lead to lower standards.

Human studies (particularly clinical trials) have the highest standards for reporting. Thus many leading biomedical journals have adopted the CONSORT statement of Moher, Schultz and Altman (2001) which outlines the requirements for reporting clinical trials. This contrasts with publications in the experimental literature where, for example, aspects of the choice of study design and justification for experimental unit numbers are often poorly substantiated.

STANDARDS

The second aspect of reporting is the standard of reporting, particularly the amount of necessary detail given in any study report. The most basic feature that has repeatedly been emphasised is to give numerical estimates (with confidence intervals) of comparisons made and not just p-values. Guidelines for referees of clinical papers have been published in several journals. These include those of the *British Medical Journal* described by Altman, Gore, Gardner and Pocock (2000). These are clearly useful for those who are designing studies, as these will eventually become the authors who are then exposed to the peer review system of the journal concerned. They would clearly benefit from knowledge of exactly what a referee will be looking for.

As indicated, the statistical guidelines referred to, and the associated checklists for statistical review of papers for international journals (Gardner, Machin, Campbell and Altman, 2000), require confidence intervals (CI) to be given for the main results. These are intended as an important prerequisite to be supplemented by the p-value from the associated hypothesis test. Methods for calculating CIs are provided in many standard statistical packages as well as the specialist software of Altman, Machin, Bryant and Gardner (2000, Chapter 17).

EVIDENCE-BASED MEDICINE

Following established guidelines and adopting a high standard of reporting of clinical studies of whatever type, clearly helps the reader to better appreciate the clinical messages suggested from the work that has been conducted. This in turn allows the reader to determine the relevance of the results to his or her clinical or research practice. What is more, this clarity facilitates those who are conducting systematic reviews to readily identify the key features of the study conducted for their overview, ultimately leading to more reliable synthesis and a firmer basis for EBM.

Key features

Review criteria for causality

Strength of the evidence is related to the choice of design

Check the local regulations for ethical approval and informed consent

A written study protocol

Cross-check the design with published guidelines and checklists

Ensure the reporting is to the highest of standards

1.10   TECHNICAL NOTES

Optimal Designs

Equation (1.1) can be generalised to situations in which there are more terms on the right-hand side, for example, $y = \beta_0 + \beta_1 x_1 + \beta_2 x_2 + \ldots + \beta_v x_v + \varepsilon$. Further the form of the variable y (or a transformation of it) can be extended to binary, categorical, ordered categorical or survival time data. These correspond to logistic regression, multilogit regression, ordinal regression and Cox proportional hazards regression models. In each case the design that minimises the determinant of the covariance matrix, consisting of all the variance and covariance terms of the estimates of the parameters $\beta_0, \beta_1, \beta_2, \ldots, \beta_v$, is termed D-optimal. For example, D-optimality allows for $\mathrm{Var}(b_0)$, $\mathrm{Var}(b_1)$ and Covariance (b_0, b_1) and not just $\mathrm{Var}(b_1)$ as we have in our exposition.

2 Measurement, Forms and Questionnaires

Summary

This chapter emphasises for all studies the importance of taking appropriate measurements. From a statistical perspective the different types of measures are described. The importance of clearly defining the measurements needed and how, when and by whom they are to be taken are underlined. The particular value of blind assessment where possible is stressed as are the importance of carefully making the observations with sufficient precision, avoiding bias and recording the data in a suitable medium. The basic structure of forms for recording data and the types of questions they may contain are reviewed. In addition, questionnaires used as instruments for measuring, for example, quality of life, are discussed. We include some general pointers to good design of forms and questionnaires.

2.1 INTRODUCTION

An important aspect of study design is the choice of measurements to be made and observations to be recorded. Once identified, details of how and when these measures are to be taken have also to be considered. This is often conveniently done using (previously designed) forms or possibly coding sheets if the data are relatively sparse, and these can be keyed directly into a database. It is important that any forms are clear, easy to complete and readily transferable to the database. In certain situations, a form may be in the format of a questionnaire to be completed by a subject recruited to the study. The distinction between a form and a questionnaire is that a questionnaire is an 'instrument' which 'measures' something, perhaps the quality of life (QoL) status of a patient, whereas a form merely records information. In practice a questionnaire instrument, may contain 'form-like' questions such as asking for gender and date of birth as well as the instrument variables themselves.

2.2 TYPES OF DATA

An integral part of the design process is the choice of endpoint measures and their corresponding data types. The type influences the final approach to analysis that will be

Design of Studies for Medical Research. D. Machin and M. J. Campbell
© 2005 John Wiley & Sons Ltd. ISBN 0 470 84495 7

necessary and this reflects back on the study size required. Thus, although we will give some general expressions for study size in Chapter 3 and further expansion in subsequent chapters, these will have to be selected and/or modified depending on the type of outcome measure chosen.

QUALITATIVE DATA

Nominal or Categorical Data

Nominal data are data that one can *name*, thus they are not measured but simply counted. They often consist of unordered 'either-or' type observations, for example, Dead or Alive; Male or Female; diagnosis of Sudden Acute Respiratory Symptoms (SARS): Yes or No. However, they can have more than two categories, for example, country of origin, ethnicity or blood group: O, A, B, AB.

Ordered Categorical or Ranked Data

If there are more than two categories it may be possible to order them in some way. For example, after treatment patients may be either improved, the same or worse; the diagnosis of SARS may be suspected, probable or definite.

In some studies, it may be appropriate to assign ranks. For example, patients with rheumatoid arthritis may be asked to order their preference for four dressing aids. Here, although numerical values are assigned to each aid, one cannot usually treat them as numerical values. They are in fact only codes for best, second-best, third choice and least preferable.

NUMERICAL OR QUANTITATIVE DATA

Numerical Discrete

Such data are counts 0, 1, 2, and so on, for example the number of SARS cases confirmed in Hong Kong on a particular day or the number of babies born on that day.

Numerical Continuous

These are measurements that can, in theory at least, take any value within a given range. Examples are maternal age (year), the birthweight of a baby (g), and height (cm). Continuous data are sometimes dichotomised to make nominal data. Thus diastolic blood pressure (DBP), which is continuous, is converted into hypertension ($>90\,\text{mmHg}$) and normotension ($\leqslant 90\,\text{mmHg}$). This clearly leads to a loss of information, but can make the data easier to summarise.

Survival Time

The measure of interest can be a time variable such as the time from randomisation into a clinical trial until the patient experiences a particular event, for example, the healing of their burn wound. The key follow-up information will be that which is necessary to determine healing. For example healing might be defined as when all the damaged body surface area finally closes. To establish this, the burn area may have to be monitored on a daily basis to determine exactly when this final closure is achieved.

For those patients in which healing occurs, the time from randomisation to healing can be determined in days by calculating the difference, t, between the date of complete healing and the date of randomisation. For those whose wound does not heal with medical treatment, but have to be excised or amputated, then the time from randomisation to this can be assessed but not then their healing time. Their data are therefore classified as *censored* at the time of operation. The time from the date of randomisation to this censoring date is termed $T+$. The eventual analysis of these 'survival' times, which involves either a t or a $T+$ for every patient, will involve Kaplan–Meier estimates of the corresponding cumulative survival curves, where 'survival' is in fact the 'healing time'.

2.3   MEASUREMENT

CONCEPTS AND INDICATORS

It is useful to clarify what is being measured and what it measures. A *concept* is what we hope to capture. It can be solid, such as a dog, or subjective, such as quality of life. An *indicator* is what we use to describe the concept. For example, the number of legs, presence of a tail and a bark are indicators of a dog. The questions in a quality of life questionnaire are indicators of Health Related Quality of Life (HRQoL).

ENDPOINTS

Assessments

The protocol for every preclinical, clinical or epidemiological study should detail the assessments to be made on the experimental or observational units involved. In all studies their objectives will usually define the endpoint or endpoints that will be used in assessing the results. Such endpoints clearly depend on the type of study concerned. They may range from simply recording variables such as gender and birthweight of babies born in a particular delivery unit, to standard clinical measures such as systolic (SBP) or diastolic blood pressure (DBP), to the date of death of patients with AIDS, to highly complex measures of tumour response in patients with juvenile leukaemia.

For each variable the method of measurement or assessment should be clearly defined. There will rarely be difficulty in determining gender at birth, but exactly when and how the baby's weight is determined may need some more thought. For example: Is the newborn baby cleaned before weighing? Are the scales of sufficient accuracy for the purposes intended? To what accuracy should weight be recorded? How often are the scales calibrated? Are the same scales used for all babies?

It is good practice to define which of the measures taken is the major endpoint of the study as this will be used to help determine study size and it will also be the main focus for the final evaluation and reporting. This needs to be observed with particular care and objectivity. In many situations, there may be several endpoints of interest, but it is important to rank them in order of priority or at least to identify those of primary and those of secondary importance.

In clinical studies some of the assessments made may focus on aspects of the day-to-day care of the patient whilst others may focus more on those measures which will be necessary in order to determine the study endpoint(s) for each subject. It is important that these assesssments are well defined and that endpoints are unambiguously defined so that they can be determined for each patient recruited to the study. Even with everyday clinical measures, such as oral temperature and BP, in the context of a study it will be necessary to define how these are to be taken. For example, a physician may only need to know if the temperature of the patient is elevated, say beyond 37.5°C, or that the BP is low or high, in order to make a diagnosis. However, in a study it may be important to record precisely the temperature, and both SBP and DBP, as the study may be investigating the change in these values following a specific intervention. In addition it will be important to specify precisely how (and when) the measure is to be taken, for example, for BP using a particular type of sphygmomanometer and after the patient has been supine for 5 minutes.

It is particularly important to assess carefully the implications of those measures which initiate a course of action if their value reaches a certain level. For example, in a clinical trial of patients with burns, one may state that 'patients are expected to be discharged from the hospital burns unit once their wound has healed to a *sufficient degree*'. However, how is 'sufficient degree' defined so that it can be unambiguously observed in each patient? In practice, it may depend more on the support available 'at home' for the patient once discharged rather than the intrinsic condition of the burn wounds themselves. In which case, this definition may lead to discharge of the patient and thereby prevent assessment of the wound for the purposes of a clinical trial to determine the relative efficacy of alternative treatments for wound management. Although such a vague definition may be informative enough if the study was designed to estimate length of hospital stay so that the (hospital) costs of treating such patients could be estimated.

If blood, urine or other samples are to be taken, once again 'when' will need to be specified but also, once obtained, the exact manner in which these are to be handled, stored and tested will need to be detailed. If these are passed to a reference laboratory for analysis then their procedures too have to be such as to satisfy the study requirements.

Single Measures

In some studies a single measure may be sufficient to determine the endpoint in each subject. For example, the endpoint may be the DBP measured at a particular time, say 28 days post-randomisation to treatment, in each patient. In this case the groups will be summarised by their respective mean DBPs. In some situations, the endpoint may be patient response, for example, the patient becomes normotensive following a period of treatment. Those who respond are termed successes and those who do not, failures. In this case, the groups will be summarised by the proportion of responders. If, on the other hand, the patients are categorised as: normotensive, still hypertensive but DBP nevertheless reduced, or still hypertensive and DBP not improved, then this would correspond to an ordered categorical variable. Alternatively, the endpoint may be defined as the time from randomisation and inception of treatment to the time when the patient becomes normotensive. In this situation repeated (say daily) measures of DBP will be made until the value recorded is normotensive (as defined in the protocol). The interval between the date of randomisation and the date of recording the first occurrence of a normotensive recording is the endpoint measure of interest.

Multiple Measures

In certain circumstances, there may be more than one possible location for the measure within a subject. For example, in determining whether or not a subject has glaucoma, the left, the right or both eyes may have the disease. Similarly, there may be evidence of failure in the left, the right or both kidneys. An extreme example is whether or not each individual tooth is affected by caries. In many cases these may be reduced to a single primary measure such as the number of teeth with caries or the ordered categorical variable, 0, 1 or 2 eyes have evidence of glaucoma, as appropriate. On the other hand, it may be advantageous to keep these aspects as distinct. For example, if we were concerned with the healing of burns then there may be more than a single (distinct) site of injury. Monitoring the progress of all sites may lead to a more efficient statistical design which then ultimately leads to fewer patients being required to enable the research question to be answered reliably. However, at the analysis stage due account that multiple sites are being monitored within each patient is essential. It is a mistake to regard these observations as independent as they come from the same individual.

Repeated Measures

In the trial taking repeated DBP assessments, these are recorded in order to determine a single outcome – 'time to becoming normotensive'. In other situations, all the successive values of DBP themselves may be utilised in making the formal comparisons. If the number of observations made on each subject is the same, and the intervals between successive observations is the same for all subjects, then the analysis may be relatively straightforward, perhaps using repeated measures of analysis of variance. On the other hand, if the numbers of observations recorded varies, or if the intervals between successive observations vary from patient to patient, or if there is occasional missing data, then the summary and analysis of such data may be quite complex.

Multiple Endpoints

If there are too many endpoints defined, the multiplicity of comparisons then made at the analysis stage may result in spurious statistical significance. This is a major concern if endpoints for HRQoL and health economic evaluations are added to the already established, more clinical, endpoints. As we have indicated, for design purposes it is essential to focus on the major (and few) key endpoints and it is these same endpoints that provide the focus at the analysis and interpretation stages once the study is complete. Any secondary level endpoints should be identified as such at the planning stage and the manner in which they are to be summarised and reported indicated. Often less formal statistical comparisons will be made of these than for the principal endpoints.

Objective Criteria

In certain situations, there is not necessarily an obvious measure to take. For example, although one may regard tumour shrinkage as a desirable property of a cytotoxic drug when given to a patient, it is not immediately apparent how this is to be measured. Were every tumour of regular spherical shape, the direction in which it is measured would be irrelevant. Furthermore the diameter, a single dimension, leads us immediately to the volume of the tumour. However, no real tumour will comply with this ideal geometrical configuration and this has led to measures such as the product of the two largest (perpendicular) diameters to describe the tumour and then a reduction in this product to indicate response.

Precisely what is the best measure to assess tumour shrinkage has been discussed by an international panel and reported in detail by Therasse, Arbuck, Eisenhauer *et al.* (2000). They offer guidelines to encourage more uniform reporting of outcomes particularly for clinical trials. Investigators of future trials may argue about the fine details, and no doubt in time these guidelines will need revision, but they would be foolish to ignore these recommendations when conducting and subsequently reporting their study.

If there are 'justifiable' reasons why other criteria should be used, or the recommendations cannot be followed for whatever reason, then before the study commences these should be reviewed by the investigating team. There is little point in conducting a study using measures not acceptable to other groups, including referees for the clinical journals, as little note will then be taken of the results. The best option is to follow the guidelines for the primary endpoint, use the 'local' measures for secondary reporting and contrast the two in any discussion.

Example – *marker lesion* – *oral lichen planus*

For patients presenting with oral lichen planus (OLP) to the trial conducted by the Asian Lichen Planus Study Group (2004) if only a single lesion was present then this was assessed. If there were multiple lesions, then the protocol defined a 'marker' lesion that was to be assessed. This was defined as the most severe and extensive OLP lesion. The assessment, with respect to the areas of erythema, reticulation and ulceration were made using the 0.5 by 0.5 cm grids of Figure 2.1 printed onto flexible transparent material placed over the affected area then traced.

In some situations less than optimal measures may have to be used. For example, although precise levels of pain experienced may be meaured in the 'laboratory' such methodology may not be practical when levels need to be assessed at the bedside. A practical method of recording pain, or variables such as strength of feeling, is by means of a *visual analogue* score (VAS). A patient completes a visual analogue scale by making a mark on either a horizontal or vertical line. It is useful for measuring aspects that may be difficult to put into words. When used to assess pain Myles, Troedel, Boquest and

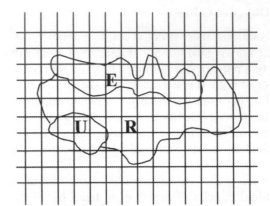

R - Reticulation
E - Erythema
U - Ulceration

Figure 2.1 Flexible transparent grid used for marking and quantifying areas of recticulation, erythema and ulceration in patients with oral lichen planus (adapted from Harpenau, Plemons and Rees, 1995. Effectiveness of low dose cyclosporine in the management of patients with oral erosive lichen planus. *Oral Surgery, Oral Medicine, Oral Pathology, Oral Radiological Endod*, **80**, 161–167. [2])

Reeves (1999) suggest that the VAS behaves as if it is approximately linear (in the sense that a score of say 4 is twice as much pain as a score of 2). Thus one advantage of the use of VAS over a closed question format is that it may give an apparently continuous variable. Nevertheless there is some suggestion that VAS do not correspond to other methods of valuing health states, and Torrance, Feeny and Furlong (2001) express doubts over their use in this particular context. Also, because individuals tend to be internally consistent, VAS are good when measuring change within individuals, they are not so good when comparing across individuals.

Example – VAS – pain assessment

Ang, Lee, Gan *et al.* (2003) in a clinical trial of patients with severe burns used a VAS to assess the pain levels experienced by the patients. It is usually preferable that the patients make such assessments themselves, marking their pain level experienced on a 10-cm VAS. However, when designing the trial the authors anticipated that some patients would have burns which affect their ability to write easily, some would be too ill to complete the task, whilst others would have language and literacy issues. As a consequence, for this trial, the responsible nurse used as necessary, the less refined verbal alternative administered in a local language or dialect familiar to the patient and assisted the patient to mark the scale when needed. An example of a typical format and wording is shown in Figure 2.2.

It is clear from this example, that the study design team need to be aware of the difficulties involved and to make adjustments to their methodology in the light of these.

*To be marked by the PATIENT after instruction. Make **ONLY ONE THIN MARKING** on the lines.)*

PAIN

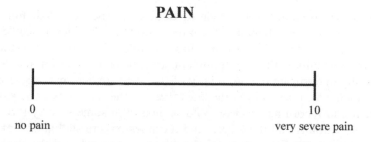

Figure 2.2   Visual analogue scale (VAS) used to assess pain

Surrogates

Sometimes it may be that the true endpoint of interest is difficult to assess for whatever reason. In this case, a surrogate may be sought. For example, when investigating the possibilities of a novel marker for prognosis it may be tempting to use disease-free survival (DFS) as a 'surrogate' endpoint for the overall survival (OS) time of patients with the cancer concerned – the reason being that, for many cancers, relapse occurs well before death and so the evaluation of the marker can occur earlier in time than would be the case if OS was to be observed.

A surrogate endpoint is a biomarker (or other indicator) which is intended to substitute for an (often) clinical endpoint and predict its behaviour. If a surrogate is to be used, then there is a real need to ensure that it is an appropriate surrogate for the (true) endpoint of concern.

TAKING THE MEASUREMENTS

Single-blind Assessment

It is clearly desirable that all observations are made as objectively as possible. However, any investigator deeply involved in a study, of whatever type, will be aware of the hypothesis under investigation and this knowledge may influence (however unintentional) the recordings he makes. Thus, knowledge of the particular intervention that the experimental unit has received may induce bias into the measurement process. Therefore, if at all possible, the assessment should be made by someone, or by some means, with no knowledge of which intervention has been given and the observer is termed 'blinded' in this circumstance.

Double-blind

If the recipient of the intervention can be blinded to the actual intervention given, for example, in a randomised placebo-controlled trial, then whoever makes the assessment cannot be informed of the specific treatment by the subject. If both the participant and the observer are blind to the therapy, then the measure is taken in a double-blind way.

Triple-blind

Clearly the above blinding from single to double can be extended. For example, in circumstances where the patient and the nurse who takes the blood sample are blind to the intervention, it is desirable that the blood sample taken and sent to the laboratory should be assessed blindly there. Although once at the laboratory for analysis there may be no difficulty in ensuring the objectivity of the measurement process, if the sample is labelled in such a way as to indicate the values of the measures anticipated then the measurement and recording process could be biased in some way by this knowledge.

The ideal situation is that the subject and the assessors are all 'blinded' or 'masked' to an appropriate extent. The extent of the blinding depends on the particular study concerned; a desirable goal is to make assessment double-blind as far as is possible. For a laboratory sample, this may be easy to achieve, while in other circumstances, such as taking the pain assessment in patients with burns, this may not be possible. In this latter case the treatments, two types of dressing, cannot be disguised from the patient or the nurse. However, swabs taken from the wounds to assess the presence of methicillin-resistant *Staphylococcus aureus* (MRSA) can be sent to the laboratory for testing in a coded format to ensure objectivity at that level.

WHICH OBSERVER

In certain circumstances, it has to be made very clear who is the observer concerned. If a QoL instrument is being used to assess patients, there are clear guidelines that have been published by Young, de Haes, Curran *et al.* (1999) for the clinical trials of the European Organization for the Research and Treatment of Cancer (EORTC). These describe the manner and circumstances in which they should be completed. For example, the patient is the 'observer' and is supposed to complete the instrument, in this case the EORTC QLQ-C30, him- or herself. Only in specific circumstances can a proxy be used for this purpose and this must then be recorded in the trial documentation.

PRECISION

A question often arises as to whether a continuous variable should or should not be recorded as a categorical variable for data recording and so for future analysis. For example, is it better to 'categorise' the variable age into three separate categories, say less than 50 (young), 50–59 (middle-aged) and 60 or more (senior), rather than bother with their individual ages? The difficulty here is that, despite the relative ease of coding, the categories are not so intuitive if recorded as 0, 1 or 2 (say) and this may increase the risk of a recording error. What is more, one is stuck with the definitions used at the outset and, should they be required to change (perhaps others have used a different categorisation), then comparisons between studies are going to be difficult. It is usually best at the recording stage to 'measure' the variable as precisely as is reasonable. Most individuals know their date of birth and the experimenter knows the date of the enquiry so that age can be easily computed at a later stage. It could then be rounded to convenient categories by creating a new variable within the database while preserving the two dates indicated. However, the direct use of the continuous variables themselves, rather than the same variable categorised, is often statistically more efficient and will keep the planned sample size to a minimum.

If the underlying variable is continuous, then the precision with which this is to be measured has to be defined. This will depend on the 'ruler' available for this process. Observers must be aware of digit preference, so that if any data set is examined one invariably sees that the last digits of a particular measure, $0, 1, \ldots, 9$, are not evenly distributed over their whole range. One solution is to ask all observers to go to 1 decimal place further than the study actually requires and leave the rounding process until the computational stage.

2.4   FORMS

In general, forms are used to record factual information, such as a subject's age, blood pressure or treatment group. They are commonly used in clinical trials to follow a patient's progress and are often completed by the investigating team. For forms, the main requirement is that each form is clearly laid out and all investigators are familiar with it. However, even if all the data are to be collected by a single investigator (say in the laboratory) it is still important that this is done in a clear and unambiguous way. Clarity of the experimental record with respect to the observations taken is becoming a routine feature of good clinical practice (GCP) that must be adhered to in clinical trials for regulatory purposes (CPMP, 1995). It is equally good practice for more basic research to utilise the same standards. In any event, variables, and their names, will need to be included in a database eventually for further analysis. Thus forms provide a good 'aide-mémoire' for a study conducted some time ago.

LAYOUT

A balance between a cramped and cluttered layout, and a well spaced but bulky series of forms has to be made. Each form should contain clear instructions about how to respond to each question. Sometimes more than one response to a question is possible. It is important to make clear whether you expect a single answer, or whether multiple replies are acceptable. It may seem obvious, but questions and possible answers should be kept together; one should avoid having the question on one page and the possible responses on another.

> **Example** – form design – randomised trial in colorectal cancer
>
> Tang, Eu, Tai et al. (2001) used the form of Figure 2.3 to register and randomise patients to their clinical trial of open versus laparoscopically assisted colectomy in patients with colorectal cancer. The top sections of the form were completed by the clinical team before contacting the central randomisation office who, once details were confirmed, provided the trial number (unique for each patient) and the allocated treatment.

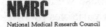

CLASICC TRIAL

REGISTRATION FORM

National Medical Research Council

Conventional versus Laparoscopic-Assisted Surgery In Colorectal Cancer

Please return this form, by post or fax, immediately after randomisation to:
NMRC Clinical Trials Office, #02-14 Bowyer Block, Singapore General Hospital, Singapore 169608. Fax: 225 3584

A patient sticker with the following information may be used for this section if available:

Patient Name_____   NRIC_____

Hospital_____   Surgeon_____

Date of birth: ☐☐ ☐☐ ☐☐
                day   month   year

Eligibility: Please tick the boxes to confirm the following:

☐ The patient has colorectal cancer.

☐ Informed consent, according to local practice, has been obtained.

What is the patient's WHO performance status? ☐
(for definition see overleaf)

NOW TELEPHONE THE NMRC CLINICAL TRIALS OFFICE (**222-7632**) TO RANDOMISE
(Monday-Friday 8.30am-5.30pm, Saturday 8.30am-12.30pm)

Trial number ☐☐☐☐   Date of randomisation: ☐☐ ☐☐ ☐☐
                                                day   month   year

Allocated Treatment: ☐   O. Open Surgery   L. Laparoscopic-Assisted Surgery

---

Signed_____   Date_____

Figure 2.3   Registration form (utilised in the trial by Tang, Eu, Tai *et al.*, 2001)

QUESTIONS

Closed Question

Closed questions can be answered by simply completing the answer in a relevant box or, as for the patient eligibility questions in Figure 2.3, ticking confirmation. When constructing responses to closed questions it is important to provide a clear range of replies. For example, this form provides a single box for the (closed) response to the

NMRC
National Medical Research Council

CLASICC TRIAL

SURGERY AND INTRA-
OPERATIVE COMPLICATIONS FORM

Conventional versus Laparoscopic-Assisted Surgery In Colorectal Cancer
Please return this form, following surgery, to:
NMRC Clinical Trials Office, #02-14 Bowyer Block, Singapore General Hospital, Singapore 169608
A patient sticker with the following information may be used for this section if available:

Patient's name_____   Trial Number ☐☐☐☐

Hospital_____   NRIC_____

To be completed by the surgeon as soon after surgery as possible

Has a liver ultrasound been carried out less than 30 days before planned surgery? ☐ 1. No
                                                                                   2. Yes

If yes, date of liver ultrasound: ☐☐ ☐☐ ☐☐   Liver metastases present? ☐ 1 No
                                day   month   year   2. Yes
Did the patient experience any of the following complications during operation?

Gross faecal contamination	☐ 1. No 2. Yes	Ureteric injury	☐ 1. No 2. Yes
Duodenal injury	☐ 1. No 2. Yes	Cardiac insufficiency/dysrhythmia	☐ 1. No 2. Yes
Pulmonary insufficiency (from pneumoperitoneum)	☐ 1. No 2. Yes	Surgical emphysema	☐ 1. No 2. Yes

Significant intra-operative haemorrhage
(ie haemorrhage that requires   ☐ 1. No
peri-operative transfusion)   2. Yes   Volume of blood lost: ☐☐☐☐ ml

Other complications (please specify)   ☐ 1. No
                                            2. Yes   Specify_____

                                              Trocar injury   Instrumentation injury
Abdominal bladder injury   ☐ 1. No   ☐   ☐
                               2. Yes

Small bowel injury   ☐ 1. No   ☐   ☐
                               2. Yes

Major vessel injury   ☐ 1. No   ☐   ☐
                               2. Yes

PLEASE TURN OVER

Figure 2.4 Surgical complications form (utilised in the trial by Tang, Eu, Tai *et al.*, 2001)

question concerning 'Allocated Treatment', with permitted responses of either 'O' or 'L' corresponding to open or laparascopically assisted surgery. Were this form in the format of a computer screen then entry procedures can be designed to prevent anything but an O or an L being entered in this space. This cannot be achieved using a paper-based system. It is more usual in forms to get a numerical answer so that in Figure 2.4, also part of the trial documentation of Tang, Eu, Tai *et al.* (2001), the responses are 1 (for No) or 2 (for Yes) to the question: 'Liver metastases present?'. This is because 'numbers', but strictly here 'codes', are easier to manipulate in a database than are alphabetical items. In fact some statistical packages cannot handle character variables and so all variables must be numeric for them. On this form, the closed question for 'Volume of blood lost' provides the unit of measure, here 'ml', required and an appropriate number of boxes for the numerical value to be recorded. Were the variable to be recorded with a decimal place then a style of boxes on the form such as, □□□•□, is a convenient reminder of this.

In most situations dates will also need to be recorded and, because of the different conventions used, and the transition over the millennium, it is important to indicate clearly the requisite (boxes) for day, month and year.

Open Questions

In general on forms, open questions are best avoided or at least kept to a minimum. In an open question respondents are asked to reply in their own words. For example, in Figure 2.4 there is also an open question: 'Other complications (please specify)'. In the context of this clinical trial any responses would be expected to be of one or two words only from the investigating team, whereas in other circumstances a full description may be expected.

2.5   QUESTIONNAIRES

A questionnaire, as opposed to a form, can be regarded as an instrument in its own right although it too may include basic demographic information, as does a form. For example, it may try to measure personal attributes such as attitudes, emotional states, levels of pain or HRQoL and is often completed by the individual concerned.

LAYOUT

As with forms, the questionnaire should have clear instructions and an attractive layout. It helps to reduce bulk by copying on both sides of a page, and reducing the size of text to fit a booklet format.

It is generally held that shorter questionnaires achieve better response rates than longer ones. However, it is hard to define what is 'too long', and if the topic is relevant to the subject concerned and if they are motivated to complete it, then length has little effect on response rates.

Example – question layout – sexual function

Jensen, Klee, Thranov and Groenvold (2004) developed a questionnaire to evaluate sexual function in women following treatment for a gynaecological malignacy as a preliminary to a longitudinal study. Part of their final questionnaire, developed after the due process described by Sprangers, Cull and Groenvold (1998) was completed, is reproduced in Figure 2.5.

Physical contact and sexual relations can be an important part of many people's lives. People who suffer from illnesses involving their pelvic region may experience changes in their sex life.

The questions below refer to this. The information you provide will remain strictly confidential. Please answer all the questions yourself by circling the number that best applies to you

PART 1
During the past month:

	Not at all	A little	Quite a bit	Very much
1. Have you been interested in close physical contact (a kiss and a cuddle)?	1	2	3	4
2. Have you had close physical contact with your family and close friends?	1	2	3	4
3. Have you had any interest in sexual relations?	1	2	3	4

	Yes	No
4. Do you have a partner? (If not, please continue to **question 8**)	1	2

Figure 2.5 Part of the questionnaire (SVQ) for self-assessment of sexual function and vaginal changes after gynaecological cancer (from Jensen, Klee, Thranov and Groenvold, 2004; reproduced by permission of John Wiley & Sons Ltd)

For questionnaires, particularly ones trying to evaluate something like HRQoL, the pragmatic advice is, if possible, do not design your own, use someone else's! There are a number of reasons for this apparently negative advice. First, use of a standardised format means that results should be comparable between studies. Secondly, it is a difficult and time-consuming process to obtain a satisfactory questionnaire.

QUESTIONS

A convenient distinction between forms and questionnaires (although by all means not always the case) is that the investigating team completes forms while the study participants themselves complete questionnaires. Thus forms can be short and snappy, and any ambiguities explained amongst the investigators, whereas questionnaires need to be very carefully designed particularly with respect to the choice of language they use to pose the questions. For example, technical jargon, like that scattered throughout the form of Figure 2.4 is suitable for a specialist surgical team but should be avoided in a questionnaire.

Closed Questions

Although a questionnaire may include some form-like closed questions, such as asking for the gender of the participant, there will be others eliciting less directly measurable information.

Example – closed question – sexual function after gynaecological cancer

Jensen, Klee, Thronav and Groenvold (2004) ask on the SVQ: 'Have you had close physical contact with your family and close friends? For this question the closed question responses offered by the questionnaire are: (1) Not at all, (2) A little, (3) Quite a bit, (4) Very much.

However, a study participant may object to being forced into a particular category, and simply not answer the question as a result. In developing the format for such questions, a useful strategy is to conduct a pilot study using an open question on a limited but representative sample of people. From their responses one can then devise suitable closed questions. In fact this type of procedure has been gone through in devising the questions of the SVQ of Figure 2.5.

One type of closed question is to make a statement and then ask whether the respondent agrees or disagrees. When a closed question has an odd number of responses, usually five or seven it is often called a *Likert* scale.

Example – Likert scale – SF36

Ware, Snow, Kosinski and Gandek (1993) use Likert-type questions in the general health section of their SF36 quality of life instrument as shown in Figure 2.6.

This format has the advantage of being compact, and there is little chance of people filling in the wrong bubble. However, some questionnaires, such as the SVQ of Figure 2.5, avoid central categories such as the 'don't know' of the SF36.

11. How TRUE or FALSE is <u>each</u> of the following statements for you?

	Definitely true	Mostly true	Don't know	Mostly false	Definitely false
a) I seem to get sick a little easier than other people	○	○	○	○	○
b) I am as health as anybody I know	○	○	○	○	○
c) I expect my health to get worse	○	○	○	○	○
d) My health is excellent	○	○	○	○	○

Figure 2.6   General health question from SF36 (after Ware, Snow, Kosinski and Gandek, 1993)

Open Questions

Just as with forms, open questions pose difficulties. Thus although they allow free rein to the participant to explain their response, this brings problems of data summary for the investigating team if the number of participants is more than a few. For certain types of investigations, such as in qualitative studies, this may be an integral part of the study design process, but for more quantitative endpoints it can be a major difficulty.

Response Bias

One problem (with possibly multiple causes) associated with asking questions is to know if the answers provided by respondents are valid. In other words, do their responses truly reflect their experiences or attitudes? If they do not, then response bias can arise in any one of a variety of ways. 'Social desirability' bias is particularly likely in respect of questions on sensitive topics, and occurs when respondents conceal their true behaviour or attitudes and instead give an answer that shows them in a good light, or is perceived to be socially acceptable. Related to this is 'sponsorship' bias, by which respondents' answers differ according to who is conducting the survey. 'Memory' bias occurs in questions involving recall of past events or behaviour and can include omission and telescoping (misplacing an event in time). Biases can also arise from the respondent mis-hearing or misunderstanding the question or accompanying instructions.

The relative threat of different types of response bias depends in part on the mode of administration. In surveys using mixed modes of administration, care is needed in interpreting findings; observed differences between respondents may be attributable to the methods of data collection, rather than to true underlying differences in experiences and attitudes. The greater anonymity afforded by a postal questionnaire, and to a lesser extent by a telephone interview, may mean that subjects are more likely to report truthfully on potentially embarrassing behaviour or experiences (for example, mental health problems). Social desirability bias is more likely in interviewer-administered surveys, since respondents may wish to 'save face'. By contrast, other forms of deception can be minimised by interviews, because some responses can be verified by observation.

Questionnaire wording and design can also induce response bias, for example through question sequencing effects (where the response given to a particular question differs according to the placement of that question relative to others), and the labelling and ordering of response categories.

2.6   DATA COLLECTION AND PROCESSING

VOLUME, COMPLEXITY AND NATURE

The desired volume, complexity and nature of data to be collected will vary from study to study. The largest volume of data can be collected in face-to-face interviews (since the burden of recording responses falls on the interviewer rather than the respondent). The downside is the temptation to collect more data than is strictly necessary for the purpose in hand. This wastes resources and may be unethical in certain circumstances.

Data of greater complexity can also be gathered in face-to-face interviews, because visual aids can be used and the interviewer can more readily provide explanations and probe and prompt for additional information. However, self-completion questionnaires are generally held to be superior to telephone surveys for collecting complex data. For example, questions involving the ranking of several items, or those using multiple response categories (for instance, a seven-point scale of satisfaction) are difficult to use in telephone surveys because there is no visual stimulus; instead, the respondent must mentally retain and process the items or categories.

Interviews facilitate the use of open-ended questions or open-ended probes, where the interviewer can record verbatim the answers given by the respondents. This may generate richer and more spontaneous information than would be possible using self-completion questionnaires. Although open-ended questions can be used in self-completion questionnaires, responses are typically less detailed since respondents tend to be less expansive in writing than in speaking.

Collecting data on 'boring' topics is easier in interviewer-administered surveys; interviewers can engage subjects' attention and interest and can use their powers of persuasion to maximise participation.

CHECKING

As already indicated, much of the data in medical studies is captured on paper-based forms, although there is an increasing trend for electronic data capture. The advantage of electronic forms is that range and cross-checks (checking the consistency of the new data with itself and with that already in the database) and value checks can be instantly applied. In addition missing values can be immediately queried, and irrelevant questions, such as asking a non-smoker for details of cigarette consumption can be skipped. However, paper forms are often used for convenience.

In spite of all precautions that may be taken in the study protocol to ensure that measurements are made according to carefully documented procedures, mistakes do occur in the recording of these values. Some of these errors may be detected by a quick check of the form on which the result has been recorded, whilst others may be missed and passed to the data file. At this stage, range and cross-checks, easy programming of which needs to be an integral feature of the database, may help to identify such problems. If problems are found, these can be checked against case-records for correction of any erroneous values identified. In some cases, this will provide confirmation that the 'apparent error' is not an 'error' at all. Some 'outlier' values may not necessarily be identified by range checks alone, but by previous or subsequent data on the same subject or by comparison with data from other subjects in the total data set. It is important that data validation occurs as soon as possible after the data item is collected so that the possibility of any correction can be maximised. It is usually a bad idea to leave such checking until the study is closed and no more new data are anticipated.

MISSING DATA

The main cause for concern is that missing data may result in bias, and that the apparent results of a preclinical, clinical or epidemiological study will not reflect the true situation. In the context of a randomised controlled trial, we will not know if the difference we observe (or lack thereof) between treatments is a truly reliable estimate of the real difference. If the proportion of missing data is small then, provided the data are analysed appropriately, one can be confident that little bias will result. However, if the proportion of missing data is not small, then a key question is: 'Are the characteristics (personal and intervention-specific) of the experimental units with missing data different from those with complete data?'. If they are not different then one can be reassured that bias may not be a serious problem. However, this is a matter of judgement, so the best solution is to make every effort at the design stage to anticipate the 'missing' eventualities and keep them to a minimum.

DATABASE

Although the choice of an optimal database will depend to an extent on the type of study planned, it is clearly important that it is reasonably easy to establish (preferably with minimal assistance from an information technology team). In particular, the variables and their type should be simple to define, make data entry and editing easy and, once entered, safe and secure. The data should be easy to access, extract, manipulate and transfer to a statistical package for analysis and the statistical package chosen must be capable of the analysis intended by the design.

Key design features

Clear definition of measures to be recorded

Clear choice of endpoints

Blind assessment whenever possible

Careful choice of data forms

Careful selection of questionnaires

Careful selection of the database

Careful selection of the statistical analysis package

Establish mechanisms to ensure 'missing data' are minimal

Establish mechanisms to ensure the data are checked for consistency

---

2.7   TECHNICAL NOTES

Just as we had equation (1.1) to indicate the model underlying structure for design purposes, we can describe aspects of the measurement process in a similar way. Thus we can express the measurement we are making in the following way,

$$x = X + \eta.$$
(T2.1)

Here X is the true value of the reading that we are about to take on an experimental unit. After we have made the measurement we record X's value as x. We know, with most measures we take, that we will not record the true value but one that we hope is close enough to this for our purpose. We also hope, over the series of measurements we take (one for each experimental unit), that the residual (or our error) $\eta = X - x$ of equation (T2.1) will average out to be small – in which case, any errors we make will have little impact on the final conclusions.

However, if there is something systematically wrong with what we are doing (possibly we are quite unaware of this), then the model we are concerned with is now

$$x = B + X + \eta. \qquad (T2.2)$$

This second model implies that even if we average out η to be close to zero over the course of the study, we are left with a consistent difference, B, beween the true value X and that we actually record, x. This is termed the bias. Thus the measurements should be taken to try to ensure that $B = 0$ from the outset.

3 Principles of Study Size Calculation

Summary

A good design is one that will answer the question posed with the minimum number of subjects possible. This chapter outlines, in general terms, the basic components required for sample size calculations. For single group studies sample size estimation is determined through the desired width of the corresponding confidence interval. For comparative studies the approach to sample size calculation, requires the concepts of the null and alternative hypotheses, significance level, power and, for the majority, the anticipated difference between groups or effect size. We stress the importance of providing a realistic estimate of the latter at the design stage. In certain circumstances, the effect size is replaced by a measure of equivalence which, if the difference between groups is less than this in magnitude, it would imply that the two groups were effectively equivalent in a predefined way. Formulae for calculating sample sizes in many situations are provided.

3.1 INTRODUCTION

A well-designed study will have formally estimated the required sample size before the study commences. Awareness of the importance of this has led to increasing numbers of medical journals demanding that full justification of the sample size chosen is provided with reports of studies. The *British Medical Journal*, the *Journal of the American Medical Association* and numerous other journals, issue checklists for authors of papers, in which there is a question relating to sample size justification. For example, the statistical guidelines for the *British Medical Journal* included in Altman, Gore, Gardner and Pocock (2000) state that: 'Authors should include information on . . . the number of subjects studied and why that number of subjects was used'. The parallel checklist for referees given by Gardner, Machin, Campbell and Altman (2000) asks: 'Is a pre-study calculation of required sample size reported?'.

Investigators, grant-awarding bodies and biotechnology companies all wish to know how much a study is likely to cost them. They would also like to be reassured that their money is well spent, by assessing the likelihood that the study will give unequivocal results. In addition, the regulatory authorities, including the Food and Drug

Design of Studies for Medical Research. D. Machin and M. J. Campbell
© 2005 John Wiley & Sons Ltd. ISBN 0 470 84495 7

Administration (FDA, 1988; Temple, 2000) in the USA and the Committee for Proprietary Medicinal Products (CPMP, 1995) in the European Union require information on planned study size. To this end many pharmaceutical and related biomedical companies provide guidelines for good clinical practice (GCP) in the conduct of their clinical trials, and these generally specify that a sample size calculation is necessary.

Providing a sample size is not simply a matter of identifying a single number from a set of tables but a process with several stages. At the preliminary stage, what is required are 'ball-park' figures that enable the investigator to judge whether or not to start the detailed planning of the study. If a decision is made to proceed, then a subsequent stage is to refine the calculations for the formal study protocol itself. For example, when a clinical trial is designed, a realistic assessment of the potential superiority (the anticipated benefit or effect size) of the proposed test therapy must be made before any further planning. The same realism applies if the purpose is to assess equivalence of the treatments under consideration. The history of clinical trials research suggests that, in certain circumstances, rather ambitious or over-optimistic views of potential benefit have been claimed at the design stage. This has led to the conduct of trials of insufficient size to answer the underlying questions posed reliably.

If too few subjects are involved, the trial may be a waste of time because realistic medical improvements are unlikely to be distinguished from chance variation. A small trial with no chance of detecting a clinically meaningful difference between treatments is unfair to all the subjects put to the risk and discomfort of the clinical trial. Too many subjects is a waste of resource and may be unfair as a larger than necessary number of subjects receive the inferior treatment if one treatment could have been shown to be more effective with fewer patients. Many of these issues have been discussed by Fayers and Machin (1995), in the context of clinical trials in cancer, and by CPMP (1995) and Julious (2004) for trials in general.

Parallel arguments apply to laboratory, preclinical and epidemiological studies. Thus Diletti, Hauschke and Steinijans (1991) detail sample size calculations for pharmacokinetic studies while Wickramaratne (1995) addresses many practical situations in epidemiology.

Computer software to assist in sample size calculations is provided by Machin, Campbell, Fayers and Pinol (1997) and Elashoff (2000).

Many medical statisticians, see for example Altman, Machin, Bryant and Gardner (2000), have suggested that there is an overemphasis on tests of hypotheses in the reporting of the results of many clinical studies. They argue that, wherever possible, confidence intervals (CIs) for the main outcome measures should be quoted. On its own, a p-value obtained from a significance test of the null hypothesis gives the reader little information if they wish to make use of the published results of a particular study. In contrast, an estimate of the effect, together with the corresponding CI, enables him or her to better judge the likely true difference between groups. Nevertheless, for the planning stages of a clinical trial, and equally for many types of studies, discussion is often more easily conducted in terms of testing hypotheses.

To estimate the number of subjects required for a study, we have to identify a single major outcome that is regarded as the primary endpoint for measuring efficacy.

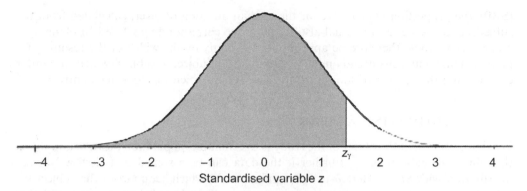

Figure 3.1 The probability density function of a standardised Normal distribution

3.2   THE NORMAL DISTRIBUTION

The Normal distribution plays a central role in statistical theory and frequency distributions resembling the Normal distribution form are often observed in practice. Of particular importance is the standardised Normal distribution, which is the Normal distribution that has a mean equal to 0 and a standard deviation (*SD*) equal to 1. The probability density function of such a Normally distributed random variable z is given by

$$\phi(z) = \frac{1}{\sqrt{2\pi}} \exp(-z^2/2). \tag{3.1}$$

The curve described by equation (3.1) is shown in Figure 3.1. For sample size purposes we shall need to calculate the area under some part of this Normal curve. To do this, use is made of the symmetrical nature of the distribution about the mean of 0, and the fact that the total area under a probability density function is unity.

Any shaded area, like that in Figure 3.1, which has area γ (here $\gamma \geqslant 0.5$), has a corresponding value of z_γ along the horizontal axis that can be calculated. For areas with $\gamma < 0.5$ we can use the symmetry of the distribution to calculate, in this case, the values for the unshaded area. For example if $\gamma = 0.5$, then one can see from Figure 3.1 that $z_\gamma = z_{0.5} = 0$. It is also useful to be able to find the value of γ for a given value of z_γ. For example, if $z_\gamma = 1.9600$ it turns out that $\gamma = 0.975$. In this case, the shaded area of Figure 3.1 is then 0.975 and the unshaded area is $1 - 0.975 = 0.025$.

For many practical purposes, it is the area in the tail, $1 - \gamma$, that is needed. We denote this by α in Table T1 which gives the value of z for differing values of α. Thus for one-sided $\alpha = 0.025$ we have $z = 1.9600$. As a consequence of the symmetry of Figure 3.1, if $z = -1.9600$ then $\alpha = 0.025$ is also in the lower tail of the distribution. Hence $z = 1.9600$ corresponds to two-sided $\alpha = 0.05$.

3.3   CONFIDENCE INTERVAL APPROACH

When studies involve a single group only, sample size calculations are couched in CI terms. That is, for the given study endpoint, for example, the mean systolic blood pressure

(SBP), the proportion hypotensive, or the median duration of fever, calculated from the subjects in a case-series it is usual also to quote the corresponding CI. When planning a case-series it would therefore be appropriate to specify ω, the width of the resulting CI desired. This width will depend on the variability from subject to subject (which we cannot control) and the number of subjects in the case-series (which we can often control).

ESTIMATING A MEAN

We first assume that the object of the study is to estimate a population mean μ, and this is thought to be close to μ_{Plan}. Further if the data can be assumed to follow a Normal distribution with SD, σ. Here σ is the population SD which summarises the subject-to-subject variation, and we anticipate its value by σ_{Plan}. Then provided we choose a relatively large sample size N, the $100(1-\alpha)\%$ CI for the population mean μ is likely to be close to

$$\mu_{Plan} - z_{1-\alpha/2}\sqrt{\frac{\sigma_{Plan}^2}{N}} \text{ to } \mu_{Plan} + z_{1-\alpha/2}\sqrt{\frac{\sigma_{Plan}^2}{N}}. \qquad (3.2)$$

The planned width, ω_{Plan}, of this CI is obtained from the difference between the upper and lower limits of equation (3.2) as

$$\omega_{Plan} = 2 \times z_{1-\alpha/2} \times \sqrt{\frac{\sigma_{Plan}^2}{N}}. \qquad (3.3)$$

Thus for a given planning value, ω_{Plan}, the number of subjects N required is obtained by reorganising equation (3.3) to give the required study size as

$$N = 4\left[\frac{\sigma_{Plan}^2}{\omega_{Plan}^2}\right]z_{1-\alpha/2}^2. \qquad (3.4)$$

In practice to calculate N_{Plan}, a value of σ_{Plan} as well as ω_{Plan} has to be provided or a value for their ratio, $\Delta_{Plan}=\omega_{Plan}/\sigma_{Plan}$. The actual value of μ_{Plan} does not feature in this calculation. Once the study is completed, the sample mean $\bar{x}$ replaces μ_{Plan} and the sample standard deviation, s, replaces σ_{Plan} in the calculation of the CI of equation (3.2).

Example – *estimating a mean* – *latency of the auditory P300 in schizophrenia*

Weir, Fiaschi and Machin (1998) give the mean latency of the auditory P300 measured in 19 right-handed patients with schizophrenia as $\bar{x}=346$ ms with SD, $s=27$ ms. Using equation (3.2), with $\bar{x}$ and s in place of μ_{Plan} and σ_{Plan} respectively, then with $\alpha=0.05$ and from Table T1, $z_{0.975}=1.9600$, the corresponding 95% CI is from 334 to 358 ms. This 95% CI has width $\omega=358-334=24$ ms.

If the study were to be repeated but in (say) left-handed patients, how many would be required to obtain a narrower CI set at a width of 20 ms? In this case, $\omega_{Plan}=20$ ms and assuming the same SD of 27 ms, $\Delta_{Plan}=\omega_{Plan}/\sigma_{Plan}=20/27=0.74$ and so equation (3.4) gives $N=4\times(1.9600)^2/(0.74)^2=28.1$ or approximately 30 left-handed patients should be studied.

ESTIMATING A PROPORTION

In a similar way, an appropriate sample size for a prevalence study can be derived using a CI approach. However, if a prevalence, π, rather than a mean, μ, is to be estimated, then σ^2 in equation (3.2) is replaced by $\pi(1-\pi)$. Thus an approximate $100(1-\alpha)\%$ CI for π is

$$\pi_{Plan} - z_{1-\alpha/2}\sqrt{\frac{\pi_{Plan}(1 - \pi_{Plan})}{N}} \text{ to } \pi_{Plan} + z_{1-\alpha/2}\sqrt{\frac{\pi_{Plan}(1 - \pi_{Plan})}{N}}. \quad (3.5)$$

Thus, similar to equation (3.4), the approximate study size required to estimate a prevalence expected to be close to π_{Plan} with width ω_{Plan} is

$$N = 4\left[\frac{\pi_{Plan}(1 - \pi_{Plan})}{\omega_{Plan}^2}\right]z_{1-\alpha/2}^2. \quad (3.6)$$

In practice to calculate N, a value of π_{Plan} as well as ω_{Plan} has to be provided for this equation. Once the study is completed, the sample proportion p replaces π_{Plan} in the calculation of the CI of equation (3.5).

Example – estimating a prevalence – glaucoma in Chinese Singaporeans

As part of a larger study of the prevalence of glaucoma in Singapore, Foster, Oen, Machin et al. (2000) identified 222 men aged 70–81 years for examination. However, of these only 142 (64%) were ultimately eligible for the study and therefore examined. From these men 15 (10.6%) were found to have glaucoma. If this study were to be repeated how many men should be examined to estimate the prevalence of glaucoma with a 95% CI of width 10%?

Here the design sets $\omega_{Plan} = 0.1$ for an anticipated value of $\pi_{Plan} \approx 0.1$. Equation (3.6) with $\alpha = 0.05$, gives

$$N = 4 \times \left[\frac{0.1 \times (1 - 0.1)}{0.1^2}\right] \times 1.9600^2 = 138.3 \text{ or } 139 \text{ men.}$$

If the anticipated prevalence is very low (less than 0.2) or high (greater than 0.8), then more exact methods described by Newcombe and Altman (2000) replace equation (3.5) for the CI – the reason being that as we get closer to the extremes of 0 or 1 then the exact CI gets less and less symmetric on either side of π_{Plan} and one consequence is that equation (3.6) can no longer be used to estimate study size as it assumes that half of the entire width of the CI is below π_{Plan} and half above. The sample sizes given in Table T2 utilise the methods for calculating CIs recommended by Newcombe and Altman (2000) for such situations.

For the example just discussed, the sample size suggested by Table T2, for $\pi_{Plan} = 0.1$ and $\omega_{Plan} = 0.1$ is $N = 141$ men, which is very close to the 139 given previously because the CIs calculated from the approximation and by the exact method are very similar. However if they are not similar, for example, when $\pi_{Plan} = 0.02$ then if we specify $\omega_{Plan} = 0.1$, this causes some difficulty as this width for the CI can no longer be divided equally above and below π_{Plan}. In such a situation, equation (3.5), and hence (3.6), should not be used and sample sizes should be obtained from Table T2. Thus for $\pi_{Plan} = 0.02$ and $\omega_{Plan} = 0.1$ Table T2 gives $N = 52$ subjects.

As sample size calculations are only guides, since they rely on the planning values stipulated which may or may not be close to those ultimately observed, then a study of 55 (or perhaps 60) subjects would be contemplated in this situation.

3.4   STATISTICAL TESTS

SIGNIFICANCE TESTS AND SAMPLE SIZE

In a clinical study we might wish to compare two or more groups with respect to a particular outcome measure. However, subjects, whether healthy volunteers or patients, vary both in their basic characteristics and (if appropriate) in their response to any intervention involved in a study. Thus, following completion of a study, an apparent difference between groups may be observed, but this may be one that is entirely due to the play of chance. In this case, such differences do not indicate *real* differences between the groups being compared.

As a consequence of the play of chance, it is customary to use a 'significance test' to assess the weight of evidence for a real difference beween groups. To do this, the probability that the observed difference could in fact have arisen purely by chance is calculated. The results of the significance test will be expressed by this 'p-value'. For example, a p-value $\leqslant 0.05$ would indicate that so extreme (or greater) an observed difference could only be expected to have arisen by *chance alone* 5% of the time or less. In consequence, therefore, it is quite likely that a *real* difference between groups is present. On the other hand the two-group comparative study may result in a p-value > 0.05 and be declared 'not statistically significant'. However, such a statement only indicates that there was insufficient weight of evidence to be able to declare that 'the observed difference between groups has *not* arisen by chance alone'. It does not imply that there is necessarily 'no (true) difference between the groups'.

However if the sample size were too small the study would be very unlikely to obtain a significant p-value even when a clinically relevant difference is truly present. Also, if only a few subjects were included in the study then, even if there is 'statistical significance' indicating a real difference between groups, the results are likely to be less convincing than if a much larger number of subjects had been assessed. Thus, the weight of evidence in favour of concluding that there is a clinically important effect will be much less in a small study than in a large one. In these circumstances, we might say that the sample size is too small for the purposes in mind.

The 'power' of a significance test is the probability that a test will produce a statistically significant result, given that a true difference between groups of a certain magnitude exists. It is of crucial importance to consider sample size and power when interpreting statements about 'non-significant' results. In particular, if the power of the study was very low in the first place, all one can conclude from a non-significant result is that the question of the presence or absence of differences between groups remains unresolved.

NULL AND ALTERNATIVE HYPOTHESES

To motivate the statistical issues relevant to sample-size calculations, we will assume that we are planning a two-group study in which subjects are allocated at random to the alternative groups and that a single endpoint has been specified in advance.

> **Example** – *difference in means – gastric emptying times*
>
> Lobo, Bostock, Neal *et al.* (2002) describe a randomised trial in which 21 patients with colonic cancer received post-operative intravenous fluids either in accordance with current hospital practice (standard treatment, *S*) or according to a restricted intake regimen (*R*). Their primary endpoints were solid-phase and liquid-phase gastric emptying times on the fourth post-operative day.

We assume the aim of the trial of Lobo, Bostock, Neal *et al.* (2002) is to estimate the true difference δ between the true mean gastric emptying time with R, μ_R, and the true corresponding time, μ_S, of S. Once the trial is completed, the observed mean emptying time with R is $\bar{x}_R$ which estimates μ_R, and the corresponding mean $\bar{x}_S$ estimates μ_S. Thus, the observed difference, $d = \bar{x}_R - \bar{x}_S$ provides an estimate of the true difference $\delta = \mu_R - \mu_S$.

The null hypothesis, termed H_0, implies that $\mu_R = \mu_S$, that is, R and S are equally effective with respect to gastric emptying time. Even when this null hypothesis is true, an observed value of d, other than zero, might well occur following completion of the trial in question. The probability of obtaining the observed difference d or a more extreme one given that $\mu_R = \mu_S$ is true, can be calculated. If under the null hypothesis this probability, termed the *p*-value, is very small then we would *reject* this null hypothesis. In which case we then conclude that the two fluid regimens do indeed differ in their effect.

Usually with statistical significance tests, by rejecting the null hypothesis, we do not specifically accept any alternative hypothesis. Hence it is usual, and good practice, to report the range of plausible population values of the true difference with a CI. However, sample-size calculations require us to provide a specific alternative hypothesis, H_A. This specifies a particular value of the effect size $\delta_{\text{Plan}} = \mu_R - \mu_S$ which is not equal to zero.

Of the parameters that have to be pre-specified before the sample size can be determined, this planning effect size is the most critical.

TYPE I ERROR, TEST SIZE AND SIGNIFICANCE LEVEL

For consistency we have to specify at the planning stage a value, α, so that once the study is completed and analysed, a *p*-value below this would lead to the null hypothesis

Table 3.1   Relationship between Type I and Type II errors and significance tests

Test statistically significant	Difference exists (H_A true)	Difference does not exist (H_0 true)
Yes	Power $(1-\beta)$	Type I error (α)
No	Type II error (β)	

being rejected. Thus if the p-value obtained from a trial is $\leqslant \alpha$, then one rejects the null hypothesis and concludes that there is a statistically significant difference beween treatments. On the other hand, if the p-value is $> \alpha$ then one does not reject the null hypothesis. Although the value of α, is arbitrary, it is often taken as 0.05 or 5%.

Even when the null hypothesis is in fact true there is still a risk of rejecting it. To reject the null hypothesis when it is true is to make a Type I error. Plainly the associated probability of rejecting the null hypothesis when it is true is equal to α. The quantity α is interchangeably termed the test size, significance level or probability of a Type I (or false-positive) error.

TYPE II ERROR AND POWER

The clinical trial could yield an observed difference $\bar{d}$ that would lead to a p-value $> \alpha$ even though the null hypothesis is really not true, that is, μ_R is indeed not equal to μ_S. In such a situation, we then accept (more correctly phrased as 'fail to reject') the null hypothesis although it is truly false. This is called a Type II (false-negative) error and the probability of this is denoted by β.

The probability of a Type II error is based on the assumption that the null hypothesis is not true, that is, $\delta = \mu_R - \mu_S \neq 0$. There are clearly many possible values of δ in this instance and each would imply a different alternative hypothesis, H_A, and a different value for the probability β.

The power is defined as one minus the probability of a Type II error, thus the power equals $1 - \beta$. That is, the *power* is the probability of obtaining a 'statistically significant' p-value when the null hypothesis is truly false.

The relationship between Type I and II errors and significance tests is given in Table 3.1.

3.5   SAMPLE SIZE FOR TWO GROUPS

It is customary to start the process of estimating sample size by specifying the size of the difference required to be detected, and then to estimate the number of subjects required to enable the study to detect this difference if it really exists. For example, Lobo, Bostock, Neal *et al.* (2002) anticipated that the mean gastric emptying time would be 30 minutes less with the restricted intake regimen *R*. Given that this is a plausible and a scientific or medically important change then, at the planning stage, the investigators should be reasonably certain to detect such a difference after completing the study. 'Detecting a difference' is usually taken to mean 'obtain a statistically significant difference with p-value $\leqslant 0.05$'. Similarly the phrase 'to be reasonably certain' is usually

interpreted to mean something like 'have a chance of at least 80% of obtaining such a
p-value' if there really is a lowering of 30 minutes by use of R as opposed to S.

ANTICIPATED (PLANNING) EFFECT SIZE

Estimates of the anticipated effect size may be obtained from the available literature,
formal meta-analyses of related studies or may be elicited from expert opinion. For
clinical trials, in circumstances where there is little prior information available, Cohen
(1988) has proposed a standardised effect size, Δ. In the case when the difference
between two groups 1 and 2 is expressed by the difference between their means
$\delta=(\mu_2-\mu_1)$ and σ is the SD of the endpoint variable which is assumed to be a
continuous measure, then $\Delta=(\mu_2-\mu_1)/\sigma=\delta/\sigma$. A value of $\Delta\leqslant0.2$ is considered a 'small'
standardised effect, $\Delta\approx0.5$ as 'moderate', and $\Delta\geqslant0.8$ as 'large'. Experience has
suggested that in many areas of clinical research these can be taken as a good practical
guide for design purposes.

THEORY AND FORMULAE

The Fundamental Equation

In a trial comparing two groups, with m subjects per group, and a continuous outcome
variable, $\bar{x}_1$ and $\bar{x}_2$ summarise the respective means of the observations taken. Further
if the data are Normally distributed with equal (population) SDs, σ, then the standard
errors are $SE(\bar{x}_1)=SE(\bar{x}_2)=\sigma/\sqrt{m}$. The two groups are compared using $\bar{d}=\bar{x}_2-\bar{x}_1$
with

$$SE(\bar{d}) = \sigma\sqrt{\frac{2}{m}}.$$

Here we assume that $SE(\bar{d})$ is the same whether the null hypothesis, H_0, of no difference
is true, or the alternative hypothesis, H_A, that there is a difference of size δ is true.

Figure 3.2 illustrates the distribution of $\bar{d}$ under the null and alternative hypotheses.
The two distributions are such that $\bar{d}$ has a Normal distribution either with mean 0 or
mean δ, respectively depending on which of the two hypotheses is true. If the observed $\bar{d}$
from a trial exceeds a critical value then the result is declared statistically significant.

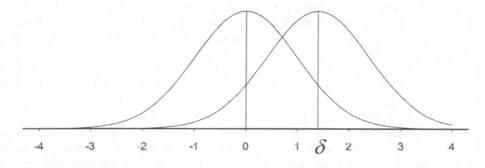

Figure 3.2   Distribution of $\bar{d}$ under the null and alternative hypotheses

For a significance level α (here assumed one-tailed for expository purposes only) we denote this critical value d_α.

Under the null hypothesis, H_0, the critical value d_α is determined by

$$\frac{d_\alpha - 0}{\sigma\sqrt{\dfrac{2}{m}}} = z_{1-\alpha}. \tag{3.7}$$

In contrast, under the assumption that the alternative hypothesis, H_A, is true, $\bar{d}$ now has mean δ but the same

$$SE(\bar{d}) = \sigma\sqrt{\frac{2}{m}}.$$

In this case the probability that $\bar{d}$ exceeds d_α must be $1 - \beta$ and this implies that

$$\frac{d_\alpha - \delta}{\sigma\sqrt{\dfrac{2}{m}}} = -z_{1-\beta}. \tag{3.8}$$

Equations (3.7) and (3.8) can be rewritten as

$$d_\alpha = z_{1-\alpha}\sigma\sqrt{\frac{2}{m}} \tag{3.9}$$

and

$$d_\alpha = \delta - z_{1-\beta}\sigma\sqrt{\frac{2}{m}}. \tag{3.10}$$

Equating the two expressions (3.9) and (3.10), and rearranging, we obtain the sample size for each group in the trial as approximately

$$m = 2\left[\frac{\sigma}{\delta}\right]^2 (z_{1-\alpha} + z_{1-\beta})^2 = \frac{2(z_{1-\alpha} + z_{1-\beta})^2}{\Delta^2}. \tag{3.11}$$

This is termed the *fundamental equation* as it arises, in one form or another, in many situations for which sample sizes are calculated.

The use of equation (3.11) for the case of a two-tailed test, rather than the one-tailed test, involves a slight approximation since $\bar{d}$ is also statistically significant if it is less than $-d_\alpha$. However, with δ positive the associated probability of observing a result smaller than $-d_\alpha$ is negligible. Thus, for the case of a two-sided test, we simply replace $z_{1-\alpha}$ in equation (3.11) by $z_{1-\alpha/2}$.

In order to calculate the sample size for the study in design the experimenter first supplies the components summarised in Table 3.2. Here, α is typically taken as small and so is β (or equivalently expressed the power, $1-\beta$, large). For example, $\alpha = 0.05$ (5%) or 0.01 (1%) and $1-\beta = 0.8$ (20%) or 0.9 (90%).

The basic equation (3.11) has to be modified to adapt to the specific experimental design, the allocation ratio (that is the possibility of the design stipulating unequal subject numbers in each group), and the particular type of endpoint under consideration.

Table 3.2 Components necessary to estimate the size of a comparative study

Effect size, δ	The anticipated (planning) size of the difference between the two groups
Type I error, α	Equivalently the test size or significance level of the statistical test to be used in the analysis
Type II error, β	Equivalently the power, $1-\beta$

ONE-SIDED AND TWO-SIDED TESTS

On biological grounds it may be plausible in the study of Lobo, Bostock, Neal *et al.* (2002) to assume that the mean gastric emptying time would be lower with regimen R. Indeed there would be little point in this replacing the standard, S, if this were not the case. Thus, the alternative hypothesis might be expressed as $\mu_R < \mu_S$. This leads to a one-sided or one-tailed test of statistical significance. On the other hand, if we cannot make any assumption about R, then the alternative hypothesis is that $\mu_R \neq \mu_S$. In general, for a given sample size, a one-sided test is more powerful than the corresponding two-sided test. However, a decision to use a one-sided significance test should never be made *after* looking at the data and observing the direction of the departure. Such decisions should be made at the design stage and made very explicit in the study protocol. In fact, one should use a one-sided test only if it is quite certain that departures in the reverse direction will always be ascribed to chance, and therefore regarded as not statistically significant, however large they happen to be. Thus Altman, Gore, Gardner and Pocock (2000) state: 'It is customary to carry out two-sided hypothesis tests. If a one-sided test is used this should be indicated and justified for the problem in hand'.

As we have indicated, sample sizes for a two-sided test merely replace $z_{1-\alpha}$ of equation (3.11) by $z_{1-\alpha/2}$. However, an improved approximation over equation (3.11) for estimating the sample size for two-group comparisons of means is

$$m = \frac{2(z_{1-\alpha/2} + z_{1-\beta})^2}{\Delta^2_{\text{Plan}}} + \frac{z^2_{1-\alpha/2}}{4}. \tag{3.12}$$

This also incorporates a two-sided test by utilising $z_{1-\alpha/2}$.

Example – difference in means – gastric emptying times

At the planning stage of the study Lobo, Bostock, Neal *et al.* (2002) specified $\alpha = 0.05$, $\beta = 0.1$ and the anticipated effect size, $\delta_{\text{Plan}} = 30 \text{ min}$. From these they calculated $m = 20$ patients per group. Although not stated this implies they used for planning purposes $\sigma_{\text{Plan}} = 29 \text{ min}$. The ratio $\Delta_{\text{Plan}} = \delta_{\text{Plan}}/\sigma_{\text{Plan}} = 30/29 = 1.03$ standard deviations, is a 'large' anticipated standardised effect size using the criteria of Cohen (1988) referred to earlier.

If we set a one-sided $\alpha = 0.05$ then from the final column of Table T1 in the row corresponding to one-sided $\alpha = 0.05$, we obtain $z_{1-\alpha} = z_{0.95} = 1.6449$. For a power of $1-\beta=0.9$, Table T1 gives in the row corresponding to one-sided $\beta=0.1$, $z_{1-\beta}=z_{0.9}=1.2816$. Substituting these in equation (3.11) we have

$$m = \frac{2(1.6449 + 1.2816)^2}{1.03^2} = 16.1$$

or approximately 17. This gives the planned study size as $N=2m=34$ patients in this case.

On the other hand, for a two-sided test with $\alpha=0.05$, and now also using the somewhat better approximation of equation (3.12) gives

$$m = \frac{2(1.9600 + 1.2816)^2}{1.03^2} + \frac{1.96^2}{4} = 19.81 + 0.96 = 20.8 \approx 21.$$

This suggests a planned study size of $N=42$ patients as was used by Lobo, Bostock, Neal et al. (2002).

In the situation of comparing two means, simple formulae for a 5% (two-sided) significance level and power 80% and 90% are respectively

$$m = \frac{16}{\Delta_{\text{Plan}}^2} \quad \text{and} \quad m = \frac{21}{\Delta_{\text{Plan}}^2}. \tag{3.13}$$

UNEQUAL GROUPS

If the variable being measured is continuous and can be assumed to have a Normal distribution, then the number of subjects m, for Group 1 when there are λm in Group 2, is obtained from equation (3.12) but modified to become

$$m = \left(1 + \frac{1}{\lambda}\right)\left[\frac{(z_{1-\alpha/2} + z_{1-\beta})^2}{\Delta_{\text{Plan}}^2} + \frac{z_{1-\alpha/2}^2}{8}\right], \lambda > 0. \tag{3.14}$$

This leads to a total study size of $N=m+n=m(1+\lambda)$ subjects.

When one group (Group 2) are patients and the others (Group 1) are normal controls but patients are scarce, then there is a statistical gain in recruiting a larger number of controls than available cases. In such situations λ may be chosen as less than 1, although if both groups of subjects are equally available the optimum ratio between them is 1:1, that is, $\lambda=1$ in equation (3.14).

Example – *difference in means* – *oscillatory potentials*

Suppose we were to repeat the study of Drasdo, Chiti, Owens and North (2002) who compared the summed oscillatory potentials in controls and patients with type 2 diabetes but confine our objective to confirming their observations that the 'during oxygen' differential of oscillatory potentials is 30 μV. We assume the *SD* from the controls is approximately the 70 μV they had observed. Thus, $\Delta_{Plan} = \delta_{Plan}/\sigma_{Plan} = 30/70 \approx 0.4$ which is a 'moderate' standardised effect size. Further we consider two options (i) equal numbers of controls and diabetic patients, that is $\lambda = 1$, and (ii) 50% more controls than diabetic patients, that is for every two patients three controls are recruited, so $\lambda = 2/3$. We further assume $\alpha = 0.05$ and power $(1 - \beta) = 0.8$.

Evaluating equation (3.14) in situation (i) gives $m = 100$, thus a total study size of $N = 2m \approx 200$ is required. Repeating the calculations under scenario (ii) gives $m = 124$ controls. However, 124 is not exactly divisible by 3 and so, to enable a randomisation in blocks of 5 (2 patients and 3 controls), this is increased to 126. Hence $n = (2/3) \times 126 = 84$ patients. This leads to a larger study size of $N = 126 + 84 = 210$ subjects in all than the 1:1 situation but now including fewer patients. In this case the reduction in the number of patients by $100 - 84 = 16$ is compensated for by a greater increase in the number of $126 - 100 = 26$ controls.

Binary Outcomes

If the outcome variable of the two-group design is binary rather than continuous, such as when a satisfactory response to treatment either is or is not observed, then the number of subjects required for Group 1, for anticipated difference $\delta = \pi_2 - \pi_1$, is obtained from

$$m = \frac{\left[z_{1-\alpha/2}\sqrt{(1+\lambda)\bar{\pi}(1-\bar{\pi})} + z_{1-\beta}\sqrt{\lambda\pi_1(1-\pi_1) + \pi_2(1-\pi_2)}\right]^2}{\lambda(\pi_2 - \pi_1)^2}. \tag{3.15}$$

Here π_1 and π_2 are the proportion who respond in the respective groups and $\bar{\pi} = (\pi_1 + \lambda\pi_2)/(1+\lambda)$. The number to be recruited to Group 2 is $n = \lambda m$, and the total number of subjects $N = m(1+\lambda)$.

An approximation to this expression, when $\lambda = 1$, is

$$m = \frac{(z_{1-\alpha/2} + z_{1-\beta})^2[\pi_1(1-\pi_1) + \pi_2(1-\pi_2)]}{(\pi_2 - \pi_1)^2}. \tag{3.16}$$

The expression in the square brackets has a maximum value of 0.5 when $\pi_1 = \pi_2 = 0.5$ and so, for a two-sided test size of 5% and power 80%, this leads to a conservative (maximal) estimate of the sample size as

$$N = \frac{8}{(\pi_2 - \pi_1)^2}. \tag{3.17}$$

Example *– difference in proportions – treatment of severe burns*

In a randomised trial by Ang, Lee, Gan *et al.* (2001), the standard wound covering (non-exposed) treatment was compared with Moist Exposed Burns Ointment (MEBO) in patients with severe burns. One object of the trial was to reduce the methicillin-resistant *Staphylococcus aureus* (MRSA) infection rate at 2 weeks post-admission in such patients from 25% to 5%.

With planning values set at $\pi_1 = 0.25$ and $\pi_2 = 0.05$, and for a two-sided test size of 5% and power 80%, equations (3.15) and (3.16) with $\lambda = 1$, both lead to $m = 50$ per treatment group, that is $N = 100$ patients. However, using the approximate calculation of equation (3.17) gives $N = 200$ patients. The very large discrepancy occurs because one of the MRSA rates is anticipated to be very low (0.05 or 5%).

In fact, as is the case when discussing equation (3.6), the approximation of equation (3.17) becomes somewhat unreliable if either one of the proportions is below (about) 0.2 or above 0.8.

Survival

If the endpoint of interest is a 'survival', then this may be the actual duration of time from the date of randomisation (to treatment) to the date of death of a cancer patient, or the time from hospital admission to some event such as contracting MRSA infection. In these cases, the 'events' are death and MRSA infection respectively. The number of subjects to be recruited to a study is set so that the requisite number of 'events' may be observed.

For subjects in whom the 'events' occur the actual survival time, t, is observed. The remainder of the subjects concerned have censored survival times, $T+$, as for them the 'event' has not (yet) occurred up to this point in their observation time. The eventual analysis of these data, which involves either t or $T+$ for every subject, will involve Kaplan–Meier estimates of the corresponding cumulative survival curves. Comparisons between groups can be made using the logrank test and the summary statistic used is the hazard ratio (HR). Methods for survival analysis are described in Machin, Cheung and Parmar (2005). The test of the null hypothesis of equality of event rates between the groups with respect to the endpoint (event) concerned provides the basis for the sample size calculations. This is expressed as H_0: $HR = 1$.

Pre-study information on the endpoint, either as the anticipated median 'survival' for each group or as the anticipated proportions 'alive' at some fixed time point, will usually form the basis of the anticipated difference between groups for planning purposes. The corresponding effect size is HR_{Plan}. If proportions π_1 and π_2 are anticipated then

$$HR_{\text{Plan}} = \frac{\log \pi_2}{\log \pi_1}. \tag{3.18}$$

Once HR_{Plan} is obtained then the number of events required to be observed in Group 1 is

$$e_1 = \frac{1}{\lambda} \left(\frac{1 + \lambda HR_{\text{Plan}}}{1 - HR_{\text{Plan}}} \right)^2 (z_{1-\alpha/2} + z_{1-\beta})^2. \tag{3.19}$$

Thus for the second group, $e_2 = \lambda e_1$ events are required or a total of $E = e_1 + e_2$ for the study as a whole.

The corresponding number of subjects needed in order to observe these events for Group 1 is

$$m = \frac{1}{\lambda} \left(\frac{1 + \lambda HR_{\text{Plan}}}{1 - HR_{\text{Plan}}} \right)^2 \frac{(z_{1-\alpha/2} + z_{1-\beta})^2}{[(1 - \pi_1) + \lambda(1 - \pi_2)]}. \tag{3.20}$$

For Group 2, $n = \lambda m$, leading to $N = m + n = m(1 + \lambda)$ subjects in all.

If the median survival time M_1 of one of the groups is given then this implies that, at that time $\pi_1 = 0.5$. Further if M_2 is given, then $HR_{\text{Plan}} = M_1/M_2$, and use of equation (3.18) gives $\pi_2 = \exp(\log 0.5/HR_{\text{Plan}}) = \exp(-0.6932/HR_{\text{Plan}})$ and, for given λ, these provide the necessary components for calculating the study size.

Example – differences in survival – gastric cancer

Cuschieri, Weeden, Fielding *et al.* (1999) compared two forms of surgical resection for patients with gastric cancer. The primary outcome (event of interest) was time to death. The authors state: 'Sample size calculations were based on a pre-study survey of 26 gastric surgeons, which indicated that the baseline 5-year survival rate of D_1 surgery was expected to be 20%, and an improvement in survival to 34% (14% change) with D_2 resection would be a realistic expectation. Thus 400 patients (200 in each arm) were to be randomized, providing 90% power to detect such a difference with $P < 0.05$'.

Here $\pi_1 = 0.2$, $\pi_2 = 0.34$ and so from equation (3.18) $HR_{\text{Plan}} = \log 0.34/\log 0.2 = (-1.078)/(-1.609) = 0.6667$. The authors set $1 - \beta = 0.9$ and imply a two-sided test size $\alpha = 0.05$ and a randomisation in equal numbers to each group, hence $\lambda = 1$. First making use of Table T1 implies $z_{1-0.025} = z_{0.975} = 1.9600$ and $z_{1-0.9} = z_{0.1} = 1.2816$, then substituting all the corresponding values in equation (3.20) gives

$$m = \left(\frac{1 + 0.6667}{1 - 0.6667} \right)^2 \frac{(1.9600 + 1.2816)^2}{[(1 - 0.2) + (1 - 0.34)]}$$

$$= 25 \times \frac{10.5080}{1.46} \approx 180 \text{ per surgical group.}$$

SUBJECT WITHDRAWALS

One aspect of a clinical trial, which can affect the number of patients recruited, is the proportion of patients who are lost to follow-up during the course of the trial. These withdrawals are a particular problem for trials in which patients are monitored over a long period of follow-up time. Any such 'lost' patients also have censored observations, as do those for whom the event of interest has not occurred at the end of the trial or more precisely at the time point when the analysis is to be conducted.

In these circumstances, as a precaution against such withdrawals, the planned number of patients is adjusted upwards to

$$N_W = N/(1 - W) \qquad (3.21)$$

where W is the anticipated withdrawal proportion. The estimated size of W can often be obtained from reports of studies conducted by others. If there is no such experience to hand, than a pragmatic value may be to take $W=0.1$.

Example – *adjusting for withdrawals* – *gastric cancer*

Thus Cuschieri, Weeden, Fielding *et al.* (1999), after allowing for some 10% for patient for withdrawals, increased $m=180$ to 198 and had a final planned trial size as $N=400$.

In the event, 400 patients were indeed recruited and the trial estimated the $HR=1.10$ (95% CI 0.87 to 1.39). Thus the trial indicated, since the observed $HR>1$, that patients were likely to do less well with the D_2 regime in contradiction to the opinions held at the design stage of the trial.

EQUIVALENCE

Implicit in a comparison between two groups is the presumption that if the null hypothesis is rejected then there is a difference between the groups being compared. Thus if this comparison involves a comparison of treatments then one concludes that one treatment is superior to the other irrespective of the magnitude of the difference observed. However, in certain situations, a new therapy may bring certain advantages over the current standard, possibly in a reduced side-effects profile, easier administration or cost, but it may not be anticipated to be better with respect to the primary efficacy variable. Under such conditions, the new approach may be required to be at least 'equivalent' to the standard in relation to efficacy if it is to replace it in future clinical use. This implies that 'equivalence' is a pre-specified maximum difference beween two groups which, if observed to be less after the clinical study is conducted, would render the two groups equivalent.

In general, having conducted a study to compare groups with respect to a particular outcome, one calculates a $100(1-\alpha)\%$ CI for the true difference, δ, between them. This CI covers the true difference with a given probability, $1-\alpha$. The concept of equivalence is illustrated in Figure 3.3 by considering the range of options possible for these CIs. In the figure the 'equivalence' limit, ε, is set to define regions beyond which, if the observed difference, $\bar{d}$, were to fall, then this would be regarded as clinically important and not indicative of equivalence. The limits are set above and below $\delta=0$, corresponding to the null hypothesis of no true difference between treatments. For this situation the effect size of Table 3.2 is replaced by the equivalence limit.

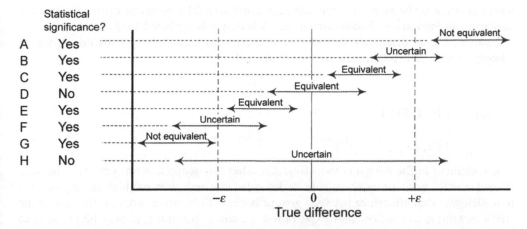

Figure 3.3 Schematic diagram to illustrate the concept of equivalence by using a series of possible comparative trial outcomes as summarised by their reported CI (after Jones, Jarvis, Lewis and Ebbutt, 1996. Trials to assess equivalence: the importance of rigorous methods. *British Medical Journal* **313**, 36 39. [3,7,9])

The CI: *A* of Figure 3.3 clearly demonstrates an important difference since even the lower limit of this CI is beyond $+\varepsilon$. If a CI crosses a boundary (CI: *B* and *F*), then one would be uncertain as to whether or not the treatments were equivalent, whereas if it were totally between the limits $-\varepsilon$ to $+\varepsilon$ (CI: *C*, *D*, *E*) then equivalence would be claimed. The uncertain outcome of CI: *H* would correspond to a trial of inadequate size.

It is quite possible to show a statistically significant difference between two treatments yet also demonstrate therapeutic equivalence (CI: *C* and *E*). These are not contradictory statements but simply a realisation that, although there is evidence that one treatment works better than another, the size of the benefit is so small that it has little or no practical advantage.

Jones, Jarvis, Lewis and Ebbutt (1996) state that when this CI approach is used to assess equivalence, two sorts of mistake can occur: we can decide that the treatments are equivalent when they are not (type I error with probability α) or we can decide the treatments are not equivalent when they are (type II error with probability β). The corresponding power of the trial, $1-\beta$, is the probability of correctly declaring equivalence when $\delta=0$. The null hypothesis H_0 is the combination of: $\delta \leqslant -\varepsilon$ and $\delta \geqslant \varepsilon$ (non-equivalence), whereas the alternative hypothesis H_A is: $-\varepsilon < \delta < \varepsilon$ (equivalence).

Continuous Outcome

For a two-sided CI approach, the sample size per group required to demonstrate the equivalence of two means in a 1:1 randomised design based on an anticipated common mean, μ, with *SD*, σ, and level of equivalence set as $-\varepsilon$ to $+\varepsilon$ is

$$m_{\text{Equivalence}} = \frac{2(z_{1-\alpha} + z_{1-\beta/2})^2}{\Delta^2}, \tag{3.22}$$

where $\Delta = \varepsilon/\sigma$ is the relevant (equivalence) effect size. The essential difference beween this and the fundamental equation of (3.11) is that β is replaced by $\beta/2$.

Equivalence is discussed further with respect to establishing bioequivalence in Chapter 8 and therapeutic equivalence trials in Chapter 9.

3.6   PRACTICE

THE EFFECT SIZE

A key element in the design is the 'effect size' that it is reasonable to plan to observe – should it exist. Sometimes there is prior knowledge which then enables an investigator to anticipate what effect size between groups is likely to be observed, and the role of the study or trial is to confirm that expectation. In some situations, it may be possible to state that, for example, only a doubling of median survival would be worthwhile to demonstrate in a planned trial. This might be because the new treatment, as compared to standard, is expected to be so toxic that only if substantial benefit could be shown would it ever be utilised. In such cases the investigator may have definite opinions about the difference that it is pertinent to detect.

In practice a range of plausible effect size options are considered before the final planning effect size is agreed. For example, an investigator might specify a scientific or clinically useful difference that it is hoped could be detected, and would then estimate the required sample size on this basis. The calculations might then indicate that an extremely large number of subjects is required. As a consequence, the investigator may next define a revised aim of detecting a rather larger difference than that originally specified. The calculations are repeated, and perhaps the sample size now becomes realistic in that new context.

One additional problem when planning comparative clinical trials is that investigators are often optimistic about the magnitude of the improvement of new treatments over the standard. This optimism is understandable, since it can take considerable effort to initiate a trial and, in many cases, the trial would only be launched if the investigator is enthusiastic about the new treatment and is sufficiently convinced about its potential efficacy. However, experience suggests that as trial succeeds trial there is often a growing realism that, even at best, the earlier expectations were optimistic. There is ample historical evidence to suggest that trials that set out to detect large treatment differences nearly always result in 'no significant difference was detected'. In such cases there may have been a true and worthwhile treatment benefit that has been missed, since the level of detectable differences set by the design was unrealistically high, and hence the sample size too small to establish the true (but less optimistic) size of benefit.

The way in which possible effect sizes are determined will depend on the specific situation under consideration. For example, if a study is a repeat of one already conducted, then very detailed information may be available on the options for the effect size suitable for planning the new study. In contrast, if very little is known, one may revert to Cohen's suggestions, gained from experience from a very wide range of studies unrelated to the one being planned, and choose (say) an effect size close to moderate at $\Delta \approx 0.5$. An intermediate possibility, for clinical trials at least, is to obtain a distribution of effect sizes as has been suggested by Spiegelhalter, Freedman and Parmar (1994). This can be obtained from a survey of the views of the clinical team, or other knowledgeable colleagues, on the likely effect size and combining their responses into a plausible effect size distribution. This prior distribution then gives a plausible range of options from which sample-size scenarios can be discussed by the planning team. An extension of this approach has been advocated by Tan, Dear, Bruzzi and Machin (2003) who suggest how information, from whatever source, may be synthesised into a prior distribution for the anticipated effect size which is then utilised for planning purposes.

For bioequivalence there has become something of an expected standard for the definition of (equivalence) effect size which we discuss in Chapter 8. However for therapeutic trials in general the limit of equivalence will be very specific to the choice of patients and therapies in question and its value will tend to be based more on clinical than statistical considerations.

LIMITED RESOURCES

A common situation is one where the number of subjects, who may be patients, that can be included in a study is governed by non-scientific forces such as time, money or human resources. Thus with a predetermined (maximal) sample size, the researcher may then wish to know what probability he or she has of detecting a certain effect size with a study confined to this size. If the resulting power is small, say $<50\%$, then the investigator may decide that the study should not go ahead. A similar situation arises if the type of subject under consideration is uncommon, as would be the case with a clinical trial in rare disease groups. In either case the sample size is constrained, and the researcher is interested in finding the size of effects which could be established for a reasonable power, say, 80%.

SEVERAL PRIMARY OUTCOMES

We have based the above discussion on the assumption that there is a single identifiable endpoint or outcome, upon which comparisons are based. Often there is more than one endpoint of interest, such as the relative survival time and response rates, as well as quality of life scores of subjects in the two groups. If one of these endpoints is regarded as more important than the others, it can be named as the primary endpoint and sample-size estimates based on that alone. A problem arises when there are several outcome measures that are all regarded as equally important. A commonly adopted approach is to repeat the sample-size estimates for each outcome measure in turn, and then select the largest of these as the sample size required to answer all the questions of interest.

However, it is well recognised that if many endpoints are included in one study and the groups are tested for statistical significance for all of these, then the p-values so obtained are distorted. To compensate for this, smaller observed p-values may be required to declare 'true' statistical significance at level α. In such cases, the sample-size calculations will be similarly affected so that to retain the level at α for all the tests conducted a value depending on the number of endpoints, k, is sometimes substituted in, for example, equations (3.14) and (3.15). A common value is simply α/k. Even when $k=2$, this substantially increases the size of the planned study.

Example – *two major endpoints – gastric emptying times*

In the randomised trial described by Lobo, Bostock, Neal *et al.* (2002) there were two primary endpoints: solid-phase and liquid-phase gastric emptying times on the fourth post-operative day. Repeating the sample-size calculations we had made earlier but with two-sided α replaced by $\alpha/2$ since $k=2$, gives from Table T1 using the two-sided column with value 0.025, $z_{1-\alpha/4}=z_{0.9875}=2.2414$. The $z_{1-\beta}=z_{0.9}=1.2816$ remains the same, and so from either equation (3.12) or equation (3.14) with $\lambda=1$, we have

$$m = \frac{2(2.2414 + 1.2816)^2}{1.03^2} + \frac{2.2414^2}{4} = 23.2 + 1.3 \approx 25.$$

This gives the planned study size with two endpoints as $N=2m\approx 50$ patients in this case. This increases the study size by 25% over the earlier calculations.

INTERNAL PILOT STUDIES

As we have indicated, in order to calculate the sample size of a study one must first have suitable background information together with some idea as to what is a realistic difference to seek. Sometimes such information is available as prior knowledge from the literature or other sources; at other times, a pilot study may be conducted.

Traditionally, a pilot study is a distinct preliminary investigation, conducted before embarking on the main trial. However, Wittes and Brittain (1990), Birkett and Day (1994) and Browne (1995) have explored the use of an internal pilot study. The idea here is to plan the clinical trial on the basis of best available information, but to regard the first patients entered as the 'internal' pilot. When data from these patients have been collected, the sample size can be re-estimated with the revised knowledge so generated.

Two vital features accompany this approach: firstly, the final sample size should only ever be adjusted upwards, *never* down; and secondly, one should only use the internal pilot in order to improve the components of the sample-size calculation which are independent of the observed difference between groups. This second point is crucial. It means that when comparing the means of two groups, it is valid to re-estimate the planning *SD*, σ_{Plan} but not the planning effect size, δ_{Plan}. Both these points should be carefully observed to avoid distortion of the subsequent significance test and a possible misleading interpretation of the final study results.

Example – *internal pilot to modify study size – gastric emptying time*

As we have discussed Lobo, Bostock, Neal *et al.* (2000) estimated their required sample size on the basis of a reduction in gastric emptying time of 30 minutes. However, after recruiting 10 patients to their study, they observed a gastric emptying time reduction of 74 minutes. As a consequence of this observed but interim value being greater than that used at the planning stage, the sample size was recalculated and *reduced* from the initial 40 patients to 20. Such a step breaks all the rules attached to the use of internal pilot studies.

The advantage of an internal pilot is that it can be relatively large – perhaps half of the anticipated patients. It provides an insurance against misjudgement regarding the baseline planning assumptions. It is, nevertheless, important that the intention to conduct an internal pilot study is recorded at the outset and the full details are given in the study protocol.

3.7 TERMINOLOGY

From a statistical perspective, when conducting a clinical study, one is estimating from a sample or samples the true or underlying population values of a particular parameter or parameters. For example, if we are concerned with estimating the mean blood sugar levels of a particular population 'at risk of diabetes', then the observations from a random sample taken from that population provide the mean $\bar{x}$. This is then the estimate of the true or population mean μ. In planning such a study, we postulate a value for μ, denoted μ_{Plan}, and the study size is based on this value. We hope that μ_{Plan} will be close to μ, but we do not know this. All we know is $\bar{x}$ as calculated from the data once collected. This too may or may not be close to μ_{Plan}. However, we nevertheless infer that it is close to μ and the associated CI provides a measure of our uncertainty with respect to the true value.

In the chapters which follow, we try to distinguish between μ_{Plan}, μ and $\bar{x}$, or their equivalents in other types of studies.

3.8 TECHNICAL NOTE

STATISTICAL MODELS

In our illustration of significance tests associated with the Lobo, Bostock, Neal *et al.* (2002) study, the parameters to estimate were described in terms of the population means, μ_R and μ_S. These represented the true mean gastric emptying times of the two fluid groups. This can also be expressed in terms of the parameters of equation (1.1). In which case, y is the gastric emptying time, $x=0$ for fluid regimen S and $x=1$ for R. With $x=0$ in equation (1.1), then $y_0=\beta_0$, whereas with $x=1$, $y_1=\beta_0+\beta_1$. Thus the difference δ, between those receiving R and S, is $y_1 - y_0 = \beta_0 + \beta_1 - \beta_0 = \beta_1$. From which $\beta_1 = \mu_R - \mu_S$ and $\beta_0 = \mu_S$ so that the two approaches are algebraically equivalent.

For single-group studies, essentially $x = 0$ for all subjects and so the model of equation (1.1) reduces to $y = \beta_0$. The aim of the study is then to estimate β_0 and the associated CI.

BAYESIAN METHODS

On occasion we refer to Bayesian methodology and so we give a very brief description of the main elements as they affect the material in this book.

In broad terms, the usual (or frequentist) approach to the estimation of the parameters β_0 and β_1 of equation (1.1) is to regard these as fixed values for the population concerned. Then once the data are collected from our study, estimates, b_0 and b_1, of these parameters are derived from only these data. In contrast, the Bayesian approach allows the estimates to incorporate information external to the study data and no longer regards the parameters as fixed.

Any external evidence, either from published data or opinions held before the study commences, can be formalised into a *prior* distribution that encapsulates an estimate of the parameter concerned and also the uncertainty about its value. This prior distribution is combined with the study data once collected, to form the *posterior* distribution of the parameter from which a probability statement can then be derived concerning the true value of the parameter. Thus we talk in Chapter 8, of the probability that the true response rate π is greater than a chosen value. This expresses the uncertainty about the true value of π following the study and replaces the CI in the frequentist approach.

4 Randomisation

Summary

The method of choice of intervention given to a particular experimental unit is an essential feature for maximising the useful information from an experimental design. We give the rationale for why a random element to the choice is desirable and describe how random numbers to assist the implementation of this may be utilised. For preclinical studies we describe how interventions may be grouped into randomised block, Latin and Graeco-Latin squares. In addition, the essential aspect of assigning experimental treatments at random, and when randomisation should be affected, in the context of comparative clinical trials is included. For cross-sectional studies, including surveys, details of how the subjects for study may be selected at random from a larger pool of available individuals are described.

4.1 INTRODUCTION

In any study where we intervene in the natural course of events a decision has to be taken as to which (experimental) intervention is given to which unit. In general whatever the basic design, one should choose the structure of the design to answer the question posed, then make the study as 'random' as possible. For example, bitter experience has shown that comparisons of treatments made by comparing non-randomised groups of patients given the alternatives are often very misleading. This does not preclude the possibility of making non-randomised comparisons in certain situations but is a reminder that they are intrinsically unreliable.

Although there is not always a clear division between the randomisation requirements of preclinical studies and clinical trials one feature usually distinguishes them. At least in the more 'experimental' type of preclinical studies the experimental units may all be available for study at the time the experiment is to begin. In contrast, for the randomised controlled trial, patients are usually recruited one at a time and over a prolonged period, so that allocation to the intervention has to be made sequentially in time and then usually patient by patient. There will be very few occasions when all the patients are recruited to a clinical trial on the same day. Thus, while for a clinical study the randomisation allocation process can be complete at the very beginning of the study, that for a clinical trial will continue until the last patient is recruited. As a

Design of Studies for Medical Research. D. Machin and M. J. Campbell
© 2005 John Wiley & Sons Ltd. ISBN 0 470 84495 7

consequence, methods such as dynamic allocation to intervention may be very useful in clinical trials but of little relevance to experiments.

4.2   RATIONALE AND MECHANICS

ESTIMATION

In essence, one purpose of any experiment is to estimate the parameters of a model analogous to equation (1.1). Thus we collect data with this purpose in mind. We would like to believe that the estimates we obtain in some way reflect the 'true' or population parameter values. In principle, if we repeated the study many times, then we would anticipate that these estimates would form a distribution that is centred on the true parameter value. If this is the case, our method of estimation is *unbiased*. For example, in a clinical trial comparing two treatments, the parameter β_1 corresponds to the true difference (if any) in efficacy between them, and the object of the trial is to obtain an unbiased estimate of this. The method of selecting which of the eligible patients are to be included in the trial does not effect this, but the way in which those patients who are recruited to the trial are then allocated to which particular treatment does. Of fundamental importance to the design of any clinical trial is the random allocation of subjects to the alternative treatments. Such allocation safeguards in particular against bias.

Randomisation also provides a sound basis for the ensuing hypothesis testing by the use of statistical tests of significance.

SIMPLE RANDOMISATION

Random Numbers

The simplest randomisation device is a coin which if tossed will land with a particular face upward with probability one-half. Repeated tossing generates a sequence of heads (H) and tails (T) such as *HHTHH TTHTH*. These can be converted to a binary sequence 00100 11001 by replacing H by 0 and T by 1. An alternative method would be to roll a six-sided die, and allocate a 0 for faces 1, 2 and 3 and 1 to 4, 5 and 6.

To avoid using a die for randomisation one can produce a table of random numbers such as Table T3. Although this table is in fact 'computer-generated', the principle is similar to that which would result from throwing a ten-sided die, with faces marked 0 to 9, on successive occasions. Thus each digit is equally likely to appear and cannot be predicted from any combination of other digits. The digits in Table T3 are grouped merely for ease of reading. The table is used by first choosing a point of entry, perhaps with a pin, but deciding in advance of this the direction of movement along the rows or down the columns. Suppose the pin chooses the entry in the 10th row and 13th column, and it had been decided to move along the rows, then the first 10 digits give the sequence 534 55425 67 (highlighted in bold and larger font in Table T3).

Random Selection

To obtain a simple random sample, it is first necessary to number all the individual members of the target population of interest through from 1 to $N_{\text{Population}}$. Simple random sampling gives each individual in the target population the same probability ($1/N_{Population}$) of being selected. Selection of one individual does not enable us to predict the next that is chosen. The next step is to generate N different random numbers in the range of the numbered list, where N is the intended study size. Any duplicate numbers are replaced at random by ones not already on the list. The numbers on this final list identify the members of the target population to be included in the study.

Example *– random sample – patients with schizoprenia*

Suppose the target population is the 100 patients with schizophrenia who are on a patient list. We then wish to choose $N=30$ at random from this $N_{Population}=100$ for inclusion in the study. First we number the patients in any order from 01 to 100 but use 00 to represent patient 100. Then using the first two digits in (say) the first column of Table T3 we find the first 30 numbers in the range 00 to 99 are successively 75, 80, 94, 67, ..., 87, 63. However, 03, 43, 50, 67, 90 and 94 are repeated in this list and so the next six random numbers are taken. These are 73, 69, 64, 31, 35 and 57, but 57 has been used previously so we choose the next which is 50. This too has to be ignored and so the next, which is 48, is taken. Now that the numbered list of 30 is complete, the corresponding patients are then identified from the list and these are examined in the study. Such a procedure is usually only practicable if the target population is not too large, although it can be quickly achieved with a suitable computer program.

Random Allocation

The first step in the simplest form of randomisation in a two-group comparative study, is to assign one intervention (say) A to even numbers, the other, B, to odd. The next step is to use the random numbers of Table T3 to generate the sequence of length $N=2m$, where m is the planned number of units in each group. For example, using the previously chosen sequence 53455 42567 generates *BBABB AABAB*. Thus the first 10 units selected will receive the interventions in this order, and once this is complete four will have received A and six B.

The method extends relatively easily to more complex designs. For example, in the case of a 2×2 factorial experimental design involving four combinations labelled A, B, C and D, each of these could be allocated the successive digit pairs: 0–1: 2–3: 4–5 and 6–7 respectively. Should an 8 or 9 occur in the random sequence then these are ignored, as there is no associated intervention for these cases. The random sequence 534 55425 would then generate *CBC CCCBC*, thus in the first eight subjects the allocation would be A 0, B 2, C 6 and D 0. This is clearly not a desirable outcome as no subject is allocated to either of the interventions A or D.

An alternative way, when there are four groups, is first to divide those members of the random sequence equal to 4 or more, by 4 and replace these by the corresponding remainder part. Thus the first number of the above sequence of 10 digits is 5, which once divided by 4 gives remainder 1, the second 3 remains as it is, while the third 4 becomes 0, and so on. The new sequence is now 13011 02123. In technical terms this is the same sequence as previously but each integer reduced modulo 4 (mod 4). If the interventions in the experiment are numbered 1 to 4, rather than 0 to 3, then for convenience we add 1 to each member of the sequence to obtain 24122 13234. The randomisation for the first eight units for the four interventions then generates *BDABB ACB*, so once completed for eight subjects, *A* is 2, *B* 4, *C* 1 and *D* 1. It is essential to choose the details of the method to be used before the randomisation process takes place.

4.3   PRECLINICAL OR LABORATORY-BASED STUDIES

Preclinical studies are usually of modest size but may be larger if the units are (say) blood samples, biopsy specimens or pathology slides. As indicated, if all units are available, or can be recruited as and when needed, then the randomisation allocation process can be completed in advance of any subject being investigated.

In preclinical experiments, the objective of the randomisation is to help ensure balance of the experimental units between the different (two or more) experimental groups in terms of their basic characteristics. This applies whether the experimental units are biopsy specimens or the human subjects themselves. Thus the objective of the randomisation is to make the final comparison of differences between experimental groups as unbiased as possible. We need to be assured that any differences observed between groups are not due to, for example, where the individual biopsy specimens from the two groups are stored in the refrigerator, but rather are due to the different experimental interventions imposed by the design.

BLOCKS

Simple randomisation will not guarantee equal numbers in the different intervention groups. To ensure equal numbers, balanced arrangements can be introduced. This is done by first generating the combinations of the intervention possibilities into blocks of an appropriate size.

The block size is taken as a convenient multiple of the number of interventions under investigation. For example, a two-group design may have block sizes 2, 4, 6 or 8, a three-group 3, 6 or 9, while for a 2×2 factorial design comprising four interventions these may be of size 4, 8 or 12. In addition, the actual block size is often also chosen as a convenient divisor of the planned study size, N. For example, if $N=64$, and with four interventions planned, a block size of 8 would be preferable to one of 12, since 8 is a divisor of 64 but 12 is not. Blocks are usually chosen as neither too small nor too large so that for two intervention groups block sizes of 4 or 6 are often used.

Suppose that equal numbers are to be allocated to *A* and *B* for successive blocks of four subjects. To do this, one can identify amongst all 16 possible combinations or permutations of *A* and *B* in blocks of four that contain two *A*s and two *B*s. Thus we are ignoring those permutations with unequal allocation, such as *AAAA* and *AAAB*. The

Table 4.1 All possible permutations of length 4 for two treatments A and B each occurring only twice

1	*AABB*	4	*BABA*
2	*ABAB*	5	*BAAB*
3	*ABBA*	6	*BBAA*

acceptable permutations are summarised in Table 4.1. These permutations are then allocated the numbers 1 to 6 and the randomisation table used to generate a sequence of digits. Suppose this sequence was again 53455 42567, then reading from left to right we generate the allocation *BAAB ABBA BABA BAAB BAAB* and *BABA* for the first 24 units.

Often, a particular digit for the sequences of Table T3 would not be used a second time until all relevant individual digits had first been used. In this case, the sequence becomes, in effect, 534– – –2–67. This generates *BAAB ABBA BABA* as previously but now followed by permutations 2 and 6 of Table 4.1, which are *ABAB* and *BBAA*. Finally we note that permutation 1 has not been used so that *AABB* completes the full 24-unit allocation sequence. Such devices ensure that for every four successive units included, balance between A and B is maintained. In this case we recruit 12 to A and 12 to B. Once again, precise details of the methods to be used have to be defined and documented before the randomisation process begins.

Experimental Designs

We also have to ensure that the measurement process itself does not lead to bias. For example, suppose all those who receive A are tested by the same experimenter I, and those who receive B by experimenter II, then observed differences between the two groups may not only reflect A versus B differences but also differences between observers I and II. We cannot eliminate differences between these experimenters (although careful training in experimental procedures may reduce this) but we can measure their differential effect by a suitable choice of experimental design, in which both experimenters test subjects from each group.

We first create the combinations *A-I*, *A-II*, *B-I* and *B-II* where (say) *A-I* is intervention A given by experimenter I. Suppose that only four subjects can be tested in 2-hour slots in one day. We can then organise these four options into four blocks of four as in Table 4.2, Panel (a).

Considering the first 16 subjects for this study, the usual way to allocate the corresponding experimental units (subjects) is to first number these from 1 to 16. Then we can assign these starting from the top left corner of the randomised block design, Table 4.2, Panel (a), and moving down successive columns (the blocks) until subject 16 is given the bottom right-hand corner intervention. This process implies that whoever assigns the numbers to the subjects is entirely ignorant of the allocation they will receive and when and by whom their 'experiment' will be conducted.

The allocation process of Table 4.2, Panel (a), implies, whilst retaining equal numbers in interventions A and B, that half the units are also allocated to experimenter I, and half to experimenter II. Each experimenter therefore conducts equal numbers of

Table 4.2 Randomised block design of two interventions (A and B) conducted by two experimenters (I and II) in 16 subjects over 4 days

Time of day	Day				Day			
	1	2	3	4	1	2	3	4
	Panel (a)				Panel (b)			
0900–1100	A-I	A-I	A-I	A-I	A-I	A-II	B-I	B-II
1100–1300	A-II	A-II	A-II	A-II	A-II	A-I	B-II	B-I
1300–1500	B-I	B-I	B-I	B-I	B-I	B-II	A-II	A-I
1500–1700	B-II	B-II	B-II	B-II	B-II	B-I	A-I	A-II
	Panel (c) Row randomised				Panel (d) Row and column randomised			
0900–1100	B-I	B-II	A-II	A-I	B-II	B-I	A-II	A-I
1100–1300	A-I	A-II	B-I	B-II	A-II	A-I	B-I	B-II
1300–1500	B-II	B-I	A-I	A-II	B-I	B-II	A-I	A-II
1500–1700	A-II	A-I	B-II	B-I	A-I	A-II	B-II	B-I

experiments (here four) with intervention A and B. This design is therefore balanced with respect to intervention and experimenter. Such a design is known as a randomised block design – here four blocks with four units per block. However, in this design intervention type A-I always occurs at the time window 0900–1100, whereas it would seem more appropriate if these were 'balanced' across all times as in Table 4.2 Panel (b). Here A-I occurs once every day and once at each time-window. Thus every row (and column) has two As, two Is, two Bs and two IIs. Now looking across each time-window, there is an equal number of interventions (here two) of each type and both experimenters have two sessions at this time. This enables variation of time of day or choice of experimenter, to be eliminated when comparing the interventions A and B, which is the purpose of the experiment.

Although the upper two panels of Table 4.2 give the basic structure of possible block designs – Panel (b) being preferable to Panel (a) – a further step is required. This is to randomise the order of the rows in the design. Thus, using the sequence (mod 4)+1 as discussed above, the rows 1, 2, 3 and 4 are reassigned to 2, 4, 1 and 3 as in Panel (c) of Table 4.2. As now becomes obvious, we should also randomise the order of the columns. This randomisation is effected, by using the remaining part of the sequence of the random series, to obtain the order 2, 1, 3 and 4. Thus Panel (d) is Panel (b) randomised first by row order, as was Panel (c), and then by column order.

The eventual experimental design will replicate the basic structure of Table 4.2, Panel (d), as many times as required to complete the experiment on the entire N (assumed a multiple of 16 here) units specified by the design. However, the randomisation process will be distinct for each of these ($N/16$) squares.

The particular design of Table 4.2(b) is termed a 4×4 Latin square. There are four such basic squares of this size and these are listed in Table T5. The squares are termed basic in the sense that one cannot obtain any one of these squares from any of the

Table 4.3 Randomised block design (RBD) for two interventions in blocks of size 4

Block	1	2	3	4	5	6
Permutation	5	3	4	2	6	1

B	A	B	A	B	A
A	B	A	B	B	A
A	B	B	A	A	B
B	A	A	B	A	B

others by reordering (permuting) the rows or columns or both. Any one of these can be taken (at random) to form the basis for the design.

The Latin square idea can be extended to include two factors which need to be balanced in an experimental design. Thus the Graeco-Latin squares of Table T6 comprise arrangements of all possible pairs of the Latin letters A, B, C and D with the four Greek characters α, β, γ and δ in any order we choose. Here there are two basic squares. One application may be when there are four interventions, the Latin letters, and four observers conducting the experiment, the Greek characters. It is clear that every observer is responsible for one observation on each intervention, and each observer tests every intervention. Rows and columns are then randomised as for the Latin square and the first of 16 experimental units assigned to the top left-hand entry, and the 16th to the bottom right-hand entry.

Randomised Block Design (RBD)

If Table 4.1 is reformatted into that shown in Table 4.3, then the (randomised) block structure of this becomes more apparent. The contents of the blocks 1 to 6 are formed by first randomising the six permutations.

Clearly the basic structure of Table 4.3 can be extended to fit the needs of the study under design. For example, if $N=48$, then the RBD is replicated a second time but with the permutations randomised again for this second time. Equally the basic structure can be adjusted to the numbers of interventions concerned. Thus Table 4.4 includes a RBD for $t=3$ interventions A, B and C conducted in blocks of size $b=3$, but over 18 units.

Table 4.4 Randomised block design for three interventions in blocks of size 3

Permutation	1	2	3	4	5	6

A	B	C	A	B	C
B	C	A	C	A	B
C	A	B	B	C	A

This design includes all possible six permutations of size 3. The eventual assignment of these permutations to the corresponding $r=6$ replicate blocks will be made at random.

Stratified Randomisation

Some imbalance in the major prognostic variables between intervention groups may arise as a result of using simple randomisation and indeed also when using blocks to balance the different intervention groups. Stratifying the randomisation by both the prognostic group as well as the intervention can reduce this imbalance. This strategy ensures that close to an equal number of units are allocated within each stratum to each of the intervention options. This may be achieved by arranging the randomisation to be balanced within predetermined blocks of units within each of the strata. In essence we have done this already when comparing experimenters I and II.

Suppose the study described in Panel (d) of Table 4.2, involved a design in which all observations were made by a single observer but of the 16 subjects, the design specified that half should be male and half female. Then relabelling I as F (for female) and II as M (for male) one achieves a design in which for each gender half receive A and half B. Thus the randomisation is now stratified by gender to ensure the intervention is balanced within each gender group.

For continuous prognostic variables, such as age, stratification can only be done when these variables are divided into categories. In general, two categories will suffice. Stratified randomisation as a method of achieving balance can become unworkable if there are too many stratification variables, because the associated number of strata cells resulting (at least two per variable) can quickly exceed the number of patients in the study.

Allocation Ratio

We have implicitly assumed that, for two interventions, a 1:1 randomisation will take place. However, the particular context may suggest other ratios. For example, if the experimental units are limited, for whatever reason, then the design team may argue that they should obtain more information within the experiment from (say) the test intervention, T, rather than the well-known control or standard, S. In such circumstances, a randomisation ratio of say 2:3 or 1:2 in favour of the test intervention may be decided. The first could be realised by use of a die with sides 1 and 2 allocated to S, and 3, 4 and 5 to T, ignoring 6. The latter ratio could be obtained by using again sides 1 and 2 for S but now 3, 4, 5 and 6 for T. However, moving from a 1:1 ratio

Table 4.5 All possible permutations of length 5 for two interventions S and T allocated in the ratio 2:3

1	SSTTT	6	TSTST
2	STSTT	7	TSTTS
3	STTST	8	TTSST
4	STTTS	9	TTSTS
5	TSSTT	0^a	TTTSS

[a]Note 0 replaces 10 to facilitate the use of random number tables.

involves some increase in study size to maintain power and this increase should be quantified before a decision on the allocation ratio is finally made.

If an allocation ratio of 2:3 for S and T is chosen, then this implies a minimum block size of 5, each comprising one of the permutations given in Table 4.5.

If a design for an experiment comprises $N=25$ subjects, then the sequence of random numbers 534 55425 67 generates from Table 4.5, the 5 blocks with the following permutations

$$TSSTT - STTST - STTTS - TSSTT - TSSTT.$$

Alternatively if we wish to avoid consecutive blocks with the same permutation we would have

$$TSSTT - STTST - STTTS - STSTT - TSTST.$$

4.4   OBSERVATIONAL STUDIES

In observational studies, say a comparison in outcome between patients with Crohn's disease and ulcerative colitis, there may be no 'intervention' involved and so the requirement for randomisation to groups is not pertinent. Nevertheless, as we illustrated in Table 4.2, different observers may be involved in the study in which case we can regard these as the 'interventions' and so randomise the patients to observers.

Further, if samples are to be taken from the experimental units, for later detailed examination and laboratory analysis, it is recommended that where they are stored and by whom they are examined should also be subject to the randomisation process. For instance, it would not seem sensible to store all the samples from one group in one location and those from the other in a second. This applies equally to proximal locations such as within a 'single' storage unit. Thus 'blocks' may correspond to the shelves of a deep-freezer.

In this way, the randomisation process extends to all levels of the experimental process and thereby as often as may be required. Only in this way can one ensure that any bias within the experimental process is reduced to a minimum. In short, if one can randomise, then do so, whether it is the appointment time to the experimenters' clinic (morning or afternoon; day of the week); the investigator, the refrigerator shelf or the laboratory testing.

Example *– bias in measurement – ciliary beat frequency*

Lyons, Djahanbakhch, Saridogan *et al.* (2002) describe a study of ciliary beat frequency (Hz) of the ampullary region of the fallopian tube epithelium in women with and without endometriosis. Although full details of, for example, how the tubal epithelium explants were incubated in peritoneal fluid for 24 h at 37°C, 100% humidity, and 5% $CO_2+95\%$ air, are included, there are no details of whether steps were taken to eliminate potential biases in the entire measurement process.

4.5   SURVEYS

If the target population is large (as will be the case for most surveys) and a convenient list is not available electronically, the process of going backwards and forwards to identify the sample can be a tedious business, although this can be facilitated by first ranking the random numbers of those chosen before beginning this process. An alternative is to use a systematic sample with a random starting point.

Suppose a list of 10 000 subjects is printed on 1000 pages of 100 per page, and a 10% sample is required. One way is to begin by choosing a number at random between 00 and 99, remembering that 00 represents 100. From Table T3 we might again start with the first two digits of the first column, so our number is 53. We then take the 53rd subject on every page as our sample. For a 0.5% sample we would take a name from every second page but first choosing a subject from the first two pages at random from 000 to 199, here 000 represents 200. If this is 103, then the third subject on each of the 500 even-numbered pages of the list is chosen as the sample.

Obviously a more convenient way is to generate the 200 random numbers by a computer program which automatically replaces any repeats and finally ranks the selected numbers for smallest to largest so that they can be identified sequentially in the target population list. If such a program is written, then it is important to retain the algorithm and the 'seed' of the random number generator so that (if necessary) the random selection can be repeated.

Example – *selecting a sample* – *Danish women*

Klee, Groenvold and Machin (1997) wished to establish population norms for aspects of Health Related Quality of Life using the EORTC QLQ-C30 instrument. Their target population was Danish women aged over 25. Their sample of 892 women was selected from the Danish Central Population Register from all those born on the same day in odd years from 1913 to 1971.

4.6   CLINICAL TRIALS

Randomisation is a key element of the design implementation for clinical trials. In fact, the randomised trial is considered the 'gold' standard against which alternative designs are compared.

As with preclinical experiments randomisation ensures (in the long run) balance between the groups in known and *unknown* prognostic factors. We have shown how balance in important (hence known) prognostic factors can be achieved by stratification but there is no other way except randomisation to ensure long-run balance of *unknown* prognostic factors.

In contrast to preclinical studies, clinical trials may require large numbers of patients. In addition, seldom will all these patients be available at the opening of the trial. Instead they will first present as and when their illness appears and so will only become available for treatment, and hence the trial, at unpredictable intervals. The intervals between patients may be lengthy if the incidence of the disease in question is low. We cannot allocate patients to the interventions before the trial is started although the 'process' for randomisation needs to be established before the first patient has consented to recruitment.

Further, as we have indicated for preclinical studies, although simple randomisation gives equal probability for each unit to receive A or B it does not ensure that by the end of recruitment to the study equal numbers of units received A and B. In fact even in relatively large studies the discrepancy from the desired equal numbers of units per intervention group can be quite large.

Example *– simple randomisation – chronic gastro-oesophageal reflux*

Csendes, Burdiles, Korn *et al.* (2002) recruited 164 patients with chronic gastro-oesophageal reflux and used a simple 1:1 randomisation to fundoplication or calibration of the cardia. This resulted in 76 randomised to fundoplication but 88 to calibration of the cardia.

SELECTING THE SUBJECTS

There will always be a clear need to identify the characteristics of potentially eligible patients for a trial. An essential element is that each patient is suitable for all the treatments or interventions on offer within the clinical trial. Thus if there are three options A, B and C, then not only must the attending physician be happy to prescribe all the options but also the patient must be happy to receive all such options. If only two of these three are acceptable then the patient should not be regarded as eligible for the trial and so should not be randomised. Also, if the physician for 'this' patient thinks one option preferable, then despite eligibility in all other respects, the patient should receive that option and so again should not be randomised to the trial.

Example *– trial eligibility – partial thickness burns*

In the randomised trial by Ang, Lee, Gan *et al.* (2001) patients with severe burns were emergency admissions into the specialist burns centre in Singapore requiring immediate treatment. Once admitted to the burns centre, only those patients with partial thickness burns were eligible for the trial. Their consent was then sought, and once given, randomisation effected by telephone to the statistical centre. Nevertheless in certain cases, the attending medical team felt that conventional therapy was more appropriate than the new therapy. For those patients, details of the clinical trial were not explained and conventional therapy commenced immediately. Clearly no randomisation took place.

WHEN TO RANDOMISE

In clinical trials, there is an additional reason to randomise the alternative interventions to patients and this is to ensure that the treatment allocation to patients is not predictable. If the allocation is predictable, then the investigating physician has knowledge that he or she may subconsciously use to influence their decision to include (or exclude) certain patients from the trial, that is, they will not judge 'fairly' if each of the treatment options is appropriate for the patient. This knowledge may also compromise the 'informed' consent procedure as it may lead to a more selective description of the options available focusing more on the option that will be given and less on the alternatives. Thus it is important that the investigating physician is not aware of the treatment to be allocated to the next patient. Also if the allocation of treatment can be predicted, then it is possible that some patients may volunteer for a trial in the hope of getting the (new) experimental therapy. On the other hand if they know they are to get the control therapy, they may withdraw consent to enter the trial. As a consequence, any prior knowledge by the clinical team or the patient of the allocation can therefore introduce bias into the allocation process, and hence lead to bias in the final estimate of the parameter β_1 at the close of the trial.

MULTICENTRE TRIALS

In clinical trials that involve recruitment in several centres, it is usual to use a stratified randomisation procedure to ensure balanced treatment allocation within each centre. In this way, one ensures that patients have the option of all treatment modalities in all centres.

BLOCKED RANDOMISATION

Randomisation can be carried out in blocks following the methods described earlier for preclinical studies. The major difference is that larger numbers of subjects are involved and so the eventual sequence of blocks may be very lengthy.

In some circumstances it may be desirable to avoid runs of the same treatment in successive patients as there could be resource implications if different medical teams are responsible for the different treatments. For example, if Permutation 1 of Table 4.5 is followed by Permutation 0 then we have *SSTTT – TTTSS*. This sequence comprises a sub-sequence within it of six consecutive patients all assigned to *T*. To avoid this happening, Permutations 1 and 0 could be removed from the list of possibilities. Alternatively, if Permutation 1 is selected, then Permutation 0 may be excluded as a possibility for the next block to be chosen.

In practice, a maximum of (say) four consecutive *B*s and three consecutive *A*s may be thought reasonable, in which case the allocation can be made using the permutations of Table 4.5 and the resulting sequence of blocks checked. Any adjacent blocks that result in sequences that are too long are removed. If removals occur, then the chosen sequence has to be extended until the randomisation list is complete.

Example *– block size – tamoxifen in inoperable hepatocellular carcinoma*

In the randomised trial conducted by Chow, Tai, Tan *et al.* (2002) of three doses of tamoxifen the authors state: 'Randomization was performed in balanced blocks of 5, stratified by center and corresponding to P, TMX60, and TMX120 in the respective ratios of 2:1:2'. In this trial, in which 329 patients were recruited, the stratification by recruiting centres, for example, those in Hong Kong, Myanmar, Singapore and elsewhere, was done to ensure that the proportions of patients receiving the different doses remained approximately constant, at all points in time, in all centres.

The investigating physician should not be aware of the block size. If they come to know, as each block of patients nears completion, guessing the next treatment to be allocated may again lead to subconscious inclusion in or exclusion from the trial of certain patients. Such a difficulty can be avoided by changing the block size (at random) as recruitment continues to reduce the possibility of a pattern being detected (even inadvertently) by the investigation team.

Clearly for the trial of Chow, Tai, Tan *et al.* (2002) this choice of block size would be between $b=5$ and 10. Sometimes the block size, perhaps between these options, is chosen at random for successive sequences of patients within a stratum of patient types.

STRATIFICATION

Just as in the more experimental types of study, it may be important in a clinical trial to ensure that the treatment options are balanced within different strata. The strata are defined in such a way that those patients within a strata are more homogeneous than those between strata with respect to the endpoint measure of concern to the clinical trial.

Example *– stratified randomisation – cranberry or apple juice for urinary symptoms*

Campbell, Pickles and D'yachkova (2003) used a simple 1:1 randomisation, within each of four strata, to assign treatment by either cranberry or apple juice to alleviate urinary symptoms during external beam radiation for prostate cancer. Their allocation into the 2×2 stratification groups of previous transurethral resection of the prostate (TURP) and International Prostate Symptom Score (IPSS) for each randomised treatment is given in Table 4.6.

Table 4.6 Stratification groups for a trial for alleviating urinary symptoms (from Campbell, Pickles and D'yachkova, 2003. A randomised trial of cranberry versus apple juice in the management of urinary symptoms during external beam radiation therapy for prostate cancer. *Clinical Oncology*, **15**, 322–328 [4]; reproduced with permission from The Royal College of Radiologists)

Juice	TURP IPSS	Negative <6	≥6	Positive <6	≥6	Total
Apple		17	27	6	7	57
Cranberry		14	27	6	8	55
	Total	32	54	12	15	112

In this trial, approximately equal numbers are randomised to apple and cranberry juice overall, and despite the different proportions in the four TURP by IPSS strata, the patients allocated are approximately equally divided between treatments.

DYNAMIC ALLOCATION

One problem with stratification is that it only works when the number of strata is few. Even three prognostic variables, each dichotomous, give eight different strata, and it soon becomes impossible to ensure balance between interventions of all the variables. A number of alternative methods, known as dynamic allocation, have been developed of which the simplest is minimisation. These replace randomisation with a (largely) deterministic method based on the characteristics of the patients already in the trial and the characteristics of the patient about to be allocated to the interventions.

Table 4.7 Distribution of patients with prostate cancer in a clinical trial according to TURP and IPSS stratification groups for a trial for alleviating urinary symptoms (data from Campbell, Pickles and D'yachkova, 2003. A randomised trial of cranberry versus apple juice in the management of urinary symptoms during external beam radiation therapy for prostate cancer. *Clinical Oncology*, **15**, 322–328 [4]; reproduced with permission from the Royal College of Radiologists)

Prognostic factor		Treatment juice Apple (A)	Cranberry (C)
TURP	Negative	44	41
	Positive	13	14
IPSS	<6	23	20
	≥6	34	35
Total randomised		57	55

To demonstrate how minimisation works, suppose that we wish to recruit an additional patient to the trial of Campbell, Pickles and D'yachkova (2003). Thus suppose we wish to allocate Patient 113, who is TURP negative with IPSS < 6, to Apple or Cranberry. First we have to construct Table 4.7 which gives the distribution of the 112 patients of Table 4.6 by each covariate and treatment allocation.

The minimisation method counts the numbers in Table 4.7 with each of these two prognostic characteristics (TURP negative or positive; IPSS < 6 or ≥ 6), in each treatment group separately. Note that patients are counted more than once – here twice. In the apple group, this count comes to $A = 44 + 23 = 67$ and in the cranberry group $C = 41 + 20 = 61$. The method then allocates the new patient to the group with the lower total. In this case Patient 113 receives cranberry juice since 61 is less than 67.

In the International Conference on Harmonisation (ICH) E9 Expert Working Group (1999) statistical principles for clinical trials, it is recommended that a random element should be incorporated into dynamic allocation procedures. Thus Scott, McPherson, Ramsay and Campbell (2002) came to the conclusion that

minimization is an effective method for allocating participants to treatment groups within a randomized controlled trial. In the majority of cases, minimization has been shown to outperform simple randomization in achieving balanced groups; this greater performance is particularly marked when trial sizes are small. Minimization has also been shown to be advantageous compared to stratified randomization methods, as it has the ability to incorporate more prognostic factors.

They advocate wider adoption of the technique within clinical trials. However, Nicholl and Campbell (2002) point out that except in extreme circumstances (when no individuals get one of the randomised treatments) the advantage of simple randomisation is that it is simpler to operate, preserves the lack of predictability, and ensures greater validity for the statistical tests.

CLUSTER TRIALS

In contrast to individually randomised trials, the cluster rather than the individuals are randomised. In addition, the number of clusters is often limited. So although randomisation may balance clusters in the long run, it does not explicitly balance individuals within clusters. Thus the main arguments for randomisation have less power for cluster designs. However, such is the overall popularity of randomisation, it would be foolish to design a cluster trial without it. Even in a trial with a very limited number of clusters (say less than six per group) where there is no possibility of balancing prognostic factors, it is worthwhile randomising so that one can claim a lack of subjective bias in intervention allocation. However, despite the limited number of clusters, it is also worthwhile stratifying by cluster size. For cluster randomised trials all the clusters are usually available at the start, so stratification and randomisation within strata can be carried out, and the clusters then informed of their allocation before beginning patient recruitment. In trials that require newly diagnosed patients, it may not be possible to specify the cluster size exactly at the start. In this case, a proxy measure of cluster size, such as the size of the clinic from which the patients are drawn, can be used instead.

Table 4.8   Advantages and disadvantages of different types of randomisation

Type	Advantages	Disadvantages
Simple	Easy to implement	May result in imbalance in numbers between groups
	Unpredictable	Does not balance prognostic factors
Blocked	Ensures (almost) equal numbers in each group even if the study stops early	Does not balance prognostic factors
		Slightly predictable
Stratified and blocked	Ensures (almost) equal numbers and balances prognostic factors in each group	Can only balance a few prognostic factors
		Slightly predictable
Minimisation	Can balance a number of prognostic factors	Needs all characteristics of previous patients to be available
		Potentially predictable, not strictly random

PRACTICALITIES

The advantages and disadvantages of the different options for randomisation are given in Table 4.8.

4.7   CARRYING OUT RANDOMISATION

If possible, a neutral party should prepare the randomisation list. For clinical trials this is usually the statistician assigned to the trial, although some of the details of this will be discussed in general terms amongst the full investigating team. In addition, once the process has been agreed the actual generation of the random sequences should be done by the statistician and should remain confidential until the study is complete. In most circumstances, it is best if the list is retained in an appropriate study or trial office that can be contacted by the responsible investigator once patient eligibility and their consent are obtained.

PRECLINICAL STUDIES

The randomisation process begins by first producing a list numbered, 1 to N, against which the particular randomised intervention is listed. Quite separately, if the experimental units are all available, the units are also numbered from 1 to N, in any order convenient. The two lists are then put together and this allows the allocation of the intervention, to the experimental units, to be made.

   In circumstances when all the experimental units are not available at the beginning of the study, then we assume they become available one at a time. Thus they are then numbered 1 to N as they present and are then assigned to the interventions planned.

One device for allocating the randomisation, which is certainly common in small-scale studies, is to prepare sequentially numbered sealed envelopes that contain the appropriate intervention inside. These can be of an opaque 'salary-slip' format, which can only be opened by destroying part of the envelope. The experimenter only prepares to open the envelope once he has decided the unit is eligible for the study. The process begins by writing the name of the unit (or a code for unique identification) on the exterior of the envelope, then tearing the envelope open to reveal the allocation. Once this is complete, the envelope and 'salary-slip' should be stored carefully and these, and any unused envelopes, retained as a check on the randomisation process.

CLINICAL TRIALS

As with preclinical studies, it is usual to generate the randomisation list in advance of recruiting the first patient. This has several advantages: it removes the possibility of the physician not randomising properly; it will usually be more efficient in that a list may be computer-generated very quickly; it also allows some difficulties with simple randomisation to be avoided.

As with preclinical studies, the randomisation can be concealed within opaque and sealed envelopes which are distributed to the centre or centres involved in advance of patient recruitment. Once a patient is deemed eligible, the envelope is taken in the order specified in a prescribed list and opened, and the treatment thereby revealed. Intrinsically, there is nothing wrong with this process but, because of the potential for abuse (envelopes can be opened and switched or disregarded), it is not regarded as entirely satisfactory. However, in some circumstances it will be unavoidable; perhaps a trial is being conducted in a remote area with poor communications. In such cases, every precaution should be taken to ensure that the process is not compromised. One simple way is to have the envelopes kept out of the clinic itself and held by someone who can give the randomisation over the telephone. The physician rings the number, gives the necessary patient details, perhaps confirming the protocol entry criteria, and is told which treatment to give, or perhaps a code number of a drug package.

Of course many of these potential problems are avoided in clinical trials in which both the attending clinician and the patient are blinded to the intervention allocated.

WHEN TO RANDOMISE

In an ideal setting, once a patient has consented to take part in a clinical trial, randomisation should take place immediately. Once the treatment allocation is known, therapy should begin immediately following that. This minimises delay and avoids the patient having the opportunity to change their mind before therapy begins. This helps to prevent the dilution that can occur if the patient switches to the comparator option in the period between randomisation and starting treatment. One consequence of any potential dilution is that it has to be offset by an increase in the number of subjects to be recruited to the trial.

However, there will be many circumstances in which therapy cannot be initiated immediately, for example, in a surgical trial. In many situations, there will be a delay until the surgery can take place (although trials have been conducted in which randomisation takes place while the patient is on the operating table). In life-threatening conditions, deaths may occur before surgery can take place. For others there is at least the possibility that their disease progresses in the intervening interval to a stage where the patient cannot be operated on. Such patients are included in the trial analysis but clearly dilute the estimate of the real difference (if any) between the interventions.

Example – *delay between randomisation and start of treatment – radiotherapy for inoperable non-small cell lung cancer*

Although full details are not provided, the delay from randomisation and commencement of radiotherapy (RT) probably resulted in three patients allocated to be treated with two fractions of radiotherapy receiving none in the trial of the Medical Research Council Lung Cancer Working Party (1996). For the 13-fraction option, six received no RT.

DOCUMENTATION

Good Clinical Practice

If a clinical trial is being conducted with a view to submission for (say) drug registration, then there may be specific regulatory requirements such as the ICH E6 Guidelines for Guidance on Good Clinical Practice of EMEA (2002) that need to be adhered to. One of these concerns study documentation of the processes involved in the trial conduct. In this respect, it is particularly important that the method of generating the randomisation is documented carefully and that it can be regenerated without difficulty. It is additionally useful should the list get lost. This makes very practical sense in the context of the randomisation for a double-blind trial in which the alternatives are packaged in such a way as to be indistinguishable.

4.8   UNACCEPTABLE METHODS

Any allocation method that is not 'random' should be avoided if at all possible. Pseudo-methods for the allocation process have often been used, such as giving successive patients the alternate treatments. This method is not random since, at least after the first patient, it is totally predictable, so the clinical team will know the intervention planned 'before' they see the patient. As we have noted, this knowledge may bias the final comparison. Similarly, if allocation is made on the basis of date of birth, then again it will always be clear which treatment is planned for which patient. Examples of these quite unacceptable methods continue to occur, but the corresponding trials would not be accepted for publication in reputable clinical journals. They contravene the CONSORT Guidelines described by Moher, Schultz, Altman *et al.* (2001).

Key design features

Random allocation of the interventions

Ensure the randomisation list cannot be compromised

Identify major (few) prognostic factors for possible stratification

Consider an appropriate 'block' size

In trials with 'one-at-a-time' recruitment consider dynamic randomisation

Commence the intervention as soon as practicable after the random allocation

5 Cross-sectional and Longitudinal Studies

Summary

This chapter describes the design of cross-sectional studies in which observations at a single time point are made on all subjects. These include designs for single groups and case-series, comparative studies for independent groups and paired two-group designs. Emphasis is placed on the manner in which subjects, particularly healthy controls, are selected for study. We also describe studies that are longitudinal in nature, typically involving repeated measurements of the same variables on the same individuals at differing times. A cross-sectional design having an endpoint that requires monitoring progress over time is also longitudinal in nature. Before-and-after and interrupted time series designs are also discussed. Methods of estimating the appropriate numbers of subjects to be recruited for each design are indicated.

5.1 INTRODUCTION

Cross-sectional designs occur in all areas of medical research, from preclinical, to clinical to epidemiological studies, although surveys, which are one type of such design, are most common in epidemiological studies. Essentially, a cross-sectional design describes a single group or compares two or more groups of subjects with respect to a particular characteristic or characteristics at one point in time. The groups themselves may be formed through an intervention on the investigators' part in an experimental type of situation or may occur naturally, for example, a comparison between male and females with respect to body weight, or between those who are sick and those who are not in terms of alkaline phosphatase levels. These latter comparisons are more observational than experimental. In observational studies the investigator has less 'control' over the design. Consequently they often raise more problems in interpretation than do experimental designs.

It is difficult to generalise but if there is a choice of which groups to compare then there is a good case to make these as distinctly different as possible. For example, in comparing patients with diabetes mellitus with healthy (non-diseased) subjects, if the choice of the diabetic patients was confined to (say) only those with a very mild form of the disease then little difference between these and the controls might be anticipated. So

Design of Studies for Medical Research. D. Machin and M. J. Campbell
© 2005 John Wiley & Sons Ltd. ISBN 0 470 84495 7

a large study would be required in order to distinguish between them. On the other hand, if these were very advanced cases, differences from controls may then be demonstrated even in a small study.

When designing a clinical study, there are certain (statistical) assumptions that one has to make and values that one has to set. Two of the latter are the test size and power of the study which are often set as $\alpha = 0.05$ and $1 - \beta = 0.8$ or 0.9. Although these values were arbitrarily chosen in the first place, because of their continual and widespread use they have now become something of a standard. Thus, if an investigator wishes to depart from these standards, it is usual to explain why. Similarly in some situations, designs have become something of a standard (although in themselves not necessarily optimal) against which future designs are compared. Once again, if alternative designs are then chosen (and there may be good reason for this) then these should be justified.

5.2   CROSS-SECTIONAL STUDIES

SINGLE GROUP

In the simplest type of cross-sectional study we look at one group and investigate the presence or absence of a particular characteristic in individuals, or record a measure from them. Since the study is describing only one group, this implies that $\beta_1 = 0$ in model (1.1). Thus we are left with estimating β_0 which may represent, for example, a population mean, μ, or a prevalence, π, depending on the context of the investigation.

Single-case-studies

By their very nature, cases that present and are worthy of a single-case-study tend to be rare, and arise unexpectedly and so such 'studies' cannot be planned. Thus, although a single-case-study avoids a formal design, there are several points that should be considered. For example, in describing a case it would often be useful to outline carefully not only the specific patient details (this is usually done as it is the primary objective of such a study) but also the number of cases seen without the features of the 'unusual' case. Thus if an atypical toxic reaction to a standard therapy is being reported, it would be useful to say how many cases with similar characteristics and diagnosis had been treated with no adverse effect of this type in (say) the year preceding the date when the index case was identified. Information should also be sought on similar (if any) cases identified in the literature.

Example – *single case study* – *Stenotrophomonas maltophilia endocarditis*

Crum, Utz and Wallace (2002) describe the case of a 56-year-old female with sickle cell disease who had been receiving red blood transfusion via a catheter. Her endocarditis was ascribed to a positive culture for *Stenotrophomonas maltophilia* in the catheter.

To contextualise this rare occurrence the authors completed a Medline search for the period 1964 to 1999 and identified reports of 24 other cases of *Stenotrophomonas* endocarditis.

Case-series

For a case-series design a justification of the sample size is required and this may be based on the desirable width of the confidence interval (CI) for the endpoint of concern. The final report should stipulate the period over which the series begins and ends.

If the design is retrospective in nature, perhaps then implying a case-notes search, care should be taken to ensure the requisite information is truly available on all (or at least the vast majority of) cases. This may be tested by a preliminary review of case-notes for some selected patients. It is particularly important to define the eligibility criteria clearly and unambiguously *before* the case-note search commences. In the event of some ambiguous cases arising, their number should be documented and reported.

Example *– case series – cutaneous anthrax*

Öncül, Özsoy, Gul *et al.* (2002) review the clinical and laboratory findings from 32 cases of cutaneous anthrax reported over a 4-year period from 1998 to 2001 in the eastern part of Turkey. They reported that swelling, redness and black eschar formation were seen in all cases and that pruritis, fatigue, fever and headache were the most common systemic manifestations.

No justification for the study size is given or equivalently why the study was confined to the 4-year period chosen.

Convenience Sample

One might anticipate that the subject pool for a cross-sectional study of patients with (say) schizophrenia is rather small. In such circumstances the study might have to 'make-do' with those patients who are available or what is termed a 'convenience' sample. The study may comprise, for example, all the current patients of the particular clinical investigator. In order for such samples to have validity we have to be convinced that no biases are likely to have occurred in the method of patient selection.

Example *– convenience sample – latency of the auditory P300 in schizophrenia*

The study of Weir, Fiaschi and Machin (1998), discussed in Section 2.3, is a typical cross-sectional study in which groups of individuals were examined for the latency of auditory P300.

In this case we need to know whether the patients with schizophrenia in this study are 'typical' of all patients with the condition? If they are, then the results of Weir, Fiaschi and Machin (1998) may be generalised to 'all' such patients and the study provides an unbiased estimate of the relevant population parameters. If they are not, then the study merely describes those included in the study.

One way of checking on this, at least partially, is to compare the demographics, for example age and gender, of the convenience sample with the same details from a relevant comparator population. If the sample subjects are similar to the comparator subjects in these respects then we may be less likely to be worried about bias. In essence a case-series is one example of a convenience sample.

Simple Random Sample

Suppose the study of Weir, Fiaschi and Machin (1998) were to be repeated, but now in 30 left-handed patients. If left-handed patients are rare, then the investigators will have to study a convenience sample. On the other hand, if left-handed patients are freely available, then the investigator should choose the 30 at random from the larger population of patients by a method such as we described in Chapter 4. In this circumstance, the estimate of β_0 obtained on completion of the study is an unbiased estimate of the mean auditory P300 for all left-handed patients with schizophrenia.

One of the astonishing facts of statistical methods is that one can make valid inferences about populations (here patients with schizophrenia who are left-handed) without having to examine every member of the population; all that is needed is a well-chosen sample. This contrasts with the convenience sample for which we do not know if the estimate is or is not biased. Thus we can rely more readily on the results established from a random sample. Thus convenience samples should be avoided if possible. When they are unavoidable in one group the members of any other (comparator) group are best selected using a random mechanism. However, even if the subjects cannot be selected at random, it may be possible to select the order in which they are examined at random or, if there are several assessors involved, to randomise the choice of assessor to the patient.

Complete Sample

In some circumstances the sample may consist of all the members of a specifically defined population. For practical reasons, this is only likely to be the case if the population of interest is not too large. Clearly complete sampling of a large population will be very expensive and time-consuming.

***Example** – complete sample – reinfection with Lyme borreliosis*

Bennet and Berglund (2002) studied all patients diagnosed with erythema migrans (EM) following vector-borne infection by *Lyme borreliosis* (LB) some 10 years earlier. They contacted all these patients and asked if they had had any new tick bites over the period May 1993 to May 1998. From the 976 infected and eligible for the study, 708 participants replied and from these a reinfection rate of 4% was computed.

In this case, since the study purpose was to investigate the long-term consequences of an infection, the choice of the population was very specifically confined to those who had been diagnosed with EM. Despite seeking a complete sample, only a proportion (but not a random sample) of this population provided the information requested. There is therefore a real possibility of bias in the estimate of the reinfection rate so obtained. However, the sample comprised a large proportion (73%) of the total and the authors checked that there were no major differences in terms of age and gender between those who participated and those who did not.

In contrast, if all members of the population can be assessed, there is no bias as the 'estimate' is the value of the population parameter itself. In this idealised situation we know all about the population as we have examined all its members. This will rarely be the case.

Study Size

The details for determining sample size, based on the desired width of the CI, in a single-group cross-sectional study are given in Chapter 3. Thus equation (3.4) gives the sample size necessary when estimating a mean and equation (3.6) for estimating a proportion or prevalence. It is worth emphasising that sample-size calculations do not provide 'exact' answers to the study size required as they are based on *anticipated* values of the parameters concerned. As we have indicated in Chapter 3, their objective is to provide a 'ball-park' figure for what the study size might be, whether 10s, 100s or 1000s. Thus investigators will usually examine a whole range of options to investigate the feasibility of the design they propose.

TWO-GROUP COMPARATIVE STUDY

In many situations, the description of the single group of a cross-sectional study may contain within-group comparisons. For example, in patients with schizophrenia, differences in mean latency of the auditory P300 between males and females may be examined. However, these comparisons are secondary to the main objective which is to describe the group as a whole. In a truly comparative study, two or more groups of subjects are identified and the examination of differences between them is the primary objective of the study. Thus Weir, Fiaschi and Machin (1998) wished to compare patients with schizophrenia with those having major depressive illness. This comparison provides the major research question and any secondary variable, such as the gender of the patients, may then be used as a covariate to see if taking this into account modifies the observed differences between groups with respect to the measures taken.

Healthy Controls and Volunteers

One important type of comparative cross-sectional study is one in which patients with a particular disease are compared with those who do not have the specific disease. In such a study, a sample of the disease population is required and also one from those not so diseased. In many circumstances, the comparator group are 'healthy' controls. However, there are particular issues with 'healthy controls' that need to be addressed. Many studies include healthy controls that are described as 'volunteers' and this is especially true of 'laboratory-type' studies. Now in defining the 'disease' group of subjects in these studies attention is rightly placed on describing them in careful detail. Unfortunately, it is not routine to describe the 'volunteers' with the same rigour, although differences between these and the index group are what the study is designed to elicit.

In fact it is well known that 'volunteers' may not be representative of the 'healthy' or 'normal' population as a whole. Rather they are chosen as laboratory or clinical staff (perhaps the investigators themselves) and so are highly selected and possibly unrepresentative for the purpose intended. What is more they may be involved in successive studies emanating from the same research group and so any inherent bias may be repeated continually.

Example – *healthy volunteers – septic shock*

Spronk, Ince, Gardien *et al.* (2002) when using orthogonal polarisation spectral imaging to visualise microcirculation merely state: 'The index was validated by testing the normal flow in ten healthy volunteers'. No details of these volunteers are given and the authors provide no justification of the sample size of 10.

Although it is relatively easy to be critical with respect to the choice of volunteers, the practice of finding such volunteers may be far from straightforward. However, their choice is critical for interpretation. We suggest that investigators should try to form a 'bank' of volunteers (healthy controls) and for a particular experiment or enquiry, draw (at random) from that bank as and when required in an appropriate way – taking care to avoid multiple use of the same individuals over a series of experiments.

The strongest evidence provided by a two-group comparison occurs when the members of each group are selected at random from the population of subjects with the relevant eligibility characteristics.

Independent Groups

The term independent implies here that the groups one is comparing comprise distinct subjects, that is, the members of one group are not members of the other. Further, neither are individual subjects of one group linked to a particular individual of another group under investigation. When considering the design of such studies, one has to decide on the definition of the groups of interest and on the possible endpoints of concern. From the latter, those of major importance to the research question posed have to be selected.

Example – *comparing independent groups – diabetic nephropathy*

Matteuci and Giampietro (2000) compared transmembrane electron transfer in 30 patients with diabetic nephropathy with the same features measured in 30 healthy volunteers. Some of their results are summarised in Table 5.1.

This study is typical of many in which two groups are compared with respect to several endpoint measures. We give details of three endpoints as summarised by the authors, and a variety of measures summarising the demographic and clinical condition

Table 5.1 Metabolic characteristics of patients with diabetic nephropathy and controls of healthy volunteers (part data from Matteuci and Giampietro, 2000. Transmembrane electron transfer in diabetic nephropathy. *Diabetes Care*, **23**, 994–999. [5])

Characteristic		Type I diabetes (D)	Controls (C)	Observed difference $d=(C-D)$	Observed standardised effect size, Δ	Reported p-value (exact)
	n	30	30			
Gender (% male)		57	47			
Age	mean	34	36			
(years)	SD	10	10			
BMI	mean	24	24			
(kg/m²)	SD	2	3			
BP	mean	92	90			
(mmHg)	SD	13	11			
GDH	mean	0.76	0.88	0.12	0.78	<0.01
(mg/ml RBC)	SD	0.12	0.18			(0.0012)
SG groups	mean	401	444	43	0.67	<0.05
(μmol/l)	SD	72	56			(0.0049)
Ferrocyanide	mean	15	13	−2	−0.40	—
(μmol ml⁻¹ h⁻¹)	SD	5	5			(0.061)

of the groups involved. Here the main purpose of the study is to compare the groups for GDH, SG and ferrocyanide levels but implicitly recognising that these levels (although they may differ *between* groups) will also differ *within* groups, depending to a greater or lesser extent on their gender, age, body mass index (BMI) or blood pressure (BP) values. The question then arises as to how much of the difference observed, for example the 43 μmol/l in SG of Table 5.1, between those with nephropathy and controls is due to the different characteristics of the subjects within the two groups. Many investigators check the demographics given in the upper panel of Table 5.1, see that there is little to choose between the means of the two groups with respect to these variables, and are then reassured that the comparisons of the lower panel are valid. In fact there are more effective ways of doing this using regression models to adjust any differences estimated by these covariates, such as age and gender here.

Consideration has to be given as to whether there are patient characteristics that are known to affect the values (apart from the major determinant of the groups or the intervention itself) of these chosen endpoints in an important way. If there are any (hopefully not too many) then recording these is an important part of the experimental design. It is wasteful of resources, and deflects from the purpose in hand to record other measures that are inessential. The temptation to measure everything 'that just might be of interest' is obvious but is best resisted.

Further, having multiple endpoints (as opposed to multiple covariates) poses several difficulties for the investigator when determining the study size, as standardised differences used for planning are not likely to be the same for each endpoint. We see from Table 5.1 that the eventual standardised effect sizes are (in absolute value) 0.40,

0.67 and 0.78. For two of these the small p-values perhaps imply that a smaller study would have been sufficient to distinguish the groups as each p-value is less than $\alpha = 0.05$. In contrast to this, the difference in mean ferrocyanide was not statistically significant, exact p-value$=0.061$. Were this the major endpoint, and a difference of $2\,\mu mol\,ml^{-1}\,h^{-1}$ is regarded as a clinically important difference, then the study was too small to establish this difference with 95% confidence. So for one outcome the study was too large and for another it was too small. In designing any study it is clear that compromises have to be made at the planning stage. Identifying the key (and few) outcome variables helps to focus on the right compromise.

Study Size

For independent groups equation (3.14) gives the sample size necessary when estimating a difference in means between two groups, equation (3.15) for comparing proportions or prevalences and equation (3.20) differences in survival times.

Limited Patients

Suppose independent investigators wished to repeat the SH measures of the study of Matteuci and Giampietro (2000) and only had a limited number (maximum 30) of patients available but could recruit controls more easily. They would first review the published results and note an observed standardised effect size for SH of 0.67. Next they may use this as the basis for planning their repeat study by setting $\Delta_{Plan} = 0.67$, keeping $\alpha = 0.05$ as in the previous study while in addition specifying a power to detect this effect of $1 - \beta = 0.8$.

If they first assume that the design will recruit equal numbers of patients and controls, then they will set $\lambda = 1$. Calculations using equation (3.14) give $m = 36$, $n = 36$ and so $N = 36 + 36 = 72$ subjects would be required. However, the number of patients suggested at 36 is above the maximum of 30 they can recruit and so the next design possibility is to reduce λ. The value for this can be obtained by expressing equation (3.14) in terms of n and λ and rearranging to give

$$\lambda = \left(n \middle/ \left[\frac{(z_{1-\alpha/2} + z_{1-\beta})^2}{\Delta^2} + \frac{z_{1-\alpha/2}^2}{4} \right] \right) - 1. \tag{5.1}$$

In this example, specifying $n = 30$, and using equation (5.1) gives $\lambda = 0.63$. This suggests that the number of controls to be recruited is $m = 30/0.63 = 48$ and $N = m + n = 48 + 30 = 78$. Thus $(48 - 36) = 12$ extra controls are required to compensate for the 6 $(30 - 36)$ fewer patients. The investigators then have to decide if this is a practical option for them.

Paired Designs

Where each individual member of one group is matched to one member of the other, adjustments have to be made to the sample-size formulae.

The 'matching' is now part of the design process, but there is often confusion both in the terms used and in what is exactly meant by 'matching'. For example, Matteuci and Giampietro (2000) refer to 30 patients with type 1 diabetes (cases) age-matched to non-diabetic subjects (controls). They analysed this using the independent groups (unpaired or umatched) form of the t-test which suggests that only the mean ages of the two groups are matched. A moment's reflection indicates that such matching could include a very wide range of ages in one group but a very narrow range in the other group yet still be matched for (mean) age. To avoid this problem 'frequency-matching' is often used. To do this, the cases may be first divided into (say) several age bands and then controls recruited in equal numbers (or of some constant proportion or multiple) as the cases. This device results in matching on mean age and will also cover the same range of ages as the cases and so both groups will then have similar SDs. Frequency matching is intended to take account of some of the within-group variability with respect to the matching characteristics to help ensure that the differences observed between groups is not materially affected by differences in within-group characteristics (here age) of the two groups.

In contrast 'pairwise-matching' on age links each case to a particular healthy control of the 'same' age. However, this 'same' age does not have to imply born on the same day but does imply that 'same' has to be defined, perhaps as not more than a year difference in age. This constrains the investigators' choice and may require extra resource to find suitable controls. A truly paired design eventually uses the difference between the patient and the control as the variable for analysis, that is, $d_i = x_i - y_i$ where x_i is the observation for case i and y_i for the corresponding (paired) control. The statistical tests then use, for example, the paired t-test. In design terms, an important consequence of 'pair-matching' over an independent group comparison may be a reduction in the sample size required to conduct the study. However, this may be offset to some extent, by the extra workload involved in the matching process or indeed the possibility of not finding a control for every case.

In certain situations, the case may have more than one matched control and so, depending on the number of matches, we describe the pair, triple or whatever as the 'Unit'. In this case, for Unit i, $d_i = x_i - \bar{y}_i$ where x_i is the observation for case i and $\bar{y}_i$ is the mean outcome for the $c = 1/\lambda$ matched controls. Here c must have a positive integer value, the choice depending on the planning context.

***Example** – matched design – TUG in children with acute lymphoblastic leukaemia (ALL)*

Marchese, Chiarello and Lange (2003) compare TUG in eight children with ALL with eight healthy age-and-gender matched controls although no details are given of how either the cases or controls were selected. TUG is a measure of time needed to stand up from a seated position in a chair, walk 3 m, turn around, return to the chair, and sit down. TUG is assessed for each ALL patient and his or her time is compared with the corresponding control in a 1:1 paired design. The corresponding time differences from these (paired) values form the units for analysis. For the day 0 assessment the time taken by those children with ALL was 5.44 sec and for the controls was 4.00 sec a difference of 1.44 sec (p-value$=0.004$). The 95% CI for this difference, using the t-statistic with 7 degrees of freedom, gives 0.62 to 2.26 sec.

Patient	Before	INTERVENTION	After	Difference
1	b_1		a_1	$b_1 - a_1$
2	b_2		a_2	$b_2 - a_2$
3	b_3		a_3	$b_3 - a_3$
...	...		...	...
m	b_m		a_m	$b_m - a_m$

Figure 5.1 Paired 'before-and-after' design

Before-and-after Designs

A 'before-and-after' design is a variation of the matched pairs design. In such a design, illustrated in Figure 5.1, the pair (of observations) is completed by a second measurement on the same subject. Thus observations are made on each subject, once before (at baseline) and once after an intervention. We denote for subject i, b_i as the baseline measurement (B), that is, the one before the intervention. The corresponding measurement after the intervention (A) is a_i. As with all studies of a paired design, the critical observations are the paired difference $d_i = b_i - a_i$.

Example *– 'before-and-after' design – whole blood clotting time*

Butenas, Cawthern, van't Meer *et al.* (2001) measured the effect of taking aspirin on whole blood clotting time in minutes in three subjects. The samples were taken before and after 3 days of aspirin (an anti-platelet drug) at 325 mg twice per day. Before aspirin the results were 4.2, 3.1 and 5.1 min and after, 3.7, 4.1 and 3.6 min respectively.

In this example, the paired differences are 0.5, −1.0 and 1.5 min from which the mean value $\bar{d} = +0.33$ min and their $SD = 1.26$ min are calculated. This gives, using the t-statistic with 2 degrees of freedom, a very wide 95% CI of from −2.80 to 3.46 min. So, after completion of the study, there remains a great deal of uncertainty about the true direction and magnitude of this difference. In their design there are three 'units', each 'unit' is formed of the pair of measures from the same individual.

Cross-over Studies

In certain situations, the type of investigation planned in the design of Figure 5.1 may be of two distinct options, both of which could be given to the 'experimental' unit or subject, although not simultaneously. In this case the two possibilities, say A and B, could be given either in the sequence A followed by B (AB) or B followed by A (BA). This would bring the advantages of a matched design to the experimental process.

In contrast to a 'before-and-after' design this enables an unbiased estimate of the difference $A - B$ to be obtained. The analysis includes 'within-subject' comparisons and these are more sensitive than 'between-subject' comparisons, implying that such trials require fewer subjects than a parallel group design comparing the same treatment options. A distinct advantage of the cross-over design over a parallel two-group study is that each subject receives both options and this may facilitate recruitment to a study if the subjects are patients.

Example – *cross-over design* – *xenobiotic enhancement of allergic response*

In an experimental study conducted by Gilliland, Li, Saxon and Diaz-Sanchez (2004) patients who were sensitive to ragweed allergen were challenged with the allergen and, in addition, either with a placebo (P) or diesel fume particles (D) both administered in a saline solution. They were randomised to the sequences PD and DP although the authors do not specify how or in what number to each sequence. Each subject received the second challenge after a 6-week wash-out period had been allowed to elapse.

We discuss more of the details of cross-over trials in Chapter 9 in the context of clinical trials, but we note here that to realise the full potential of such a design, equal numbers of subjects should be allocated to the sequences (here DP and PD) which was not the case in this study which describes 19 patients. One should also note that the measure of difference for both those receiving sequences DP and PD is $d = y_D - y_P$. This is the first period observation minus the second for one half the subjects and the second period minus the first observation for the other half.

Study Size

For sample-size calculations for paired designs one also has to specify an anticipated standardised effect size. Here we postulate the value δ_{Pair} as the anticipated difference in outcome between the paired measures. In addition, we must also specify the SD of the paired data, σ_{Pair}. In this case, this is the anticipated SD of the d_i and not that of the x_i or the ys. Together these then define the standardised effect size as $\Delta_{\text{Pair}} = \delta_{\text{Pair}}/\sigma_{\text{Pair}}$. Alternatively the small, medium and large standardised effects suggested by Cohen (1988) may be used at this stage.

If the variable d_i being measured is continuous and can be assumed to have a Normal distribution then the number of 'Units' U, comprising 1 case and λ controls, is estimated by

$$U = \frac{1}{2}\left(1 + \frac{1}{\lambda}\right)\left[\frac{(z_{1-\alpha/2} + z_{1-\beta})^2}{\Delta_{Pair}^2} + \frac{z_{1-\alpha/2}^2}{2}\right].$$ (5.2)

We can see from equation (5.2) that as λ increases, $1/\lambda$ gets closer to zero and so U gets smaller and hence the number of cases (equal to the number of units) required becomes fewer. However, the number of subjects studied, $N_{Subjects} = U(1+\lambda)$ increases as there is now more than one control per case.

For an approximate calculation of sample size with $\lambda=1$, test size 5% and power 80%, equation (5.2) can be approximated by

$$U = N_{Pairs} = 2 + \frac{8}{\Delta_{Pair}^2}.$$ (5.3)

***Example** – sample size – whole blood clotting time*

If we were to repeat the study of Butenas, Cawthern, van't Meer *et al.* (2001), then using the values they obtained of $\bar{d} = +0.33$ and $SD = 1.26$ as planning values for δ_{Plan} and σ_{Plan} respectively, then these give $\Delta_{Plan} = 0.33/1.26 \approx 0.25$. Substituting this into equation (5.2) with $\lambda = 1$, two-sided test size $\alpha = 0.05$ and power, $1-\beta = 0.8$ gives

$$U = N_{Pairs} = \frac{1}{2} \times \left(1 + \frac{1}{1}\right) \times \left[\frac{(1.96 + 0.8416)^2}{0.25^2} + \frac{1.96^2}{2}\right]$$

$$= 128 \text{ or approximately } 130 \text{ pairs.}$$

However, if we were only interested in establishing whether there was a major decrease in clotting times with the use of aspirin we might set $\delta_{Plan} = 1$ min, then $\Delta_{Plan} = 1/1.26 \approx 0.8$ and the study size calculations using equation (5.3) lead to $U = N_{Pairs} = 15$. By any reasonable standards, the choice of only three subjects for the study conducted by Butenas, Cawthern, van't Meer *et al.* (2001) was far too small.

To calculate the sample size of a cross-over trial, use can be made of equation (5.2) also. However, in this instance λ is constrained by the design to be 1, since the first and second observations on the individual subject make the (matched) pair.

MORE THAN TWO GROUPS

In cross-sectional studies there may be more than two groups to compare. However, in this case, the design situation is more complex. This is because there is no longer one, clear alternative hypothesis. Thus, for example, with a three-group design the null hypothesis that the population means are all equal remains comparable to that for a two-group design, but there are several potential alternative hypotheses. These include one which postulates that two of the group means are equal but these differ from the third, or one for which the means are ordered in a ranking in some way.

Once a g-group study has been completed, the resulting analysis (and reporting) is somewhat more complex than for a simple two-group comparison. However, it is the importance of the questions posed, rather than the ease of analysis and reporting, which should determine the design chosen.

In general the null hypothesis for a g-group design is, H_0: $\mu_1 = \mu_2 = \ldots = \mu_g$ and one possible alternative hypothesis is the global alternative hypothesis that all the means differ, each from the other, that is, H_A: $\mu_1 \neq \mu_2 \neq \ldots \neq \mu_g$.

***Example** – comparison of three groups – mitochondrial dysfunction*

Brealey, Brand, Hargreaves *et al.* (2002) conducted a study that measured phosphocreatine content (nmol/mg dry weight) in skeletal muscle in controls (*C*), comprising otherwise healthy patients undergoing elective total hip replacement, and septic shock patients ultimately surviving (*A*) and those ultimately not surviving (*B*). A section of their results is summarised in Table 5.2, Panel (a).

Here there are three groups to compare and the test of the null hypothesis was made using the Kruskal–Wallis test. This gave a p-value$=0.02$ which suggests that there are indeed real (not just chance) differences between the groups. However, from this it is not entirely clear where the differences arise. The difference $C - B$ is the most extreme,

Table 5.2 Median and interquartile range (IQR) concentrations of phosphocreatine content (nmol/mg dry weight) in skeletal muscle (after Brealey, Brand, Hargreaves *et al.*, 2002, Table 2; reproduced by permission of the *Lancet*)

	Panel (a)			Panel (b)		
	Septic survivors (*A*)	Septic non-survivors (*B*)	Controls (*C*)	Septic non-survivors (*B*)	Septic survivors (*A*)	Controls (*C*)
				$x = -1$	$x = 0$	$x = +1$
m	12	9	8	9	12	8
Median	47.1	36.1	62.4	36.1	47.1	62.4
IQR	47.1[a]–65.3	28.4–45.7	56.8–63.9	28.4–45.7	47.1–65.3	56.8–63.9

[a]This value, equal to the median, is quoted in the original article.

and this must make the major contribution to the statistical signficance. However, the 'global' test outcome says little in respect to the statistical significance of the differences between $A - B$ and $C - A$.

In general, g-group studies broadly divide into those in which the groups do not have any formal structure and those that do. In the sense used here, a comparison of birthweights of children born in three different locations is unstructured whereas a preclinical study comparing the effect of three doses of the same compound on human cell growth is structured.

Unordered Groups

Unordered group designs comprise comparisons of $g=3$ or more groups: A, B, $C, \ldots$, G and these groups are arbitrarily labelled as such. In contrast to the two-group design in which only one comparison is made, there are now $g(g-1)/2$ possible pairwise comparisons. For example, with $g=3$ groups A, B and C, the three comparisons are A versus B, B versus C and finally C versus A. For $g=4$ groups there are six comparisons and for $g=5$ there are 10.

At the design stage of such a study, it is essential to define which of the possible comparisons is of primary importance. For example, in the study of Table 5.2 the authors' principal interest may have been to compare patients with sepsis and healthy controls – in which case the alternative hypothesis may be expressed as: $(\mu_A = \mu_B) \neq \mu_C$. To test this an optimal design would be observe m_1 patients with sepsis (irrespective of whether they survived or not) and m_1 controls, thus recruiting $N=2m_1$ subjects in total.

However, a secondary question may be to see if there are differences between those with sepsis who survive and those who do not. Thus the alternative hypothesis for this secondary question is: $\mu_A \neq \mu_B$ and the healthy group are not involved. To test this, an optimal design would be to recruit m_2 patients with sepsis who survived and m_2 with sepsis who did not! Clearly if $m_2 + m_2 = m_1$ then the design is complete since the total study size remains at $N=2m_1$. On the other hand if $m_2 + m_2 > m_1$ then this second question cannot be reliably addressed without increasing m_1 at least for those with sepsis. This might be compensated for by decreasing the sample size of the control group and thereby maintaining the same total sample size. However, the investigators cannot determine in advance the numbers who will die of their sepsis and so have to make a judgement concerning their relative proportion. This will then impact on the final choice of design.

Study Size

If a global test that uses the analysis of variance (ANOVA) is required for the comparison of means from a g-group design, then Day and Graham (1991) give the nomogram of Figure 5.2 for this purpose. To use their nomogram the method depends on first identifying anticipated or planning values for each of the g means, then calculating

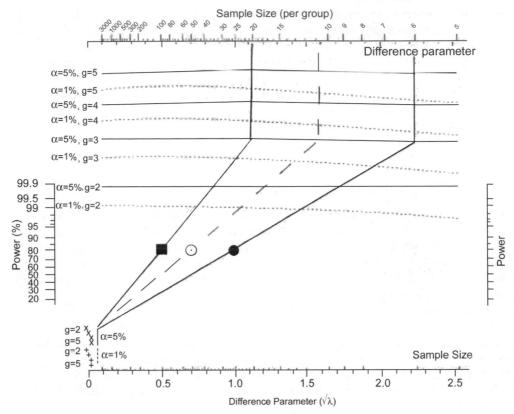

Figure 5.2 Nomogram for a comparison of up to five independent samples of a continuous variable relating power, $(1-\beta)$, group sample size, difference parameter ψ and significance level, α (from Day and Graham, 1991; reproduced by permission of John Wiley & Sons Ltd)

$$\psi_{\text{Plan}} = \sqrt{\frac{\sum(\mu_i - \bar{\mu})^2}{(g-1)\sigma^2_{\text{Plan}}}}. \tag{5.4}$$

Here $\bar{\mu}$ is the mean of the g anticipated planning means with values $\mu_1, \mu_2, \ldots, \mu_g$, and σ_{Plan} is the anticipated *SD* of the measurements which is assumed the same within each group.

To use the nomogram one begins by first identifying the point with coordinates $(\psi, 1-\beta)$ and then joining this to the point (g, α) of the lower left-hand corner of Figure 5.2. The straight-line trajectory between these points is then extended until it cuts the horizontal (but slightly curved) line of (g, α). At this point a new line is extended vertically upwards to cut the sample-size scale at m. The final study size is then $N = g \times m$. In Figure 5.2 the steeper the initial trajectory, the greater the sample size will be required.

Example – *sample size for a three-group comparison* – *phospocreatine in skeletal muscle*

Suppose we wished to repeat the study of Brealey, Brand, Hargreaves *et al.* (2002) and decided to use their results as the basis for the planning. Although they do not give the mean values in each group, we take the medians as a guide to their value and set for our planning purpose, $\mu_A = 50$, $\mu_B = 40$ and $\mu_C = 60$. These give $\bar{\mu} = (50 + 40 + 60)/3 = 50$. The width of the interquartile range is often about 2 *SDs*, suggesting a value for $\sigma_{Plan} \approx 10$. Substituting these in equation (5.4) with $g = 3$ gives $\psi_{Plan} \approx 1$. Using Figure 5.2 with $g = 3$, $\alpha = 5\%$ and a power of 80% gives the lower continuous line trajectory shown to cut at $m \approx 6$ per group. This implies a total study size of $N = g \times m = 18$ subjects.

However, this calculation is based on an uncertain planning value of the *SD*. So the investigators prudently repeat their calculations with σ_{Plan} taking values of 15 and 20, leading to $\psi_{Plan} \approx 0.7$ and 0.5 respectively. The corresponding trajectories are also shown in Figure 5.2 and lead to estimates for m of 11 and 20, and finally total sample sizes of 33 and 60 respectively. Discussion of all three of these options then follows, and practicalities suggest (perhaps) that the repeat study should be of a similar size to the original but with equal numbers per group set at (say) 12.

Although the change in *SD* makes quite a difference to the estimated sample size, as will a change in the values of the means at the extremes, a change in the position of that mean in the 'centre' changes ψ_{Plan} to a lesser extent. However, if this mean is at the mid-point of the interval, then ψ_{Plan} is at its minimum and this will result in a maximum sample size amongst the many possible scenarios for this 'central' mean.

Factorial Designs

In some circumstances there may be two principal study questions that are posed. In some such cases both questions may be answered within a single study by use of a factorial design. In a 2×2 factorial design, the two factors A and B are each studied at two levels. Factor A could represent two types of subjects such as those with disease and those that are healthy (not diseased), while Factor B may represent giving them (or not) an intervention of some kind. Thus we can think of a subject as either 'not-sick', denoted by (1), or 'sick' denoted by (*s*). Further we can think of giving each subject either 'intervention – no', (1), or 'intervention – yes', denoted (*i*). There are therefore four subject groups formed by (1)(1), (1)(*i*), (*s*)(1) and (*s*)(*i*) or more briefly denoted (1), (*i*), (*s*) and (*si*). Such a design is termed a 2×2 factorial design and the two factors are I and S. Patients eligible for such trials are randomised to one of the four treatment options in equal numbers, often in blocks of size $b = 4$ or 8.

Example – 2 × 2 factorial design – anaemia in children: iron, sulfadoxine-pyrimethamine, neither or both

In a study conducted by Verhoef, West, Nzyuko *et al.* (2002) anaemic but symptom-free infants were randomised to either iron alone, sulfadoxine-pyrimethamine alone, both or neither (placebo) to investigate their influence on haemoglobin levels after 12 weeks. This study takes the form of 2 × 2 factorial design of no treatment (**1**), iron alone (***i***), sulfadoxine-pyrimethamine alone (***s***) or both iron and sulfadoxine-pyrimethamine (***is***). These alternative options are summarised in Figure 5.3. An important feature of this trial was the use of a double-blind placebo for each supplement; thus, for example, infants of Group I receive both the placebos.

The two questions posed simultaneously are the value of iron and the value of sulfadoxine-pyrimethamine supplementation in symptom-free children at high risk of anaemia. In addition, this factorial design allows an estimate of the iron by sulfadoxine-pyrimethamine interaction. For example, the effect of iron supplementation alone raised haemoglobin concentrations by an estimated 1.5 g/L over placebo while with sulfadoxine-pyrimethamine alone it was greater at 8.5 g/L. On this basis, if the two supplements act independently of each other, then both given together as supplements should raise levels by $1.5 + 8.5 = 10.0$ g/L. In fact, the levels were raised by 9.1 g/L which is quite close to this value. Had a substantial interaction been present, the combination treatment iron and sulfadoxine-pyrimethamine (if synergistic) would have given a value in excess of 10.0 or considerably lower if the reverse was the case.

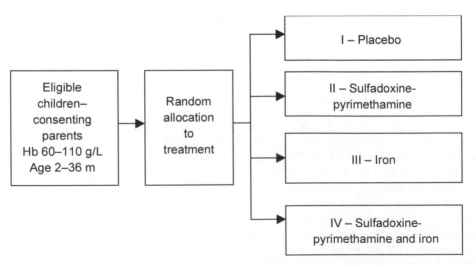

Figure 5.3 Randomised 2 × 2 factorial trial of intermittent iron and sulfadoxine-pyrimethamine on subsequent haemoglobin levels in infants at high risk of anaemia (Verhoef, West, Nzyuko *et al.*, 2002; **360**, 908–914, reproduced by permission of the *Lancet*)

Study Size

Although the 2×2 factorial design consists of four groups, comparisons are made pairwise. However, a central issue is whether we are willing to assume that the interaction term is zero or not. If assumed zero then smaller sample sizes are required for each comparison of the main effects. If not assumed zero, then one has to consider whether we wish to have a sufficiently large study size to enable a reasonable power for detecting an interaction. For example, in a 2×2 factorial study there are four means to be compared with m subjects per group. However, for efficient use of such a design and on the assumption of no interaction between the factors, the two main effect comparisons each reduce to comparing two means with $2m$ subjects in each group, and so one is back to two, two-group comparisons.

Suppose the 2×2 factorial study compares two factors, A and B, then we recommend planning in several stages. The first step would be to consider the sample size for factor A. The second step would be to consider the sample size for factor B which may have a different effect size, test size and power, from the factor A comparison. Clearly, if the sample sizes are similar then there is no difficulty in choosing, perhaps, the larger as the required sample size. If the sample sizes are very disparate then a discussion would ensue as to the most important comparison and perhaps a reasonable compromise reached.

Example – 2 × 2 factorial design – heart rates

Dodd, Day, Goldhill *et al.* (1989), in a 2×2 factorial design including low ($5\,\mu g\,kg^{-1}$) and high ($10\,\mu g\,kg^{-1}$) doses of glycopyrronium, G, administered either 1 minute before, or simultaneously with, edrophonium, E, to 60 subjects and measured their heart rates after 10 minutes. Thus the four options in this case, are (1), (g), (e) and (eg) and the corresponding mean heart ratess based on 15 subjects in each group were 71.3, 93.9, 77.1 and 93.3 beats per minute respectively, with $SD \approx 12$.

Day and Graham (1991) use these data to illustrate the sample-size calculations as made by use of Figure 5.2. The estimated effect of dose of glycopyrronium is the difference in mean heart rate from the 30 subjects on high dose (93.6) with the corresponding mean for those 30 on low dose (74.2), that is $93.6 - 74.2 = 19.4$ beats per minute, ignoring time of administration. This difference has

$$SE = SD\sqrt{\frac{2}{m}}.$$

The corresponding difference for the simultaneous compared to prior administration of edrophonium is 2.6 beats per minute, with the same SE.

If the smallest difference of clinical importance is $\delta = 5$ beats per minute, then a replication of this trial may consider $\Delta_{\text{Plan}} = \delta_{\text{Plan}}/\sigma_{\text{Plan}} = 5/12 \approx 0.4$. Further use of equation (3.12) for comparing two means with test size $\alpha = 0.05$ and $1 - \beta = 0.8$, gives

$m=100$ or $N=200$ subjects in total. These would then be allocated at random into the four groups, 25 in each. Such a trial would be of more than sufficient size to demonstrate an increase of 19.4 beats per minute with high dose glycopyrronium but would not be sufficient to reliably demonstrate a difference due to when the administration of edrophonium was made of 2.6 beats per minute.

If one was concerned to estimate reliably the interaction (if any) between edrophonium and glycopyrronium, then this is equivalent to estimating: Interaction $=(93.9-71.3)-(93.3-77.1)=6.4$ beats per minute but this has

$$SE = SD\sqrt{\frac{4}{m}} = \sqrt{2}SD\sqrt{\frac{2}{m}}.$$

Now if the smallest interaction of clinical importance is 5 beats per minute, this makes the corresponding $\Delta_{\text{Plan}}=\delta_{\text{Plan}}/\sigma_{\text{Plan}}=5/[12\times\sqrt{2}]=5/16.97\approx0.3$.

Using equation (3.12) once more with test size $\alpha=0.05$ and $1-\beta=0.8$, gives $m=176$ or $N=352$ subjects in total. These would then be allocated at random into the four groups, 89 or rounded to 90 in each. So a much bigger study would be required with this object in mind.

Ordered Groups

In Table 5.2 we have assumed that the groups described there as A, B and C, are essentially unstructured. However, if they are structured in some way, then note of this structure may change the approach to design and hence their eventual analysis. Thus studies with g (>2) groups may involve a comparison of different doses of the same drug or some other type of ordered groups. In such cases, although the null hypothesis would still be that all population means are equal, the alternative will now be H_{Ordered} in the form of either $\mu_1<\mu_2<\ldots<\mu_g$ or $\mu_1>\mu_2>\ldots>\mu_g$.

Although Brealey, Brand, Hargreaves et al. (2002) include in their three-group design, controls (C), septic shock patients ultimately surviving (A) and septic shock ultimately non-surviving (B), they ignore an intrinsic ordering of the severity of the condition as is evidenced by the latter group of those who die. To emphasise this, their results are summarised again in the right-hand columns of Table 5.2, Panel (b), but there the groups are now ordered in terms of increasing severity of their 'disease' status. The corresponding median values now show a decline following the order of severity.

If the groups are formed by g doses of the same drug, then the alternative hypothesis, H_{Ordered}, may be expressed by the equivalent of equation (1.1) in which case the model is $\mu=\beta_0+\beta_1$ (dose). This implies that the relationship between the amount of drug given and the measure observed is linear. In which case, the purpose of the study will be to estimate the regression coefficient, β_1. Thus the null hypothesis is H_0: $\beta_1=0$, which implies, if it were true, that the dose has no influence on the outcome measure and so all dose groups have the same mean value β_0. The alternative hypothesis is clearly H_1: $\beta_1\neq0$.

In comparing two, of three, groups in a situation similar to that of Table 5.2, the corresponding mean differences $\bar{d}$ have variance,

$$\text{Var}(\bar{d}) = \sigma^2\left[\frac{1}{m}+\frac{1}{m}\right] = \frac{2\sigma^2}{m}. \tag{5.5}$$

Here for convenience we assume the groups are of the same size m and have common SD, σ. Alternatively, if the g-groups are ordered in some way, and these are associated with a value of an underlying 'dose-like' variable x, then the parameter of interest is the slope β_1 estimated by b_1.

We have indicated in equation (1.2) that

$$\text{Var}(b_1) = \frac{\sigma^2}{\sum_i^N (x_i - \bar{x})^2},$$

where in the situation here $N=gm$. However, with m subjects in each dose group j, and hence with the same value of x_j, this can be expressed as

$$\text{Var}(b_1) = \frac{\sigma^2}{m \sum_j^g (x_j - \bar{x})^2}. \qquad (5.6)$$

For a $g=3$ group design of equally spaced values of x, this becomes

$$\text{Var}(b_1) = \frac{\sigma^2}{2m}.$$

Thus the design effect, DE, defined by equation (1.6) for comparing two design options, gives

$$DE = \frac{1/\text{Var}(b_1)}{1/\text{Var}(\bar{d})} = \frac{1/[\sigma^2/2m]}{1/[2\sigma^2/m]} = \frac{2m}{\sigma^2} \cdot \frac{2\sigma^2}{m} = 4.$$

This suggests that the regression model design is statistically more efficient than the three possible two-group comparisons in this situation. However, it does assume, which we have not verified by experiment, that there is a linear relationship. In practice, the assumption of linearity will be checked using the experimental results once obtained.

It is important to emphasise, that the choice of the values for x will be under the direct control of the experimenter in a dose-finding study and so represent real values. In the more observational type of design of Brealey, Brand, Hargreaves et al. (2002) the values of x set at -1, 0 and $+1$ only rank the groups in order and so their quantities do not represent real numerical values. However, these can often be regarded as real values for design and analysis purposes although some care is needed.

Study Size

In this (ordered categorical) situation we are estimating β_1 and so one method of calculating an appropriate study size is to define the desired width of the corresponding CI as we did in deriving equation (3.3) and hence (3.4). By analogy with equation (3.3) we have

$$\omega_{\text{Plan}} = 2 \times z_{1-\alpha/2} \sqrt{\frac{\sigma^2_{\text{Plan}}}{m \sum (x - \bar{x})^2}}$$

and from this we obtain

$$m = 4 \left[\frac{\sigma_{Plan}^2}{\omega_{Plan}^2 \sum (x - \bar{x})^2} \right] z_{1-\alpha/2}^2. \tag{5.7}$$

In Table 5.2(b), the estimate of the change in phosphocreatine content between groups C $(x=1)$ and B $(x=-1)$ gives an estimate of the slope as $b_1=(62.4-36.1)/[1-(-1)]=26.3/2 \approx 13$. So if we then specify that the width of the 95% CI should be 10 nmol/mg dry weight, we are planning for a final CI of from approximately 8 to 18 nmol/mg dry weight. Thus setting $\alpha=0.05$, $\omega_{Plan}=10$, $\sigma_{Plan}=10$ as previously, and with $g=3$, using $x=-1$, 0 and 1, equation (5.7) gives

$$m = 4 \left[\frac{10^2}{10^2 \times 2} \right] \times 1.96^2 \approx 8$$

per group and total study size of $N=3 \times 8 = 24$.

Alternatively to estimate a linear regression slope, Day and Graham (1991) show how equation (5.4) can be modified and the nomogram of Figure 5.2 utilised. Essentially, equation (5.4) is modified to become

$$\psi_{Linear} = \sqrt{\frac{\sum (\mu_i - \bar{\mu})^2}{\sigma_{Plan}^2}}, \tag{5.8}$$

and Figure 5.2 entered as if for a $g=2$ group comparison with this value of ψ_{Linear}. The reason for the value of value $g=2$ here is because the slope of a regression line is estimated with 1 degree of freedom (df). This is the same as the between groups df for a two-group ANOVA.

Example – linear response – phosphocreatine in skeletal muscle

We review the possibility of a repeat of the study of Brealey, Brand, Hargreaves *et al.* (2002) and, for our planning purpose, $\mu_A=50$, $\mu_B=40$ and $\mu_C=60$ but this time we will assume a linear response to x rather than just a three-group comparison as previously. In this case equation (5.8) gives $\psi_{Linear} \approx 1.4$. Using Figure 5.2 with $g=2$, $\alpha=5\%$ and a power of 80% then the trajectory leads to a cut at $m \approx 5$ per group. This implies a total study size of $N=g \times m=15$ subjects is required. This is less than the 24 using the CI indicated above, and the 18 when no structure to the three means was implied.

CHANGES OVER TIME

A cross-sectional study can be repeated on the same population type at different time points to assess changes. However, in this case the new population sampled does not comprise those same individuals but rather an entirely different sample.

Example – *repeated cross-sectional study obesity in adolescents*

McCarthy, Ellis and Cole (2003) conducted a cross-sectional study investigating measures of potential obesity in 776 adolescents aged 11–16 in the UK in 1997. This was a repeat of similar studies that had been conducted in 1977 in boys and one in 1987 in girls. In these studies waist measurement was taken of each child. Comparisons between the two dates suggested that waist circumference had increased by an average of 6.9 cm in boys over the 20-year period and 6.2 cm in girls over the 10-year period.

In this case, all members of the 1997 population are clearly different individuals to those in the 1977 and 1987 cohorts. This contrasts with a longitudinal study in which the same individuals are assessed a second or further times.

COVARIATES

Although it is difficult to be precise in this respect, the careful recording of subject characteristics that are known to modify the outcome measures should be made. These are variables that, over and above any intrinsic effect of the different interventions or group definitions, influence the value of the endpoint measures for an individual. For example, there may be major differences in healing time of burns dependent on the cause of the injury. Taking such characteristics into account (often using regression methods) may then lead to a more sensitive final comparison of groups. Essentially this is because some of the variability is ascribed to these characteristics so that the resulting, and reduced, *SD* is more purely a measure of the random variation. Thus a key aspect of the experimental design is the identification of such measures. However, investigators should guard against the recording of too many 'possible' (modifier) variables that may only affect outcome in a marginal way but focus on those that are 'known' to be influential.

At the end of a study, the estimated difference beween groups may be changed to some extent by taking account of such covariates. In addition, even in circumstances where there is little change in the estimate, the width of the corresponding CI may be reduced, since the *SD* may be reduced, thereby providing more reliable information with respect to the study question.

Design features – cross-sectional

Specify the study objectives

Identify the groups to be compared or the intervention proposed

Ensure a representative sample

Select the endpoints

Choice of covariates

Explore the options for study size

5.3 LONGITUDINAL STUDIES

REPEATED MEASURES

In longitudinal studies a subject once recruited will be followed over time and successive measurements taken. For example, the study may involve patients admitted to hospital with suspected dengue fever for care during which time their platelets are monitored on a daily basis. Once the platelet level recovers to (say) $100 \times 10^9/L$ or more then the patient is discharged. Such a repeated measures study investigating platelet changes is longitudinal rather than cross-sectional in nature. It is a 'repeated measures' design as platelets are monitored daily and there is also a 'survival-time' endpoint which is the time from their admission to hospital to the time when their platelets recover sufficiently for discharge.

This is a typical (laboratory-based) repeated-measures design using clinical material. These often have repeated measures at convenient intervals during the 'working 8-hour day' followed by an observation when getting back to work the next morning!

Example – *repeated measures* – *ciliary beat frequency*

The study of Lyons, Djahanbakhch, Saridogan *et al.* (2002) is a repeated measures study in that the ciliary beat frequency (Hz) of the ampullary region was recorded at 0.5, 2, 4, 8 and 24 hours. The results are summarised in Figure 5.4 where the bars show the standard error (*SE*) at each point. These indicate the need for an appropriate analysis of a longitudinal study which would consist of a comparison of the *whole* patterns over time (or some important features), not just a series of repeated statistical tests at every observation point.

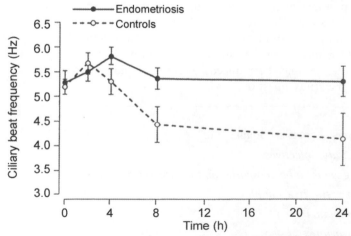

Figure 5.4 Effect of duration of incubation on the between-group difference in ciliary beat frequency (from Lyons, Djahanbakhch, Saridogan *et al.*, 2002, **360**, 1221–1222, Figure 1; reproduced by permission of the *Lancet*)

Clearly, this is an 'experimental' situation for which material for study is strictly limited and difficult to obtain. However, in such situations, even more care has to be taken in selecting the best design to answer the question posed as repeating such an experiment may not be feasible. In less 'difficult situations' a badly chosen design can always be repeated but this too is best avoided if at all possible as it is clearly wasteful of resources. In this example, the choice of design is entirely in the hands of the investigators, as the 'experimental' material, once collected from the donor women, is freely available to sample at times stipulated by the design team. In fact a better choice of design may have been to take more observations when the curves appear to separate, at about 4 hours, but the design team may not have anticipated this feature. Alternatively a choice of observations times taken on a logarithmic scale at 0.5, 1, 2, 4, 8 and 16 hours may have been closer to optimal.

In other situations, the investigators may be more limited in their range of options as the subjects may not be able or willing to provide unlimited samples on repeated occasions.

Example – *repeated measures – creatinine levels post renal transplant*

Calne, Moffatt, Friend, *et al.* (1999) studied the mean creatinine levels (μmol/L) in 31 cadaveric renal allograft recipients with values observed at transplant and then at 1, 3, 6, 9 and 12 months. Their results are summarised in Figure 5.5 but in this case the bars shown around each point are not defined.

In this situation, although the design team will determine when the samples are taken, exigencies of the clinical situation will have to be considered when choosing the frequency and spacing of these repeat observations. Also individual patients may refuse to participate on certain occasions. Here it is more difficult to be optimal with the statistical design.

Example – *repeated measures – sexual function after radiotherapy for cervical cancer*

In the longitudinal study of Jensen, Groenwold, Klee *et al.* (2003) investigating sexual function after radiotherapy for early-stage cervical cancer, 118 women who were disease-free following external beam radiotherapy (EBRT) were asked to complete an SVQ, part of which we described in Figure 2.5. Consenting patients were given the first questionnaire, with a stamped addressed envelope, to be completed at the termination of their EBRT. Thereafter, they received identical, mailed questionnaires at 1, 3, 6, 12, 18 and 24 months after RT but only if they remained disease-free. This repeated measures study is dependent on the women remaining disease-free, returning the fully completed questionnaires and on time. So, in comparison to the designs summarised in Figures 5.4 and 5.5, there is a real challenge for the investigators to maintain the basic stucture of the design throughout the course of the study.

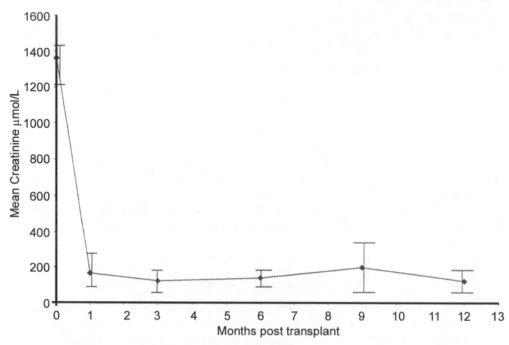

Figure 5.5 Campath 1H mean creatinine after transplant (from Calne, Moffatt, Friend *et al.*, 1999, Figure 1; reproduced by permission of Lippincott, Williams & Wilkins)

AUTOCORRELATION

One important aspect of longitudinal data with repeated measures on the same subject is that successive observations are unlikely to be independent. This contrasts with cross-sectional designs in which there is, for the particular endpoint under consideration, a single variable whose value in a subject will not depend on the magnitude of the corresponding value in other subjects.

A key consideration then in planning a study involving repeated measures is the nature and strength of this correlation. Correlation coefficients are a measure of the degree of association between two variables and that for measuring the association between successive measures in time is

$$\rho_T(1,2) = \frac{\sum(y_1 - \bar{y}_1)(y_2 - \bar{y}_2)}{\sqrt{\sum(y_1 - \bar{y}_1)^2 \sum(y_2 - \bar{y}_2)^2}} \ . \tag{5.9}$$

Here y_1 and y_2 represent the values of two successive assessments of the same measure made on the same subject (or on specimens taken from the subject). For example, these may be the different ciliary beat frequencies (Hz) of the ampullary region of the fallopian tubes taken over time. Equation (5.9) is termed the *auto-* or *serial-correlation*. The expression is symmetric in terms of y_1 and y_2, and hence $\rho_T(1, 2) = \rho_T(2, 1)$; the T is included here to emphasise the time element.

The problem for the investigators is that the properties of a repeated measures design depend on ρ_T. The value of this, and how it changes with the time interval between observations, may be hard to pinpoint. Despite this, simplifying assumptions can often be made to facilitate the design process. For example, it is often assumed that the serial correlation between measurements made on any two arbitrarily chosen times, say time t and time t', have the same value of $\rho_T(t, t')$ whatever values of t and t' we happen to choose. In this case we can write $\rho_T(t, t') = \rho$ since it does not depend on the choice of these times. When this form of autocorrelation structure applies this is termed as 'compound symmetry'.

'Before-and-after' Design

Now we can extend the simple 'before-and-after' design of Figure 5.1 both backwards in time and forwards in time, to make v repeated observations on each subject before the intervention, and w observations after. Thus the options for this 'repeated-measures' design relate to the choice of v and w. For the study of Lyons, Djahanbakhch, Saridogan *et al.* (2002) there can be no observations made before the specimens are collected, $v = 0$, and they set $w = 5$. Thus there is no other design option than to set $v = 0$. On the other hand the first creatinine value is taken from patients of Calne, Moffatt, Friend *et al.* (1999) at baseline, that is at a time just before the renal allograft, in which case $v = 1$ and they also set $w = 5$.

In the simplest form of design, the intervention is assumed to change the level of the outcome variable by a fixed amount (which may be zero and so has no effect), and the new level is then maintained over the post-intervention observation period. One statistical summary measure for such a design is to compute the mean of the 'before-intervention' observations of each subject, and then the corresponding means of the 'after-intervention' observations. The difference between these two forms the unit of analysis. Thus for subject i, this difference is $d_i = \bar{y}_{wi} - \bar{x}_{vi}$ where $\bar{y}_{wi}$ and $\bar{x}_{vi}$ are the respective post- and pre-intervention means for that subject. In a single-group study, the null hypothesis is that the mean of these differences is zero.

This repeated format for pre- and post-intervention measurements can be utilised in, for example, a parallel two-group study. In this case, the model for comparing the two groups may be written as

$$d_i = \beta_0 + \beta_1 \tau + \varepsilon_i, \tag{5.10}$$

where $\tau = 0$ for one group and $\tau = 1$ for the other. The object of the study is to estimate β_1. Since d_i is a difference, β_1 estimates a difference of differences. A more flexible alternative to equation (5.10) is

$$\bar{y}_{wi} = \beta_0 + \beta_1 \tau + \beta_2 \bar{x}_{vi} + \varepsilon_i, \tag{5.11}$$

where $\bar{x}_{vi}$ is the covariate. If β_2 is set at 1 then equation (5.11) becomes (5.10), an analysis of differences. However, if we allow the regression coefficient, β_2, to be estimated from the data (rather than imposing a specific value for it of unity) then an analysis of covariance can be conducted leading to a more efficient analysis. In addition

β_1 now represents the difference between the means of the $\bar{y}_{wi}$ obtained from each (intervention) group, adjusted for values of $\bar{x}_{vi}$.

Study Size

For planning purposes we assume that the observations taken in a proposed repeated measures design are equally spaced in time, both before and after the intervention and there is compound symmetry. For a parallel two-group design for continuous observations from a Normal distribution, and anticipated standardised effect size Δ_{Plan}, the sample size for each group required for two-sided test size α and power $1-\beta$ is

$$m_{Repeated} = R\left[\left(1 + \frac{1}{\lambda}\right)^2 \frac{(z_{1-\alpha/2} + z_{1-\beta})^2}{\Delta_{Plan}^2} + \frac{z_{1-\alpha/2}^2}{4}\right]. \qquad (5.12)$$

This is the same as equation (3.14) except for the multiplier R, where

$$R = \left[\frac{1 + (w-1)\rho_T}{w} - \frac{v\rho_T^2}{[1 + (v-1)\rho_T]}\right] \qquad (5.13)$$

and $v \geqslant 0$ and $w \geqslant 1$.

From these equations $n_{Repeated} = \lambda m_{Repeated}$ and the total study size is $N_{Repeated} = m_{Repeated} + n_{Repeated}$.

Table T7 gives the values of the multiplier R of equation (5.13) for use in equation (5.12) to determine study size. It can be seen that sample size in a repeated measures design depends critically on each of v, w and ρ_T. In general R decreases as v, the number of pre-intervention observations, increases. It also decreases quite rapidly as the number of post-intervention observations w increases. However, the pattern with increasing ρ_T is a little more complex, but with a general decline in R for $\rho_T > 0.3$.

If no pre-intervention measures are taken, then $v = 0$ and R comprises only the first term in equation (5.13). If in addition $w = 1$, then there are no repeated measures and so $R = 1$.

An important situation is when $v = 1$ and $w = 1$, that is when a baseline measure is taken immediately before the intervention, followed by a single observation after – this is now a cross-sectional design. In this case $R = 1 - \rho_T^2$ and unless $\rho_T = 0$, R is always less than 1. This therefore implies that compared to equation (3.14) the number of subjects required is less. From this one can conclude that for a given fixed study size, including a baseline measure of the endpoint (if possible) will improve the statistical efficiency of the design. In effect, the width of the relevant CIs will be reduced.

The calculation of R requires that an anticipated value for the correlation coefficient ρ_T needs to be specified. Experience suggests that these correlations are often between 0.60 and 0.75. For example, Draper, Brodaty, Low et al. (2002) reported $\rho_T = 0.63$ for the autocorrelation between morning and evening total scores of the Harmful Behaviour Scale, obtained approximately 12 hours apart, amongst residents of nursing homes.

An exploratory approach when making sample-size calculations is to try out various values of ρ_T to see what influence these will have on the proposed sample size. It is unlikely that ρ_T would be negative, consequently, if we set $\rho_T=0$ in this exploration, we obtain a minimum estimate of the required sample size.

Example – *sample size for a repeated measures design – ciliary beat frequency*

Suppose we had been planning a study similar to that conducted by Lyons, Djahanbakhch, Saridogan *et al.* (2002) of Figure 5.4, and thought the mean ciliary beat frequency in controls, averaged out over a 24-hour incubation period, would be 5 Hz, with *SD* of approximately 0.75 Hz. Further we anticipate this may be higher in those with endometriosis by approximately 0.5 Hz. Assuming two-sided $\alpha=0.05$ and $1-\beta=0.8$, the investigators wish to review the design options with respect to the number of repeated measures w and the effect of the autocorrelation ρ_T.

First using $R-1$, with $\alpha=0.05$, $1-\beta=0.8$ and anticipated standardised effect size $\Delta_{Plan}=0.5/0.75=0.67$, equation (5.10) with $\lambda=1$, gives $m=36$. Their usual design is to have $v=0$, $w=5$, so $R=(1+4\rho_T)/5$ which with $\rho_T=0.5$, 0.6 and 0.7 gives $R=0.60$, 0.68 and 0.76 which can also be obtained from Table T7. This range of ρ_T then suggests that the sample sizes per group to consider are $0.60 \times 36 \approx 22$, $0.68 \times 36 \approx 25$ and $0.76 \times 36 \approx 28$. After discussion, a compromise sample size may be set as $m_{Repeated} \approx 25$ and hence set $N_{Repeated}=50$.

Suppose we wish to design a repeated measures trial of a blood-sugar-level-reducing drug against a placebo control in which two pre-randomisation measures were planned but it was not clear how many were to be taken post-randomisation. We assume compound symmetry with $\rho=0.7$ and a standardised effect size of $\Delta_{Plan}=0.4$, two-sided $\alpha=0.05$ and $1-\beta=0.8$.

Table T7 gives for $\rho=0.7$, $v=2$ and $w=1$, 2, 3 and 4 the successive values for R as 0.42, 0.27, 0.22 and 0.20. This immediately suggests that little will be gained in terms of reducing the sample size by having more than $w=3$ for the design. From equation (5.12) with $R=1$ gives $m_{Repeated}=100$ then different designs reduce this to $100 \times 0.42=42$, 27, 22 and 20 respectively with total sample size, N, of twice this number. Thus if we finally choose the design with $v=2$, $w=3$ and $N=44$ patients, the number of *observations* that are required is $T=N \times (v+w)=44 \times 5=220$. This is not very different from 200, the number of patients that would be required if only a single observation had been made per patient. So this design would be very attractive if patients were not easy to recruit but once recruited would be happy to undergo investigation on five separate occasions.

Even if compound symmetry cannot be assumed, calculations made on the above basis will provide a guide to appropriate study size. A pragmatic approach would then be to inflate the sample size by (say) 10% to account for the unknown influence of the autocorrelation structure. If a programme of studies is planned then as experience is accumulated this cautious approach may be refined.

Interrupted-time-series Design

An interrupted-time-series design takes the same form as a 'before-and-after' design but the type of 'events' recorded are not necessarily amongst individuals directly recruited to the study and the endpoints are usually counts. Such a design was used to test the efficacy of introducing compulsory seat-belt wearing in cars – comparing injury rates and severity before and after the change of law. Thus the design includes all the members of a national population (some of whom may never travel by car) and records the numbers who have a severe injury before and after the change in the legislation. In theory at least, an individual member of the population could have several accidents prior to the law change and several afterwards. As a consequence the observations may be correlated to some extent although the injuries will in general occur in different individuals at the different times. Clearly this design is longitudinal and assessments are repeated over time but it is not a 'repeated-measures' design in the sense we have used the term previously.

Example – *interrupted-time-series design – air-pollution control*

Clancy, Goodman, Sinclair and Dockerty (2002) showed reductions in respiratory and cardiovascular death rates in Dublin, Ireland. This reduction followed the control of particulate air pollution after the sale of coal for burning on domestic fires was prohibited by law. They showed, for example, that the age-standardised death rate for respiratory deaths fell after the ban by 15.5% (95% CI 12 to 19%). The structure of their design is given in Figure 5.6.

The main design aspects for an interrupted-time-series are: What period of time constitutes a unit? and: How long should we measure before and after the intervention? Clancy, Goodman, Sinclair and Dockerty (2002) used death rates that are reported annually. They chose an equal number of units before and after the intervention. In general balancing the number of units in this way will optimise the statistical efficiency of the design. Finally there is the question of how many units. Usually this will depend on data availability, but it is wise to choose at least three before and three after, so that the variance of the outcome can be estimated. One could apparently increase the number of units by reducing the time interval of each unit. Thus Clancy, Goodman, Sinclair and Dockerty (2002) could have doubled the number of units by measuring over 6 months (and totalling) rather than once a year (and totalling). However, this can introduce greater fluctuations into the data and is unlikely to improve statistical efficiency.

Before	Intervention	After
Pre-ban 6 years	Ban on	Post-ban 6 years
01 Sep 1984–31 Aug 1990	coal sales	01 Sep 1990–31 Aug 1996

Figure 5.6 Interrupted-time-series 'before-and-after' design (based on Clancy, Goodman, Sinclair and Dockery, 2002, **360**, 1210–1214; reproduced by permission of the *Lancet*)

Design features – longitudinal studies

Specify the study objectives

Identify the groups to be compared or the intervention proposed

Achieve a representative sample

Select the endpoints

Choice of covariates

Choice of numbers of baseline and longitudinal measures

Explore the options for study size

Choice of suitable autocorrelation structure

Choice of the number of repeated measures

5.4   TECHNICAL DETAIL

COMPOUND SYMMETRY

In fact equation (5.10) is a rather simplified version of the model for a repeated measure design. In some instances the error structure represented by ε_i in that model is more complex, and so are some of the regression coefficients themselves. In particular β_0, instead of being thought of as a fixed quantity representing the common and fixed value for all subjects should $\beta_1 = 0$, is considered to have a different or random value for each individual, termed α_i, with its own *SD*, σ_α. This leads to the following random effects model

$$y_{ij} = \alpha_i + \beta x_{ij} + \varepsilon_{ij}, \tag{T5.1}$$

where y_{ij} is the *j*th observation on subject *i*, α_i is the random effect of subject *i* and ε_{ij} are random error terms with *SD*, σ. If the ε_{ij} are all independent then it can be shown that the correlation between two measurements y_{ij} and y_{ik} made on the same individual is

$$\rho = \frac{\sigma_\alpha^2}{\sigma_\alpha^2 + \sigma^2}. \tag{T5.2}$$

Thus one implication from model (T5.1) is that observations have the same correlation irrespective of how far apart in time the observations are made. This is known as compound symmetry.

AUTOREGRESSIVE MODEL

There are occasions when the assumption that the ε_{ij} of equation (T5.1) are not independent. For example, in interrupted-time-series it would seem sensible to allow a model where the autocorrelation reduced as the time gap increased. The most common one is to allow for what is termed a first-order autoregressive model. In this case, we assume

$$\varepsilon_{ij} = \rho \varepsilon_{ij-1} + \eta_{ij}, \tag{T5.3}$$

where the η_{ij} are independently identically distributed error terms and ρ is the autocorrelation which must lie beween -1 and $+1$. The term 'first order' is used since equation (T5.3) connects the observation at time $(j-1)$ with the next after it, at observation time, j.

6 Surveys, Cohort and Case–Control Studies

Summary

In this chapter we discuss the design of surveys, cohort studies, case–control studies and case–crossover designs. Aspects of surveys include the specification of the target population for the survey and the identification of the sampling frame. The ways in which subjects are drawn from the sampling frame are described. Emphasis is placed on alleviating problems associated with the failure to obtain the requisite information from subjects selected for a survey. In a cohort study groups of individuals, often those who are exposed to what may be deemed a particular risk, are followed in time and compared with a parallel group of those not so exposed. The object of the study is to quantify the risk that may result from the exposure, often with respect to developing a particular disease. In contrast, case–control studies consider patients with a particular disease or condition and a suitable control group. These are investigated (retrospectively) in time to help establish any causative agents or risk factors. Methods of estimating the appropriate numbers of subjects to be recruited are indicated. Finally, we discuss case-crossover designs which are longitudinal in nature but in which a subject acts as their own control.

6.1 INTRODUCTION

The feature that often distinguishes surveys from other cross-sectional studies is that they are population-based. The populations surveyed are large, which contrasts with a cross-sectional study recording details of patients attending a particular clinic when numbers may be small. In many circumstances in a survey the investigator does not make the observations directly on the selected survey participants. Rather the participants themselves are asked to self-report, perhaps by completing a questionnaire. At the other extreme, a survey may involve very specialist measures that require highly trained observers. Thus a survey might intend to describe the sexual health of women which requires the women to return a self-completed questionnaire, or to determine the prevalence of glaucoma in the community which requires the presence of a suitably experienced ophthalmologist to take specialist measurements.

If a longitudinal study is purely observational in nature, and there is no planned intervention by an investigator, then it is often described as a cohort study. Over the

Design of Studies for Medical Research. D. Machin and M. J. Campbell
© 2005 John Wiley & Sons Ltd. ISBN 0 470 84495 7

follow-up time, some individuals will be exposed to a potential risk factor. However, just as we reserved the term 'survey' for large, population-based cross-sectional studies the term 'cohort' usually refers to large, population-based and longitudinal studies also. Thus the pregnant women living in Chernobyl at the time of the disaster are a 'cohort' who could be then followed over time. In many cohort studies a second (unexposed) group of individuals are also identified and followed in the same way and so an investigator may choose a second group of women living away from Chernobyl at the time of the disaster. The object is to see, for example, if the women from Chernobyl have a higher rate of birth defects amongst their babies than the non-exposed women.

In contrast, a case–control study starts with the identification of persons with the disease of interest, and a suitable control (reference) group of persons without the disease. The relationship of the disease with the potential risk factor for the disease is examined by comparing the diseased and non-diseased with regard to how frequently the risk factor was present in each group before the disease manifested itself. Thus case–control studies are retrospective in nature.

Case–control studies may be relatively modest undertakings of a short time span, whereas cohort studies are intrinsically large with considerable follow-up of the individuals recruited usually entailed.

We also described case-crossover designs which can be useful if it is difficult to obtain controls. Here a subject acts as their own control and it is assumed the effect of exposure on risk is immediate.

6.2 SURVEYS

Surveys are just one type of cross-sectional study but are treated differently because they are large and, for example, involve self-completed questionnaires; they often have problems associated with low response rates. Broadly speaking there are three main types of survey: self-completed; interviewer-assisted or completed; and those that require specialist examination by a clinical team. In a self-completed questionnaire survey, the types of questions asked and/or the responses required can only be of limited complexity as no direct assistance is given to the potential respondent except that provided on the questionnaire itself. In interviewer-administered or -assisted surveys, the investigator is part of the interview process and their role will be clearly defined by the research team. By its very nature a survey that requires specialist assessment of the individual participants will be expensive to conduct and may involve the participants attending special centres for examination, bringing logistical difficulties.

TYPES OF SURVEY

The type of survey chosen will depend on the primary research question in mind. This is clearly the prime focus for the research team at the design stage as it will have a major influence on the size and complexity of the survey undertaken.

Postal Survey

This type of design is one in which an unsolicited questionnaire arrives either through the post, or via email, which the targeted individual is asked to complete and return.

The clear advantage is that a 'postal' survey can be very large and spread over a very wide geographical area. The spread brings little or no extra cost as a single price of a postage stamp usually brings national coverage. Postal surveys require few personnel and need minimal equipment. However, questionnaires have to be returned through the post; if successive rounds of reminders are required for those who fail to respond, the interval between first dispatch and subsequent return of questionnaires can be prolonged.

A postal survey requires least effort for the participants. For example, they do not have to decline participation in a face-to-face situation but can refuse to comply merely by ignoring the postal request. They can also only partially comply by failing to follow instructions on the questionnaire, or by omitting responses to those questions which are difficult or perhaps embarrassing to complete. Their only discomfort may be a postal reminder from the investigators if they do not return the questionnaire by a certain date.

For the investigator the likelihood of a low response rate is a real possibility. In addition, a postal survey will tend to have a lower response rate from certain specific groups, such as those with low levels of literacy. Also if errors or omissions are made when completing the questionnaire then it not usually possible to return to check these with the respondent. Neither can one be certain that it is the target individual who actually completes the questionnaire, and not a relative or carer.

Example – *postal survey   sexual function in Danish women*

As part of a larger study of sexual functioning, Jensen, Groenwold, Klee *et al.* (2003) surveyed a group of women selected from the Danish general population. The women received the questionnaire through the post and returned it in the same way. Questions ranged from asking whether or not they had a partner, to quite intimate details concerning their sexual health. The eventual response rate achieved, after one reminder (Danish law permits only one) was 49% from 892 women contacted.

Interview

Interviewer-administered surveys are generally more expensive than postal surveys. This derives mainly from the costs of training and paying interviewers and of their travel costs. Face-to-face interviews also generally require an initial contact (by letter, telephone or in person) to set up an appointment for the interview; and multiple contacts may be needed to agree a convenient time. Alternatively one can conduct the interview by telephone, although again multiple contacts may also be required to find a convenient time. Telephone surveys have low cost, their geographical spread can be very wide, they are a speedy method of data collection and they can give a higher response rate than other types of survey. However, costs increase with the number of attempts required to contact subjects who are not available at the first call, and with the number of long-distance calls required. The costs of all interviewer-based surveys increase significantly with geographical dispersal of the sample members.

Example – *interview survey* – *Health Related Quality of Life (HRQoL)*

In the survey of adult residents in Singapore conducted by Thumboo, Fong, Machin *et al.* (2002) fieldworkers identified all eligible subjects on the basis of gender, age and literacy. They visited them at their home within 7 days after an introductory letter was sent, invited them to complete the SF-36 of Ware, Snow, Kosinski and Gandek (1993) and checked returned questionnaires for completeness. In addition they obtained information on ethnicity, social economic status and other potential determinants of HRQoL through a structured interview. Subjects were deemed 'uncontactable' if they were not contacted after three visits, each 3 days apart.

Interviewer-administered surveys are generally more appropriate whenever a large number of open-ended questions are included. However, coding responses to such open-ended questions to facilitate summary and analysis can be both difficult and time-consuming. As a result, interviewer-administered surveys may take longer to produce results than postal surveys. Balanced against this, however, there is no need to wait for questionnaires to be returned and data processing can begin once the interview is completed. The speed with which data are available for analysis can be increased by the use of computer-assisted techniques, such as 'touch-screen' questionnaires, which minimise the need for subsequent data entry and checking. This is also the case in 'captive-audience' self-completion surveys, for example, those administered to a group of patients in a waiting room. In these data can be collected simultaneously from a large number of respondents, and checked and verified on the spot.

Face-to-face interviews generally require highly trained and motivated interviewers, since they must work autonomously. Less experienced interviewers may be used in telephone surveys, since stricter control and closer supervision is possible by the design team. This greater control can also help to reduce inter-interviewer variability.

Clinical Examination

If a clinical examination is required, perhaps if one is studying the prevalence of a particular disease and attempting to find associated aetiological factors, then a clear protocol outlining the diagnostic process is required. Since a survey is designed to identify rather than treat cases, care has to be taken that the survey participants (particularly those who do not have the disease) are not subjected to unnecessary and lengthy examinations to determine diagnosis.

So there has to be a balance set between unequivocal diagnosis and the exigencies of the logistical situation. Care has also to be taken in making provision for subsequent action when a subject is found to have the disease. Of course, one incentive for the participants may be that the survey provides an early screen for the presence (or absence) of the disease or condition in question.

ENDPOINTS

As with any study, the major endpoints have to be identified at the design stage. This is particularly important in surveys when a large number and wide-ranging series of endpoints may be of interest. Nevertheless it is necessary to choose key endpoints for sample-size purposes and to define the principal groups between which comparisons are to be made. The ease with which the endpoint can be deduced from the responses is particularly important in large surveys.

Example – *endpoints* – *sexual activity in secondary school children*

Slap, Lot, Huang *et al.* (2003) conducted a questionnaire survey of 4000 school attendees in Nigeria. The objectives of the study were to determine the prevalence of sexual activity and so the secondary school children were asked via a self-administered questionnaire: 'Have you ever had sexual intercourse (sex with another person)?'. The children would be required to be literate and understand the meaning of the question. In this example, for some 'sexual intercourse' and 'sex with another person' are not necessarily the same so there may be some ambiguity here.

In order to compare the levels of sexual activity amongst those coming from monogamous and polygamous family structures the design team had to ensure that sufficient children were identified from each group.

If the endpoint concerns the presence or absence of a particular disease, then a precise definition of the corresponding diagnostic criteria need to be specified together with the clinical investigations that have to be used to determine the diagnosis. However, in many surveys no one endpoint is paramount so that many questions are asked and endpoints recorded. For example, Jensen, Groenvold, Klee *et al.* (2003), in their postal survey described earlier, asked women a whole range of questions on sexual function after radiotherapy for cervical cancer and their publication reported on 20 of these.

It is worth noting that different methods of data collection can produce different results. Thus Dillman (2004) reports that a self-administered survey of respondents resulted in 15% rating their health as 'very good', whereas a survey of the same respondents by personal interview shortly after resulted in 27% answering 'very good'.

TARGET AND SAMPLE POPULATIONS

Just as for any cross-sectional study, one must define precisely the population of subjects of interest. As a survey is such a large undertaking this population must be defined with considerable care. The survey or *target* population, more formally defined in Figure 6.1, is the population for whom the results of the survey will apply. The target population for a survey is often so large that, except in cases of a national census, it is impractical to assess all its members. As a consequence, only a *sample* of the actual target population is surveyed.

Survey feature	Definition
Survey or target population	All the units (individuals, households, organisations) to which one desires to generalise the survey results
Coverage	The subjects in the population that are to be covered by the sampling frame
Sampling frame	The list from which a sample is to be drawn for inclusion in the survey
Sample	The units of the population drawn for inclusion in the survey
Completed sample	All the units that completed questionnaires.

Figure 6.1   Definitions of terms used when designing surveys (part based on Dillman, 2004; reproduced by permission of John Wiley & Sons Ltd)

The *sampling frame* is the list of subjects of the target population from which the sample can be selected. For large, population-based studies, many countries have adults listed on an Electoral Register and this is often reasonably complete in its coverage. This Register may be available for use and hence provides the basic sampling frame. In a health context, other sources of potential subjects are hospital and primary care records. Thus the list of all patients admitted to a hospital with a specific diagnosis over a 10-year interval might comprise the sampling frame for a survey. However, the population listed is clearly not the 'general' population at large in such cases.

ACHIEVING A REPRESENTATIVE SAMPLE

Once the sampling frame is established, a key element is then to draw the sample from it using a method that involves a random component. Depending on the particular survey in mind, the sampling process can be single- or multi-stage and may or may not involve dividing the population into subpopulations or strata.

Single-stage Sampling

A single-stage sample takes a sample directly from the sampling frame corresponding to the entire target population. The method, although it may change depending on how the target population is compiled, involves selecting (at random) from a numbered list those subjects chosen for the survey.

Multi-stage Sampling

In surveys that are planned to cover a whole nation or perhaps a large geographical area with a large or dispersed population, the sampling can be done by stages. For example, first a list of regions within a country is obtained and then one region selected from this list at random. For this region, and this region alone, the districts are then identified, and (say) two of these selected at random. This process can continue for as often as necessary until the primary sampling frames are identified. Then random samples are taken from these sampling frames.

Example – *multi-stage sampling* – *glaucoma in Mongolia*

In an investigation of the prevalence of glaucoma in the field survey conducted in Mongolia by Devereux, Foster, Baasanhu *et al.* (2000) the sampling strategy first involved the selection of two provinces, Hövsgöl and Ömnögobi. From each province urban and rural communities were then selected. Thus for Ömnögobi, Dalanzadgad, the regional capital, was chosen for the urban community while for the rural component, Sevrei was randomly selected from a total of 15 districts. Within each of the chosen districts the handwritten census data were then used to identify the individuals for examination.

Stratification

Prior knowledge of the determinants of, for example, prevalence can improve the design of a survey. Thus previous experience in other populations might suggest that more cases would be identified if the sample were structured to favour the older citizens.

Stratification can be either proportionate or disproportionate. Suppose we wished to survey patient opinion in a particular hospital and we know there were 100 medical patients and 200 surgical patients. A proportionate sample of 1 in 10 would take 10 medical and 20 surgical patients. Suppose further that of the medical patients 10 were under the age of 45. A disproportionate sample may take all those under 45 years of age and a 1 in 10 sample of those 45 or more. The purpose of stratifying is to get more homogeneous responses from within the strata. If one felt that age was more likely to influence patient opinion than whether presenting at a medical or surgical department then, with these two options, age would be chosen as the strata for the survey design.

One reason for stratifying is to increase the precision of the estimate. A technical explanation is given in section 6.6, but briefly: the variability of an estimate is made up of between strata variability and within strata variability. By stratifying in the design, between strata variability is removed and, by making units within strata more homogeneous, the within-strata variability is reduced.

In the following example, the reduction in *SE* using stratification appears very small. However, this is because the comparison made here is not strictly between the results from a simple random design against those from a stratified design, but is rather analysing a stratified design as if it were a simple random design. As a consequence, the reduction in *SE* using a stratified design will usually be greater than this example indicates. In general the ease of using a roughly proportional sampling scheme outweighs any slight efficiency gains that may be had from disproportionate sampling.

Example – *stratified sampling* – *prevalence of glaucoma*

As it is well known that prevalence of glaucoma increases with age and it is higher in men than women, Foster, Oen, Machin *et al.* (2000) carried out a survey of ethnic Chinese living in Singapore stratified on the basis of these two factors. The target population was first divided into four age-group strata and then each of these age-specific subpopulations was then further divided but in favour of the females, according to their ratio in the area of the survey. The final numbers selected, approximately 500 from each age stratum, and the numbers subsequently examined for glaucoma are given in Table 6.1.

Table 6.1 Details of population, sample selected, cases examined and numbers found to have glaucoma in Chinese residents of Singapore (part data from Foster, Oen, Machin *et al.*, 2000, Table 1. The prevalence of glaucoma in Chinese residents of Singapore: a cross-sectional population survey of the Tanjong Pagar District. *Archives Ophthalmology*, **118**, 1105–1111. [3,6])

Gender	Age (years)	Sample size selected	Number examined m_i (%)	Number with glaucoma r_i	Proportion with glaucoma p_i	$m_i p_i \times (1-p_i)$
Male	40–49	229	125 (55)	1	0.0080	0.9920
	50–59	203	117 (58)	2	0.0171	1.9665
	60–69	249	173 (69)	9	0.0520	8.5282
	70+	222	142 (64)	15	0.1056	13.4117
Female	40–49	251	151 (60)	0	0.0000	0.0000
	50–59	297	189 (64)	1	0.0053	0.9964
	60–69	259	170 (66)	3	0.0176	2.9393
	70+	290	165 (57)	14	0.0848	12.8055
	Total	2000	$N_{\text{Sample}} =$ 1232 (62)		$r = 45$	

From this the estimate of the prevalence is 45/1232 or 3.65%. Ignoring the stratification this has standard error,

$$SE = \sqrt{\frac{p(1-p)}{N_{\text{Sample}}}} = \sqrt{\frac{0.0365 \times 0.9635}{1232}} = \sqrt{\frac{0.035167}{1232}} = 0.005343 \text{ or } 0.53\%.$$

Taking the stratification into account uses the values in the last column of Table 6.1 to give

$$SE_{\text{Stratified}} = \sqrt{\frac{\sum m_i p_i (1-p_i)}{N_{\text{Sample}}^2}} = \sqrt{\frac{41.6396}{1232^2}} = 0.005238 \text{ or } 0.52\%.$$

By sampling a greater proportion in older age groups one can improve efficiency and, provided due care is taken, the design can still estimate (say) the adult prevalence of the

1. Improves the precision of the estimates
2. Ensures subgroups which form the strata are adequately represented
3. Convenience

Figure 6.2   Reasons for the use of stratified sampling

condition. This is calculated by taking a weighted average of the prevalences observed within each of the strata. If the objective is to catalogue the changes in the ageing eye (perhaps the change in grade of glaucoma through successive decades) then it may be that a larger proportion of the young need to be examined in order to obtain sufficient cases within this group for examination. Thus with the planned total study size preserved, the sampling fractions for the respective age groups may be rebalanced to achieve this. Figure 6.2 lists the reasons for using stratified sampling.

PRACTICALITIES

Figure 6.3 lists the main sources of survey error.

Coverage Error

Care has to be taken to ensure that the sampling frame really includes all the subjects of interest. In certain countries, those confined to prison are removed from the Electoral Register. In this case, should the Register be taken as the sampling frame, these individuals clearly could not be surveyed. Thus any shortcomings of the chosen sampling frame in their coverage of the desired population need to be noted by the design team.

Response Rates

A well-designed survey will attempt to have as high a response rate as possible. Inevitably, in questionnaire surveys there will be non-responders. An important principle is that, by virtue of not replying, the non-responders are different from the responders. Hence it is useful to obtain and report as much information on the non-responders as possible. If the population were sampled from an age–sex register, it would be possible to give the age and gender distribution of both the responders and non-responders.

Example – response rates – HRQoL

In the survey of Thumboo, Fong, Machin *et al.* (2002) a randomly selected sample of those subjects previously deemed uncontactable were later surveyed to determine their demographic characteristics and SF-36 scores. These initial non-respondents did not differ substantially from study participants in their summary characteristics and so they and their responses were consequently included in the full analysis.

Type of error	Definition
Coverage error	Applies if some units in the survey population have a zero probability of being included in the sample
Sampling error	Result of collecting data from only a subset, rather than from all members of the sampling frame
Non-response	Not all subjects in the sample are in the completed sample. Non-responders may differ from responders
Sampling	Random variation means that a small sample is less precise than a large one
Measurement	Subjects may misunderstand questions, or deliberately give false replies

Figure 6.3   The main sources of survey error (part-based on Dillman, 2004; reproduced by permission of John Wiley & Sons Ltd)

Surveys with a low response rate will have relatively low precision and the confidence intervals (CI) around any estimates of population parameters will be wider than planned. For postal surveys a response rate in excess of 70% is thought desirable, although Asch, Jedrziewski and Christiakis (1997) report that rates for postal surveys actually published in the medical literature are often lower than this.

Important reasons for non-response in surveys have been identified as: subjects not literate; moved from their listed address; away from home for the duration of the survey; not at home when an interviewer tries to make contact; and refusals. Thus for example Jensen, Groenwold, Klee *et al.* (2003) not surprisingly found in their survey that women who were non-Danish-speaking were more likely to be non-responders. The relative importance of each of these non-response reasons will depend on a range of factors specific to the planned survey itself.

Improving Response Rates

As a proportion of non-responders may be anticipated, it is very important at the design stage of a survey to review methods that may reduce the size of this proportion. Some pointers to how this may be achieved have been discussed in Chapter 2. In addition to those mentioned there, response rates may be improved by inclusion of a covering letter explaining the purposes of the research, why it is important and why the recipient has been selected. The letter might also mention what steps have been taken to guarantee confidentiality (an important consideration for some respondents) and what organisation is responsible for conducting the research.

Once the questionnaires have been distributed and replies are scheduled to arrive, then a time should be set to activate follow-up of individuals who do not reply. Campbell and Waters (1990) showed that one follow-up increased the response rate from 50% to 70%. A common approach is to send a letter (say) 2 weeks after the original, reminding and emphasising the recipient of the importance of returning the questionnaire. A new copy of the questionnaire can be included with this first reminder,

Questionnaire	Clear focus
	Clear design and simple layout
	Appealing to look at
	Thoroughly piloted and tested
Conduct	Participants notified about the study in advance with a personalised invitation
	Aims of the study and means of completing the questionnaire are clearly explained
	Researcher available to answer questions and collect completed questionnaires
	Researcher presentation
Participants	Feel they are stakeholders in the study
	Offered incentives or prizes in return for completion
Postal survey	Enclosure of a stamped addressed envelope for returning the completed questionnaire
Electronic survey	

Figure 6.4 Evidence-based suggestions for increasing response rates (based on Edwards, Roberts, Clarke *et al.*, 2002, and Boynton, 2004)

or if necessary this can be sent with a further (second) reminder. For ease of the survey team, one can also use different colours for questionnaires on the second and subsequent mailings to distinguish waves of responses.

A disadvantage of an anonymously completed survey design, in which even the survey team do not know from whom the response comes, is that non-responders cannot be identified and therefore reminded at a later date. However, this anonymity, rather than just confidentiality as would be routine in most clinical studies, might improve the overall response rate. The advantages and disadvantages have to be weighed by the survey design team.

Response rates have been improved by providing a monetary incentive. Thus Shaw, Beebe, Jensen and Adlis (2001) showed that a US$2 incentive achieved a 67% response rate whereas a US$5 increased this by 7% to a 74% response. Kalantar and Talley (1999) showed that recipients promised a lottery ticket were more likely to respond than those who were not. However Gattellari and Ward (2001) surprisingly showed that a promise to make a donation to a relevant professional organisation actually decreased participation rates!

Figure 6.4 gives suggestions for increasing response rates.

Bias

Very importantly, poor response rates are likely to result in a major bias in the estimates of the appropriate population parameters. This is because non-respondents tend to differ from respondents in important and systematic ways. Further a significant disadvantage of interviewer-administered surveys is that the interviewers themselves can introduce errors both in a random and a systematic way. Random errors are more likely to be due to interviewer inaccuracy, for example recording answers incorrectly or occasionally altering the wording of a question by mistake. Examples of systematic effects are: selective recording of subjects' responses; differences in the extent to which interviewers probe for a substantive response or accept 'don't know' answers; and consistent re-wording of the questions as they are posed.

Systematic bias can occur even when there is only one interviewer, if the interviewer does not accurately record the respondent's answers, but instead is consistently selective in what he or she records. It is an even greater problem where a survey requires multiple interviewers since observed differences across groups of respondents may be an artefact of the way in which different interviewers have posed questions or recorded answers. Computer-assisted personal interviewing may prevent routine errors and omissions, but this method requires high levels of investment for implementation.

Personal characteristics of the interviewer, such as age, gender or level of experience and training, may also affect both response rates and the nature of the responses given. Similarly, the setting in which data is collected may affect responses. For example, it has been shown that responses to physical function items on a health status measure may be confounded by place of administration, with higher scores for hospital inpatients resulting from restrictions caused by the hospital care regime rather than by their impaired health.

Procedures

The survey protocol should highlight a plan for preserving the confidentiality of the data during collection, processing, and analysis, if individually identifiable data are to be collected. The protocol should also include an outline of a plan for quality assurance during each phase of the survey process to facilitate monitoring and assessing operational performance during survey implementation. The plan must include contingencies to modify the survey procedures, if design parameters appear unlikely to meet expectations, for example, if a lower than anticipated response rate is becoming apparent.

Survey Size

Usually the investigators will wish to compare groups with a survey, such as the comparison of those with partners and those without in the Danish survey of women. Thus the survey now divides into two groups although not necessarily of equal size. These women may then be further divided into those from rural or urban locations, and of high or low educational achievement. Membership of these, $2^3 = 8$ categories is expected to affect individual responses to an important degree. In design terms we can now think that the object of the survey is to estimate the parameters of each of these subpopulations. We can do this by setting the width of the corresponding 95% CI and using equations (3.4) for estimating a mean or equation (3.6) for a prevalence.

To calculate sample size using equation (3.4) the width, ω, of the CI has to be pre-specified and so too has σ. However, in some circumstances, knowledge of the latter may be difficult to obtain. To circumvent this difficulty, one possibility is not to set the CI to have fixed width, ω, but to have this width as a fixed proportion, ε, of the mean value, μ, that is by setting $\omega_{\text{Plan}} = \varepsilon_{\text{Plan}} \times \mu_{\text{Plan}}$. Substituting in equation (3.4) then gives the planned study size as

$$N_{\text{Plan}} = 4\left[\frac{\sigma_{\text{Plan}}^2}{\varepsilon_{\text{Plan}}^2 \mu_{\text{Plan}}^2}\right] z_{1-\alpha/2}^2 = 4\left[\frac{\Omega_{\text{Plan}}^2}{\varepsilon_{\text{Plan}}^2}\right] z_{1-\alpha/2}^2, \tag{6.1}$$

where $\Omega_{\text{Plan}} = \sigma_{\text{Plan}}/\mu_{\text{Plan}}$ is termed the coefficient of variation (CV).

Sample sizes determined in this way are given in Table T8. As Ω increases the SD becomes larger as a proportion of the mean and hence the sample size increases. However, as ε increases we are permitting the width of the final CI to be wider and hence the sample size required becomes smaller.

Example – *survey size*

Suppose we were planning a survey in which eight important subgroups of individuals are to be surveyed, then considering any one of these groups, the investigators might choose $\Omega_{\text{Plan}} = 0.3$ and $\varepsilon_{\text{Plan}} = 0.1$. Then, for a 95% CI, Table T8 gives the number of subjects to be surveyed from one such group as $m_{\text{Plan}} = 140$. Careful examination of the entries surrounding these values suggest that study size is quite sensitive to the choices of Ω_{Plan} and $\varepsilon_{\text{Plan}}$.

However, the planned study has $g = 8$ such groups, so a preliminary estimate of the total survey size is $N_{\text{Total}} = g \times m = 1120$. Now factoring in a potential non-response rate, often at least 20%, may be prudent and so they increase their numbers per strata to give a revised $N_{\text{Total}} = 8 \times 140 \times 1.2 = 1344$ or approximately 1400 subjects.

Further the design team has identified five major endpoints from their survey questionnaire and are conscious that multiple testing may produce spuriously significant results. The Bonferroni correction with $k = 5$, suggests replacing $\alpha = 0.05$ by $0.05/k = 0.01$. As a consequence $m_{\text{Plan}} = 140$ is replaced by the entry of Table T8 with $\alpha = 0.01$ giving $m_{\text{Plan}} = 240$. Thus for the eight subpopulation survey design, and taking into account a 20% failure-to-respond rate, a suggested survey size is $N_{\text{Total}} = 8 \times 240 \times 1.2 = 2304$ or approximately 2500 subjects would be sent questionnaires.

If the numbers of endpoints were (say) 20 rather than eight, then this process would imply replacing $\alpha = 0.05$ by $0.05/20 = 0.0025$. However, with such a small value for the test size the resulting sample sizes will be very large. So a pragmatic design (if there are five or more endpoints) is to set the test at $\alpha = 0.01$, rather than 0.05, to calculate survey size. Once the survey is conducted and the results collated, the corresponding p-values are then first multiplied by k ($\geqslant 5$) before interpretation commences. Alternatively or additionally, the results might be expressed with 99% rather than 95% CIs.

REPORTING

It is particularly important when reporting the results of a survey to describe in careful detail the choice of population concerned and the sampling frame utilised for the sample selected. Any known deficiencies of the sampling frame should be described. It is clearly important to detail the steps taken in obtaining the final sample, such as the various stages in a multistage or stratified sampling scheme. This should include details of how the final (random) selection was made. Any difficulties encountered in this process should be detailed. For example, Devereux, Foster, Baasanhu *et al.* (2000) noted that operational difficulties had led to an additional 107 community-based subjects being included inadvertently in their study. The numbers of units in the various stages need to be given. As a preliminary to the actual results of the survey with regard to the endpoints chosen, details of the sample size chosen, the numbers completing the survey and response rates need to be specified.

Design features – surveys

Define the key research question(s) and associated endpoints

Define the target population and the sampling frame

Choosing between a postal-, telephone- or interview-based survey

Type of sample: simple random. multistage, stratified

Consider how to maximise response rates

Survey size

6.3   COHORT STUDIES

The key feature of a cohort study is that the same subjects are observed longitudinally in time over an extended (sometimes lengthy) period but may involve no direct measurements by the investigator who is just waiting for a particular event to occur. One outcome may the occurrence or not of the event itself or the time from recruitment for this event to manifest itself. For example, all those pregnant women who happened to live close to the Chernobyl Nuclear Reactor when it failed could have been followed until the baby was born in order to discover any untoward events with respect to their babies' health at birth. Any monitoring of the women over time may be to ensure that, for example, any spontaneous abortions are recorded.

Example – cohort study – type 1 diabetes

Hovind, Tarnow, Rossing *et al.* (2004) established a cohort of 286 patients with type 1 diabetes and followed these by means of an outpatient diabetic clinic until the development of micro- and macro-albuminuria. The object of the study was to establish baseline predictors for these outcomes. Their study suggested that an increased risk was related to, for example, male gender and increase in mean arterial blood pressure. Prognostic factor studies such as this are discussed in more detail in Chapter 11.

A common purpose of a cohort study is to quantify the risk (often an exposure of some kind) in a specific target population of getting the outcome of interest and to compare this with a control population not exposed to the risk in question. The outcome concerned is often the development of a particular disease.

There are two types of cohort design, *prospective* and *retrospective*. A prospective study chooses a group of patients and then waits for events to occur. Obviously this has the disadvantage of taking a long time to complete; even a relatively short duration cohort might take as long as 5 years.

Thus a prospective cohort study begins by defining both the exposure and the consequent disease of interest. In establishing, for example, the 'at-risk' women the eligibility requirements for the cohort study would have to be carefully specified. For example, the exposure may be the use of one type of oral contraceptive (OC) and the disease ovarian cancer. In which case, the women would all have been at some stage users of the OC in question, perhaps be of a certain age range and parity and, very importantly, they would have to be deemed *free* of ovarian cancer. The cohort of 'control' women would be 'never-users' of the OC but otherwise defined in exactly the same way. However, since the choice of the 'ever' or 'never' use of the OC women for the cohort study is not determined by a random process, great care has to be taken in ensuring that the two groups of women are as comparable as possible. Once the two cohorts are established, then the women are followed for a certain, often lengthy, period of time. This will be long enough to ensure that a sufficient number of ovarian cancers will develop in both the exposed and non-exposed groups.

Sometimes it may be unclear what measurements will be required in the future. Thus an important type of design is one where, at the time of screening a population for a particular condition, blood samples are taken, frozen and stored. After a number of years, certain genes may have been identified as possible risk factors for a particular disease. This can be investigated if aliquots of the blood are thawed and the presence or absence of the gene identified. These results then define the 'exposed' and the 'non-exposed' cohorts.

Cohort studies follow subjects from exposure to outcome and so are suitable for identifying causality according to the Bradford-Hill criteria of Figure 1.1. A cohort

---

Example – prospective cohort – residual neurological symptoms after neuroborreliosis

Berglund, Stjernberg, Ornstein *et al.* (2002) identified, from a population-based survey, 349 cases of suspected neuroborreliosis, a vector-borne infection transmitted by ticks, who had been treated with antibiotics at the time. Of these, the diagnosis of neuroborreliosis was confirmed by the medical records in 130 of whom 114 completed the follow-up of 5 years. Amongst them 28 showed some signs of residual neurological symptoms.

Thus there is a single outcome in this cohort study, which is the estimated proportion of patients at 5 years still exhibiting signs of neurological symptoms. Their prevalence is estimated by $p_{Residual} = 28/114 = 0.25$ or 25%.

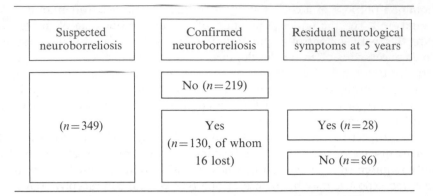

Suspected neuroborreliosis	Confirmed neuroborreliosis	Residual neurological symptoms at 5 years
	No (n=219)	
(n=349)	Yes (n=130, of whom 16 lost)	Yes (n=28)
		No (n=86)

Figure 6.5   Design of the prospective cohort study conducted by Berglund, Stjernberg, Ornstein *et al.* (2002) to identify those with residual neurological symptoms 5 years after a diagnosis of confirmed borreliosis. (Reproduced by permission of Taylor & Francis)

design is usually not suitable to study the potential development of a rare disease, since in order to have enough cases of the disease a very large cohort and/or a very extended follow-up period would be required. In such circumstances a case–control design may be an option.

The design and progress of this (typical) single-group cohort study is summarised in Figure 6.5. Thus this cohort of patients with a particular disease was established by first examining a larger group to target those of particular interest, this group was then followed for a specific period of time at which the necessary endpoint measure(s) was taken.

A retrospective cohort, on the other hand identifies a group of subjects in the past. Their fate up to the present can be ascertained using population registers. Relative to prospective cohort studies, retrospective studies are cheap and quick to complete. However, they do require the existence of longstanding records and are limited to variables contained in those records.

> ***Example** – retrospective study – babies*
>
> Barker, Forsén, Uutela *et al.* (2001) identified a group of male babies born in Helsinki, Finland, between 1933 and 1944 who had had their birth weight recorded. They established that, among those who were thin at birth, the risk of coronary heart disease is further increased if they had poor living standards in adult life.

Cohort studies are not usually thought of as repeated measures designs as they are often designed with a single endpoint in mind, although once a prospective cohort is established it is tempting to examine it in detail from time to time so it may then develop into a repeated measures study.

Data Collection

There are special issues relating to data collected for cohort studies as some of the information required might not be available prospectively. For example, in establishing the exposed group, although it may be relatively easy to determine if a woman 'ever' used a particular OC, it may be much more difficult to ascertain the total period of use in order to obtain a more precise estimate of her exposure. On a related issue, care is needed to ensure that the controls were 'never' users. As cohort studies are longitudinal in nature often requiring extensive follow-up, it is self-evident that very careful planning at the design stage is essential to determine when observations are to be taken and to ensure the necessary mechanisms are in place.

Disease Data

Precise definition of the disease(s) to be identified, as the cohort is followed in time, must be made and one must be as sure as possible that those who apparently do not have the disease are truly free of the disease in question. If the definition is not precise, there is scope for misclassification and this may dilute the differences between the exposed and non-exposed cohorts and thereby diminish the estimate of risk.

INTERPRETATION

Bias

Cohort studies are subject to a number of biases including those caused by treatment selection and differential follow-up. An example of treatment selection bias is if the purpose of a cohort study is to estimate the rate of cardiovascular disease in men sterilised by vasectomy, it is necessary to have a comparison group of non-vasectomised men. However, as we have noted with 'ever' users of OCs, comparisons between such groups may be biased as it is not feasible to randomise men to 'sterilisation' or 'no-sterilisation' groups. It is clear that men who are seeking sterilisation would certainly not accept the 'no-sterilisation' option. As a consequence, the final comparison is made between those men who *opt for sterilisation* against *those who do not*. This may introduce inherent biases as, for example, the vasectomised men may be fitter than the non-vasectomised men and this may influence their cardiovascular disease rates.

Follow-up bias can arise when follow-up is poor, or when it is more complete for one group than for the other. Thus it is possible that, for example, subjects exposed to radiation are more likely to be carefully monitored than subjects not exposed.

Healthy Worker Effect

Studies of occupational cohorts are bedevilled by the *healthy worker* effect, whereby people in work are, by nature, healthier than people out of work, since many illnesses prevent people working. Thus even if an occupation is truly hazardous to health, when comparisons are made between workers (the healthy) and the non-working (potentially less healthy) population, it may not be obvious that there is indeed a risk present.

Covariates

In the design of a cohort study, careful consideration must be given to identifying and subsequently measuring important prognostic variables that may differ between the cohorts. Provided they are recorded, differences in these baseline characteristics between groups can be used to adjust the associated risk estimates to better reflect the true difference between the unexposed and exposed groups.

Study Size

Commonly, a cohort study is summarised by the relative risk (RR) when the endpoints of interest are the proportion with the disease in the exposed, E, and unexposed groups, U, after a particular time, T, has elapsed from when the cohort is established. The RR is estimated by

$$RR = \frac{p_E}{p_U},$$ (6.2)

where $p_E = r_E/m_E$ and $p_U = r_U/m_U$ are the proportions of those who develop the disease amongst the exposed and unexposed groups respectively.

At the design stage the anticipated proportion with the disease in the unexposed groups by the projected observation time, π_U, is usually required. This will depend on both the magnitude of the underlying (annual) risk, θ_U, and the proposed length of follow-up, T. If these are known or can be anticipated, then $\pi_U = \theta_U T$. The design team then have to postulate a corresponding π_E, usually greater than π_U, which, if indeed present, would be a clinically important finding to report.

Then, if the unexposed and exposed cohorts are of relative size $1:\lambda$, the sample size of the control cohort group, with two-sided test size α and power $1-\beta$, is given by Prentice (1995) as

$$m_U = \left(1 + \frac{1}{\lambda}\right) \frac{\left(z_{1-\alpha/2} + z_{1-\beta}\sqrt{\dfrac{\lambda}{1+\lambda} + \dfrac{(1-\pi_U+\varphi\pi_U)^2}{(1+\lambda)\varphi}}\right)^2}{\pi_U(1-\pi_U)(\log \varphi)^2},$$ (6.3)

where

$$\varphi = \frac{\pi_E(1-\pi_U)}{(1-\pi_E)\pi_U}.$$ (6.4)

Here φ is the exposed versus unexposed odds ratio (OR). If both π_E and π_U are small then φ and the RR of equation (6.2) are very close numerically. Equation (6.3) leads to the sample size for the exposed cohort as $m_E = \lambda m_U$ and finally the total study size, $N = m_U + m_E$.

In many applications the numbers available for the exposed group may be limited. This may be offset to some extent by increasing the proportion of controls (non-exposed) in the design. Thus the statistical efficiency of the design may be maintained by choosing $\lambda < 1$. In planning in such a situation, the numerical value of m_E is set by the resource limitations to M_E say, and this then implies the numbers of the controls would then have to be set at $M_U = M_E/\lambda$. We now have to choose λ, by substituting a range of values for λ into equation (6.3) and identify that value which gives an m_U close to M_U. The corresponding value of λ then gives the number of controls for every case to be recruited.

Example – *cohort size*

Suppose we are planning a cohort study in which the subjects will be followed for $T=6$ years and the annual incidence rate is expected to be $\theta_U = 1$ per thousand in the unexposed group. It is thought that an increased risk comparable to a $RR=1.25$ might be present in the exposed group. Further the cohorts are set to be of the same size, that is, $\lambda=1$.

These assumptions lead to planning values of

$$\pi_U = \theta_U T = \frac{1}{1000} \times 6 = 0.006$$

and, using the equivalent of equation (6.2), $\pi_E = \pi_U \times RR = 0.006 \times 1.25 = 0.0075$. From these, equation (6.4) gives $\psi = [0.0075 \times (1 - 0.006)]/ [(1 - 0.0075) \times 0.006] = 1.25$ which, in this case, is numerically equal to the RR. With these assumptions and 5% significance and 80% power, then equation (6.3) and Table T1 give the number in the control cohort as

$$m_U = \frac{1}{2} \frac{\left(1.9600 + 0.8416 \sqrt{0.5 + \dfrac{(1 - 0.006 + 1.25 \times 0.006)^2}{2 \times 1.25}}\right)^2}{0.006 \times 0.994 \times (\log 1.25)^2} = 51\,253.$$

Thus the number for the exposed cohort is $m_E = \lambda m_U = 51\,263$ also. Finally $N = 2 \times 51\,263$ or approximately $100\,000$ individuals are required.

A more pragmatic approach is to base the sample size on previous cohorts that have yielded useful information. Cohort studies on cardiovascular risk factors are commonly between 5000 and 20 000 people. For example the Framingham study, which has had a major effect on the understanding of heart disease, was started in 1948 with 5209 residents in the town of Framingham, Massachusetts, USA. Studies of elderly people, where events are more common, can be smaller than those of young people. Cohorts of between 80 000 and 100 000 may be adequate to detect modest associations (odds ratios of 1.5 or greater) within 6 years. Studies looking at the relationship between diet and cancer have been in the range 50 000 and 100 000 but there has been some work to suggest that the relative risks are only about 1.1 to 1.2, which require cohorts of upwards of 400 000. Clearly planning studies of such size requires a very experienced team of investigators with considerable resources at their disposal.

REPORTING

Key aspects of reporting cohort studies that impact on the basic design are very clear definitions of how the members of the retrospective cohorts are identified and the respective exposure or non-exposure ascertained. If the cohorts are then followed until a particular disease develops, clear definitions of the disease and the corresponding diagnostic procedures have to be provided. This implies a careful description of the intended follow-up schedule and procedures. Clearly, the numbers recruited will need to be reported and, as will be the case in most cohort studies, the progress of the patients so recruited should be charted. This charting includes reporting the events (with dates) as they occur, but also subject losses, for example those who move away from the study area and can no longer be examined or traced, those who no longer agree to participate, and those who may have experienced a competing event (say, have died) before the endpoint of interest could be observed. Finally the numbers of events in the exposed and non-exposed groups must be unambiguously reported.

Design features – cohort studies

Identify the key research question(s) and associated endpoints

Consider the choice between a cohort and a case–control study

Careful choice of eligibility criteria for membership of the cohort(s)

Make sure the disease is clearly defined

Determine the period of follow-up necessary

Ensure cases and controls have similar periods of exposure

Provide a clear definition of the endpoint(s)

Minimise potential bias in the ascertainment of risk factors

Determine cohort size(s)

6.4   CASE–CONTROL STUDIES

The use of the term 'case–control' study is usually restricted to designs in which one is trying to identify the risks of having become a case. They are not the same as cross-sectional studies comparing cases and (say) healthy volunteers, which are trying to discover current risk factors. In contrast, the objective of a case–control study is to establish whether there were differences (in the past) between the groups (as they have now become over the passage of time) at a time before they were ever formed. That is at a time before the 'case' became a 'case'. The cross-sectional investigation is, for example, for potential use in diagnosis (how is a diseased patient distinguished from one that is not diseased?) and the case–control to identify items for possible use in 'prevention' of possible future cases.

    Thus, in contrast to a cohort study, a case–control study starts with the identification of persons with the disease (or other outcome) of interest, and a suitable control

	Advantages	Disadvantages
Case–control	Cheap	No estimates of absolute risk
	Relatively small	Only approximate estimates of relative risk
	Results available quickly	Potential biases, such as recall bias
Prospective cohort study	Estimates of relative and absolute risk	Large and expensive
	Less susceptible to bias than a case–control study	Potential biases, such as selection bias and healthy worker effect
		Results available slowly
Retrospective cohort study	Estimates of relative and absolute risk	Prognostic factors limited to what has been measured in the past
	Results available quite quickly	

Figure 6.6   Choice between a case–control, a prospective cohort and a retrospective cohort study

(reference) group of persons without the disease. The object of the study then is to find the equivalent of previous exposures to risk factors like those investigated in a cohort study, or (perhaps genetic) characteristics of the subjects themselves that might have precipitated the disease in question. The strength of the potential risk factor to the disease is estimated by calculating the OR.

The relative merits of a case–control and cohort designs are summarised in Figure 6.6.

SOURCES OF DATA

The special issues relating to data collected for a cohort study may be more acute with a case–control design, as much of the information required will only be available retrospectively. Thus its completeness and reliability of these data may be of considerable concern.

Disease Data

Precise definition of the disease(s) to be studied must be made. If the definition is not precise, there is scope for misclassification and this may dilute the differences between cases and controls and thereby diminish the estimate of risk. A failure to get all the cases over the defined period can lead to bias when the exposure of interest is related to the probability of being included in the study.

Exposure Data

Exposure data should be obtained in an identical fashion from both cases and controls. Clearly it helps if the data are objective records rather than personal reflections. A major source of bias in case–control studies is *recall* bias. This arises because cases, having been defined by their disease, often have a major interest in it, and will try and recall anything that may be associated with it. In contrast the controls may have no particular interest in the disease in question and may consequently not be so motivated. For example, women with cervical cancer, knowing possible links with the number of sexual partners, may recall more precisely the number of casual partners concerned whereas the controls who are patients with (say) appendicitis may not be so willing to reveal such highly personal detail.

Selection of Controls

The choice of controls for any study requires careful consideration. In particular controls should be free of the disease at the time they are serving as controls. Consider a case–control study looking at the risk of hormone replacement therapy (HRT) for cervical cancer. Women taking HRT may be required to have an annual cervical smear. Other women, not on HRT, may be required to have a smear only every 3 years and they may also have less incentive to turn up for screen. Thus women on HRT may be more likely to have a cervical cancer detected, whereas some of the controls may have cervical cancer, but it has not been detected yet. One of the major difficulties with case–control studies is in the selection of a suitable control group, and this has often been a major source of criticism of published case–control studies. This has led some investigators to regard them purely as a hypothesis-generating tool, to be corroborated subsequently by a cohort study.

Since a case–control study is designed to estimate relative, and not absolute, risks, it is not essential that the controls be representative of all those subjects without the disease.

Hospital or Community Controls

Since cases often arise from hospital records, it makes sense to recruit controls from hospitals. Hospitals are a convenient and cheap source of controls, especially in situations where a clinical procedure, such as a blood sample is required. There are two major risks of bias in the use of hospital controls.

A risk factor for the study disease may be a risk factor for admission to hospital for the controls. For example, in a study of lung cancer and smoking, the cases are incident lung cancer patients, and the control patients entering the hospital without lung cancer. However, controls may have come to hospital for smoking-related diseases such as heart disease and so an estimate of the risk for lung cancer will be too low.

In general, people with multiple diseases or conditions become over-represented in a hospital population, which in turn affects the distribution of risk factors as well. For example, obese patients with high BP are much more likely to be admitted to hospital than those patients with high BP who are not obese. Thus a case–control study, which looked at risks of high blood pressure using hospital cases and controls, is then likely to overestimate the risk due to obesity.

Controls drawn from the community have the great advantage of being drawn from the true population of those without the disease. They are best when the cases also arise in the community. The main disadvantage of community controls is that they may be inconvenient to find, and their data may be of inferior quality.

Other sources of controls are often dictated by matching criteria. For example, friends, relatives or neighbours of the case can be used. Clearly there can be problems with overmatching in a shared environment, if for example the study was investigating the risks of passive smoking.

A useful compromise, especially if the cases arise naturally from the medical system, is to use both hospital and community controls.

UNMATCHED AND MATCHED DESIGNS

There are two variations in the design corresponding to whether the controls are a sample from a suitable non-diseased population, leading to an unmatched design, or are chosen to match individual cases for certain characteristics.

Unmatched Design

In an unmatched design the eligible cases will be first identified, and then often an equal number of controls selected. In selecting the controls, no note of the individual characteristics of the cases is taken, although, for example, the same general age range and gender composition will often be taken overall or sometimes in a frequency matching (but not paired) design.

Example – unmatched case–control study – vehicle driver sleeplessness

In a study to investigate the influence of vehicle driver sleepiness on risk of serious injury in road traffic accidents, Connor, Norton, Ameratunga *et al.* (2002) used a case–control design. The cases were all drivers involved in crashes where there had been at least one occupant admitted to hospital or killed. If the driver had been killed or was too ill to participate, data were obtained by proxy interview.

A total of 615 eligible cases were identified, involving 63 deaths, from which information was obtained from 571. The 746 potential controls, of whom 588 agreed to participate, were drivers recruited on public roads, representative of all drivers in the specific region during the study period but these were not individually matched with the cases. The basic design of this study is summarised in Figure 6.7.

The *OR* for having less than 5 hours sleep in the 24 hours prior to the accident was 2.7 (95% CI 1.4 to 5.4) from which the authors concluded that acute sleepiness in car drivers increases the risk of a crash in which a car occupant is killed or injured.

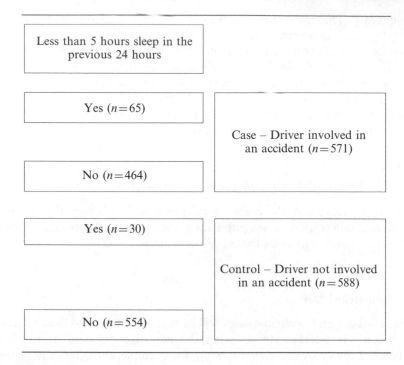

Figure 6.7 Progress of an unmatched case–control study (based on Connor, Norton, Ameratunga *et al.*, 2002. Driver sleepiness and risk of serious injury to car occupants: population based case-control study. *British Medical Journal*, **324**, 1125–1128. [6])

Study Size

In this situation the anticipated effect size is $\delta = \pi_1 - \pi_2$, where π_1 and π_2 are the proportions who experience the event in the respective groups. On this basis the number of subjects to be recruited to a study for equal-sized groups of size m, is given by equation (3.16). Alternatively, the same difference between groups may be expressed through the OR which is defined as

$$OR_{\text{Binary}} = \frac{\pi_2(1 - \pi_1)}{\pi_1(1 - \pi_2)}.$$ (6.5)

This formulation leads to an alternative to equation (3.16) for the sample size. Thus, for the total study size, cases and controls $N_{\text{Odds-Ratio}}$, this is

$$N_{\text{Odds-Ratio}} = \frac{4(z_{1-\alpha/2} + z_{1-\beta})^2 / (\log OR_{\text{Binary}})^2}{\bar{\pi}(1 - \bar{\pi})}$$ (6.6)

where $\bar{\pi} = (\pi_2 + \pi_1)/2$. This equation is quite different in form to (3.16), but for all practical purposes, gives very similar sample sizes, with divergent results only occurring for relatively large (or small) OR_{Binary}.

This expression is very useful when planning a study if an anticipated value of an OR is provided. If then the anticipated prevalence of the potential risk factor, π_1, is available for one group then

$$\pi_2 = \frac{OR\pi_1}{(1 - \pi_1 + OR\pi_1)}. \tag{6.7}$$

This then provides the components for the sample size to be determined by use of equation (6.6).

Matched Design

Matching can either be 1:1 or with more controls than cases. Thus in contrast to the unmatched design, every control is now linked to a corresponding case.

The main purpose of *matching* is to permit the use of efficient analytical methods to control for confounding variables that might influence the case–control comparison. In addition, it can lead to a more careful consideration of appropriate controls. Despite these advantages, matching can be wasteful and costly if the matching criteria lead to many available controls being discarded because they fail the matching criteria. Usually it is worthwhile matching only on, at most, two or three variables that are known to influence outcome but whose influence is not one objective of the study in design. This is because with this design one cannot determine the risk for the matching variables. For example, if we match cases and controls for age, we cannot determine the effect of age on risk.

We also have to avoid 'over-matching' in a paired case–control design. This would occur if, for the above example of the case–control study looking at the risk of hormone replacement therapy (HRT) on cervical cancer, cases and controls were both drawn from women who had been evaluated by uterine dilatation and curettage. Such a control group is inappropriate because agents that cause one disease in an organ often cause other diseases or symptoms in that organ. In this case it is *possible* that oestrogens cause other diseases of the endometrium, which have required the women to have dilatation and curettage and so present as possible controls.

Example – matched case–control study – suicides

King, Baldwin, Sinclair *et al.* (2001) used a matched case–control study to investigate social factors involved in suicides by patients following recent discharge from psychiatric inpatient treatment. Each discharged index patient was matched with two control patients with respect to: gender, age within 10 years, psychiatric diagnosis, type of ward and date of admission. Importantly the follow-up period for each control was the same number of days as the number of days from discharge to the event leading to death for the index patient. A key exposure variable was whether there had been a break in continuity of contact with the mental health services.

The authors succeeded in matching 1:2 for 197 of the cases while only a single match was found for the remaining 37. They established that an increased risk of suicide was associated with: 'when a significant professional was on leave, or about to go on leave, at the time of the fatal act'; $OR = 18.5$ (95% CI 4.5 to 76.3). The OR was calculated after adjustment for history of self-harm (Yes or No) and other covariates.

Study Size

In the situation where the case–control study is of a 1:1 matched design, then the risk factor under investigation, will be present (indicated 1) or absent (indicated 0) respectively amongst the case–control pair in one of the following four possibilities, (0,0), (0,1), (1,0) and (1,1). In the first and last of these pairs there is 'agreement' amongst the pair, while for the other two alternatives there is 'disagreement' or 'discordance'. At the analysis stage it is the ratio of the number of discordant pairs, s, of one type compared to the numbers, t, of the other type that estimates the $OR\ (=s/t)$. Thus the design team need to specify a planned value for this, which we denote by ξ. Further, the observed discordance rate is calculated by $p_{\text{Discordant}}=(s+t)/N_{\text{Pairs}}$. Again the design team need to specify a planned value for this, which we denote by $\pi_{\text{Discordant}}$. The number of case–control pairs to be recruited to a case–control study with test size α and power, $1-\beta$ is

$$N_{\text{Pairs}} = \frac{\left[z_{1-\alpha/2}(\xi+1) + z_{1-\beta}\sqrt{(\xi+1)^2 - (\xi-1)^2\pi_{\text{Discordant}}}\right]^2}{(\xi-1)^2\pi_{\text{Discordant}}}. \tag{6.8}$$

Example – sample size – suicides

Suppose we were to repeat the format of the case–control study of King, Baldwin, Sinclair *et al.* (2001) but in another locality, and since the previously observed association with the risk factor of 'an absent carer' was so strong, a 1:1 rather than a 1:2 matching was planned. However, there is some concern that the observed OR was perhaps somewhat high, so a value of $\xi_{\text{Plan}}=5$ is set. They were also unsure of the value for the proportion of discordant pairs and so consider the options of π_{Plan} of 0.1, 0.2 and 0.3. The three calculations using equation (6.8) with test size $\alpha=0.05$ and $1-\beta=0.8$, give N_{Pairs} of 175, 86 and 57. With this information, the investigators may then decide to conduct a 1:1 case–control study with 100 pairs but also ensure that the covariates of the earlier study are also recorded.

Often the problem at the design stage is to anticipate the proportion of discordant pairs. However, King, Baldwin, Sinclair *et al.* (2001) show that in the control group about 1% of subjects, have a key carer on leave or leaving, compared to about 5% in the cases. If we assume these two proportions are independent, then the proportion of pairs in which the case had the factor and the control did not is $0.01 \times (1-0.05)=0.095$. Similarly, the number of pairs in which the control has the factor and the case did not is $(1-0.01) \times 0.05=0.0495$. Thus a planning estimate of $\pi_{\text{Discordant}}$ is $0.095+0.0495=0.1445\approx0.15$.

Thus, using equation (6.8) for the same design specification as before, but $\pi_{\text{Discordant}}=0.15$, gives $N_{\text{Pairs}}=116\approx120$.

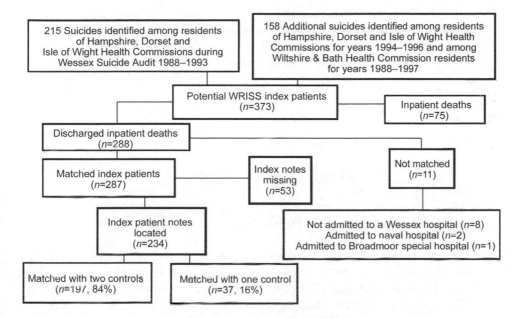

Figure 6.8   Identification of 234 Wessex Recent In-Patient Suicide Study (WRISS) index recently discharged inpatient suicides (from King, Baldwin, Sinclair *et al.*, 2001; reproduced by permission of the *British Journal of Psychiatry*)

REPORTING

As case–control studies are retrospective in nature, and there are many potential difficulties associated with them, it is particularly important that the reporting process is detailed. In particular the flow of cases and controls throughout the various stages of the study needs to be outlined. A very clear indication of this reporting process is given by King, Baldwin, Sinclair *et al.* (2001) in Figure 6.8, which follows the format of the guidelines suggested for reporting randomised controlled trial.

Design features – case–control studies

Identify the key research question(s)

Consider the choice between a case–control or a cohort study

Think of the cohort that has generated the cases and try to ensure controls come from the same cohort

Choice of controls

Beware of biases particularly recall bias

Think about choosing more than one control per case

When cases are from hospitals, think of having both hospital and community controls

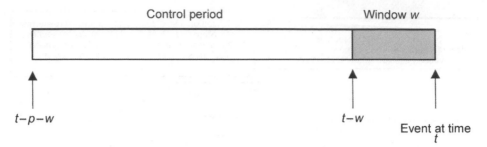

Figure 6.9   Case–crossover design

6.5   CASE–CROSSOVER DESIGNS

Case–crossover designs are ones in which subjects are followed up over time, and act as their own controls. There are two types of case–crossover design (Farrington, 2004). The first is based on the idea of a case–control study. Suppose we believe that, if someone is exposed to a hazard, then there is a 'window' with a period, w, in which any adverse events can be seen. After that period, any events are unlikely to be caused by that particular hazard. The idea is illustrated in Figure 6.9. We assume that the event occurs in N subjects each at an individual time t. We then look backwards in time from that particular t to see when the intervention (the hazard) had occurred in that subject. We know that all subjects had been exposed to the hazard at some time. This would either be in the window period, w, or in the control period, p. Noting this for all patients gives m interventions in w, and n in p, where $m+n=N$. The odds ratio estimating the risk of the intervention depends on the values of w and p and can be calculated using a Mantel–Haenszel estimator (see Park, Ki and Yi, 2004).

***Example** – case–crossover design – MMR vaccine and aseptic meningitis*

Park, Ki and Yi (2004) describe a study looking at the link between the mumps-measles-rubella vaccine and the occurrence of aseptic meningitis. From 420 confirmed cases, they eventually found 39 with accurate vaccination records. They chose the window period to be $w=42$ days and the control period the year preceding the event, excluding the window period, i.e. $365-42=323$ days. Among the 39, they found 11 vaccinated during the window (hazard) period and 28 during the control. Since the control period is the same for each subject, the odds ratio for the risk of meningitis due to MMR is simply the ratio of the two incidences $(11/42)/(28/323)=3.0$ (95% CI 1.5 to 6.1).

An alternative design is based on the idea of a cohort study (Farrington, 1995), who termed it a self-controlled case-series method. The design is illustrated in Figure 6.10.

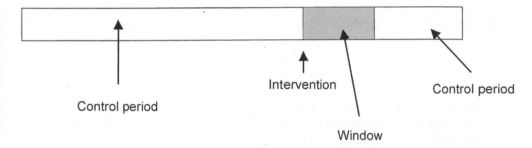

Figure 6.10 Self-controlled case-series design

Here we know the time of the interventions and we observe whether events occur during the 'window' period, and during a control period.

Maclure and Mittleman (2000) discuss the use of case–crossover studies and state that the design applies best if the exposure is intermittent, the effect on risk is immediate and transient and the outcome is abrupt. Farrington (2004) points out that the requirement of constant underlying exposure probability is fundamental to the case–crossover design. Thus, for example, if a study is being used to look at the side effects of a vaccine, and the vaccine is not given below a certain age, control periods which overlap that age would not be equivalent to control periods in which there was a high probability of being vaccinated. The self-controlled case-series does not suffer this problem, and full adjustment for age and time is possible.

Example – self-controlled case series – MMR vaccine and convulsions

Farrington (1995) also examined the effects of the MMR vaccine, this time on the risk of convulsions. All children had had at least one convulsion. There were two hazard periods, 6–11 days after vaccine, and 15–35 days after vaccine. There were 336 events in 329 children. There were 183 events after the vaccine, of which 13 occurred 6–11 days after the vaccine and 12 occurred 15–35 days after the vaccine. The results showed a relative incidence of 2.11 (95% CI 1.21 to 3.69) for the 6–11-day window, and 0.58 (95% CI 0.33 to 1.03) for the 15–35-day window.

6.6   TECHNICAL DETAIL

STRATIFIED SAMPLING

Suppose in a particular survey there are k strata and $m_1, m_2, \ldots, m_i, \ldots, m_k$ subjects are recruited to each strata, then the total sample size is

$$N_{\text{Sample}} = \sum_{i=1}^{k} m_i.$$

Suppose that r_i of those selected in each strata have the characteristic of interest (say, glaucoma) so that $p_i = r_i/n_i$ is the corresponding proportion observed. In this case the (weighted) estimated proportion with the characteristic in the whole population is

$$p_{\text{Stratified}} = \frac{\sum m_i p_i}{N_{\text{Sample}}} = \frac{\sum r_i}{N_{\text{Sample}}}. \tag{T6.1}$$

The individual values of m_i do not appear in this expression. As a consequence this overall proportion is an unbiased estimator of the true proportion in the population at large or, equivalently, β_0 of equation (1.1).

However, the principal reason for stratifying is that the stratified estimate of the prevalence usually has a smaller standard error (SE) than an estimate derived from a purely random sample. The reason is that the variation in any estimate from a survey can be divided into two elements: that between strata and that within each stratum. In stratified sampling the variation between strata does not enter into the SE, since the method ensures that this component of variation in the population is exactly reflected in the sample. Thus the best choice of strata is to choose ones that differ as much as possible from each other.

The standard error of a proportion, from a proportionate stratified sample, is approximately

$$SE(p_{\text{Stratified}}) = \sqrt{\frac{\sum m_i p_i (1 - p_i)}{N_{\text{Sample}}^2}}. \tag{T6.2}$$

However, if a study of the same size had come from a random sample of size N_{Sample}, then the SE is

$$SE(p_{\text{Random}}) = \sqrt{\frac{p_{\text{Random}}(1 - p_{\text{Random}})}{N_{\text{Sample}}}} \tag{T6.3}$$

where $p_{\text{Random}} = R_{\text{Random}}/N_{\text{Sample}}$ and R_{Random} is the total number in the random sample with the characteristic in question.

The Design Effect (DE), corresponding to that of equation (1.6), is

$$DE = \frac{\text{Var}(p_{\text{Stratified}})}{\text{Var}(p_{\text{Random}})} = \frac{\sum m_i p_i (1 - p_i)}{N_{\text{Sample}} p_{\text{Random}}(1 - p_{\text{Random}})} = \frac{\sum m_i p_i (1 - p_i)}{p_{\text{Random}}(1 - p_{\text{Random}}) \sum m_i}. \tag{T6.4}$$

It can be shown, except in some cases where there is only a trivial difference, that the DE is always less than one. Thus a stratified sample gives a more precise estimate of a parameter. These results also hold if a mean is being estimated rather than a proportion.

7 Clinical Trials – General Issues

Summary

This chapter gives an overview of the broad types of clinical trials, ranging from designs appropriate to the first use of a new drug or procedure in humans to public health intervention trials. The chapter focuses on those issues common to all trials, such as subject or patient eligibility, informed consent, the therapeutic options, equipoise and uncertainty, and other practicalities. We also draw attention to the desirability of formally registering each trial before it commences and ensuring that all subjects entering these trials are also registered. The roles of the committees responsible for ethical approval of the trial and their data and safety monitoring are discussed.

7.1   INTRODUCTION

Technical (statistical) aspects of experimental design can be used in a whole variety of settings; nevertheless there are specific problems associated with implementing these designs in practice in the field of clinical trials. These problems mainly arise because the 'experimental' units are human and, in many instances, patients suffering some kind of disease. A critical feature here is that subject (patient) consent to participate in studies must be obtained following a due process that is often determined by national laws, and the trial must have ethical approval. This 'consent' process may inhibit the type of trial that one may wish to conduct. The problems may occur at three levels: the Ethics Committee may refuse permission for the trial, the clinicians may not agree to refer patients to the trial and the patients themselves may refuse to enter.

Designing any clinical trial, of whatever size, is a major undertaking and we should warn that it is necessary to bring together a skilled statistical and multidisciplinary team to ensure that an optimal design is chosen. In some cases, the 'best' experimental design may not be a practical option for the investigation and so a balance has to be struck between what is statistically optimal and what is practicably achievable.

Three key terms that are often confused when describing clinical trials are *efficacy*, *effectiveness* and *efficiency*. Efficacy relates to how the treatment works in a trial, effectiveness relates to whether it works in real life, and efficiency relates to whether it is the best treatment for the purpose.

Design of Studies for Medical Research. D. Machin and M. J. Campbell
© 2005 John Wiley & Sons Ltd. ISBN 0 470 84495 7

Phase	Objective
Preclinical	To investigate pharmacokinetics and types and level of toxicity usually in healthy volunteers.
I	To estimate the maximum tolerated dose (MTD) of a proposed agent or combination, using a cautious dose-escalation strategy in patients.
II	To establish clinical activity and to roughly estimate clinical response rate in patients.
III	A randomised comparison of efficacy of the candidate treatment against a currently accepted standard in patients.

Figure 7.1 Objectives of preclinical studies and clinical trials of the different phases in the development of a drug (part based on Bryant and Day, 1995; reproduced by permission of Blackwell Publishers Ltd)

7.2   TYPES OF TRIALS

The objectives of each phase, in a somewhat idealised pathway, of a typical development programme for a new drug are summarised in Figure 7.1 and range from studies to determine the pharmacokinetic profile of a drug in healthy volunteers to large-scale randomised comparative trials. However, some of these steps may be taken in parallel and even simultaneously in the same subjects.

The nomenclature of Phase I, II and III has been developed for drug development but they essentially apply (although modifications may be necessary) to new approaches to surgery, radiotherapy, medical devices and combinations of such procedures. They also extend beyond merely therapeutic trials to planning, for example, trials comparing alternative forms of contraception in women, and trials evaluating alternative health promotion interventions. However, in some instances, such as in trials comparing educational packages, they may start at the Phase III stage without involving the earlier phases.

Although there is not always a clear division between preclinical studies and clinical trials, the essential difference is that in the latter there is usually some therapeutic intent. As a consequence, even in a very early dose-escalation Phase I trial in a patient with a malignancy, there is a concern not to give too little of a drug as such a dose would be extremely unlikely to bring any (anti-tumour) benefit to the patient. Thus an early stage clinical trial may include in the design some assessment of response as for a Phase II trial.

If these trials are concerned with patients, as opposed to 'healthy' controls, then careful note of this fact must play a role in determining those who are eligible for the trial. These considerations will differ from phase to phase in the drug development process, the particular treatment modality under consideration, the severity of the disease and many other factors.

PHARMACOKINETIC STUDIES

At some stage in the drug development process a new compound moves from the laboratory and is then usually tested in animals prior to its introduction in humans. A first step into humans may be to determine the pharmacokinetic properties of the drug in healthy volunteers. Studies carried out primarily to address pharmacokinetic issues are often referred to as ADME studies, since they are designed to characterise four fundamental aspects of a drug's kinetics: Absorption, Distribution, Metabolism, and Excretion. In some circumstances the profile may need to be determined in patients, rather than in healthy volunteers, as the disease itself may affect the pharmacokinetic properties in an important way. These studies may be comparative in nature when assessing the bioequivalence of a new compound as compared to a previous standard.

Example – *PK profile of sumatriptan tablets – migraine relief*

Walls, Lewis, Bullman *et al.* (2004) describe the PK profile of a new form of sumatriptan tablets for potential use for patients with migraine. In their study healthy subjects were used. They concluded that the new form was bioequivalent to sumatriptan conventional tablets and was absorbed more quickly.

PHASE I TRIALS

After the ADME studies, or in parallel, a Phase I clinical trial commences in patients. Typically a Phase I trial takes the form of testing a range of doses suggested by studies in the laboratory animal or by comparison with those drugs with similar properties. The trial aims to determine which of these chosen doses (if any) should be passed to the next phase of development to determine its activity. The dose is often chosen on the basis of the highest feasible with an acceptable toxicity profile. The definition of 'acceptable toxicity' and how it is to be assessed is crucial to this phase.

Example – *Phase I trial – unresectable pancreatic cancer*

Muler, McGinn, Normolle *et al.* (2004) describe a Phase I trial in which 19 patients with pancreatic cancer were treated with cisplatin combined with gemcitabine and radiation therapy (RT). They concluded that cisplatin doses up to $40\,\text{mg/m}^2$ could be safely added to full-dose gemcitabine and conformal RT.

PHASE II TRIALS

Once the dose of a compound is recommended from a Phase I study, then activity at that dose may be tested in a Phase II trial. Such studies, although not generally comparative in nature, will often be designed with the knowledge that other compounds are active for the disease in question, so that evidence of at least this minimum activity may be sought. The definitions of how 'activity' is defined and assessed are crucial to this phase. If sufficient activity is demonstrated then this may suggest testing for efficacy in a randomised Phase III comparative trial.

Example *– Phase II trial – carcinosarcoma of the female genital tract*

Van Rijswijk, Vermorken, Reed *et al.* (2003) conducted a Phase II trial in 48 women with carcinosarcoma of the genital tract. Although the activity of the combination of cisplatin, doxorubicin and ifosfamide was established (overall response rate 56%), they did not recommend this treatment combination but suggested that those 'with more favourable toxicity profiles should be explored'.

It is clear from this example that Phase II trials are not confined to those testing a single agent.

PHASE III TRIALS

Randomised

Phase III trials are comparative in nature so that a typical structure is to compare the drug suggested as active with the standard treatment for the disease in question. This usually takes the form of a randomised controlled trial (RCT) and this design is regarded as the design 'gold standard' for this evaluation. This does not imply that it is the only type of trial worthy of conduct but rather that it provides a benchmark against which other trial designs are measured. The standard or control treatment used in the comparison may have been a compound that had arisen from a previous drug development programme. The earlier phases for the new drug in question will have utilised only indirect measures of efficacy, perhaps tumour response, so it is now important to define the efficacy measure to be used for this evaluation. In any new drug development programme we may hope that the contender drug will outperform the standard but we will not know this until the trial is complete. Measures of efficacy might be the survival of the patient, time to resolution of their disease, pain relief or health related quality of life (HRQoL), or a combination of several of these.

In some cases, the 'best' experimental design may not be a practical option for the trial. For example, in the context of a planned 2×2 factorial trial of (say) two drugs A and B, against a placebo for each, there are four combinations (1), a, b, and ab. (We discuss placebo treatment in more detail in section 7.5.) With these combinations there is the intention that one in four of the patients receive both placebos, with therefore no chance of activity. Equally patients may receive both *A* and *B*, perhaps associated with feared unacceptably high toxicity. These considerations may reduce the optimal four-group parallel design to a practical three-group design of either [(1), *a*, *b*] or [*a*, *b*, *ab*] configuration depending on the circumstances. Both these designs are less (statistically) efficient than the full factorial so may require more patients than the full design to answer the less complete range of questions.

In general one may be looking for superiority of the test over the standard, but there are circumstances where a satisfactory outcome for the new drug is that the test does not perform worse than the standard to a predefined extent. Such non-inferiority designs imply that, although some compromise may be conceded on the main outcome variable, these other factors favouring the new therapy will offset this. For example, if the new compound was equally effective (not better) but had a better toxicity profile, then this would be useful.

In this context, it is important to make the distinction between randomisation and a random sample used in, for example, a population survey. Patients in a randomised trial are seldom, if ever, a random sample of the population of patients with the disease in question. As a consequence, trials have good *internal* validity, but may be difficult to generalise. Thus, for example, there is a paucity of trials of drugs in children, and it is unclear sometimes whether results obtained from trials in adults can be generalised to children.

Non-randomised

In certain circumstances, when a new treatment has been proposed for evaluation, investigators have recruited patients into a single-arm study. The results from these patients are then compared with information on similar patients having (usually in the past) received a relevant standard therapy for the disease in question. However, such historical comparisons may well be biased in many possible ways but to an unknown extent, so that it will not be reasonable to ascribe the difference (if any) observed entirely to the treatments themselves. Similar problems arise if all patients are recruited prospectively but allocation to treatment is not made at random. Again in such cases the comparisons made will be biased and hence are unreliable. Of course, in either case there will be situations when one of these designs is the only option available. In such cases, a detailed justification for not using the 'gold standard' of the randomised controlled trial is required.

Understandably, in this era of EBM, information from non-randomised comparative studies is categorised as providing weaker evidence than that from randomised trials.

Example – *non-randomised design* – *glioblastoma in the elderly*

Brandes, Vastola, Basso *et al.* (2003) describe a study comparing radiotherapy alone (Group A), radiotherapy and the combination of procarbazine, lomustine and vincristine (Group B), and radiotherapy with temozolomide (Group C) in 79 elderly patients with glioblastoma.

The authors state: 'The first group (Group A) was enrolled in the period from March 1993 to August 1995.... The second group (Group B) was enrolled from September 1995 to September 1997.... The third group (Group C) was enrolled from September 1997 to August 2000 and...'.

The authors conclude: 'Overall survival was better in Group C compared with Group A (14.9 months v 11.2 months, $P=0.002$), but there were no statistical differences found between Groups A and B or between Groups B and C'.

However, since patients have not been randomised to groups, we cannot be sure that the differences (and lack of differences) truly reflect the relative efficacy of the three treatments concerned.

7.3   ELIGIBILITY

Common to all phases of clinical trials is the necessity to define precisely who are eligible subjects. If healthy volunteers are required then a definition of 'healthy' is required. This definition may be relatively brief or complex depending on the substance under test. At the very early stage of the process it is very understandable that great care is taken in subject and, particularly, patient choice. In these situations, perhaps involving the very first use of the compound in humans, all the possible adverse eventualities have to be considered. These usually result in a very restricted definition for those that can be recruited.

Example – *eligibility to a pharmacokinetic study* – *bioavailability of telithromycin*

Bhargava, Lenfant, Perret *et al.* (2002) in a bioavailability study of the antibacterial telithromycin define the subjects to be recruited as follows: 'Male subjects aged between 18 and 45 y were recruited. Subjects were eligible for inclusion in the study if they were judged to be free of clinically significant disease on the basis of complete medical history and physical examination, standard clinical laboratory tests, a 12-lead electrocardiogram (ECG) (QTc $\leqslant 400$ ms) and vital sign assessments (heart rate $\geqslant 40$ beats/min). Liver function tests, aspartate aminotransferase (AST) and alanine aminotransferase (ALT) had to be strictly within the normal range'.

Example – *eligibility to a Phase I trial* – *unresectable pancreatic cancer*

In the Phase I trial of Muler, McGinn, Normolle *et al.* (2004), to be eligible patients were deemed to have unresectable pancreatic cancer, with or without metastases, based on helical computed tomography scan, endoscopic ultrasound and surgical consultation. In addition, their age was to be greater than 18 years, Zubrod performance status $\leqslant 2$, estimated life expectancy of at least 12 weeks and adequate organ function defined as: absolute neutrophil count $\geqslant 1500\,cm^3$, platelets $\geqslant 100\,000/cm^3$, serum creatinine $< 1.5\,mg/dL$, bilirubin $< 3\,mg/dL$, and AST < 5 times upper limit of normal. Further they had to have no prior history of abdominal irradiation or chemotherapy for pancreatic cancer.

Once the possibility of some activity (and hence potential efficacy) becomes indicated then there is at least a prospect of therapeutic gain for the patient. In this case, the investigators may expand the horizon of eligible patients but simultaneously confine them to those in which a measurable response to the disease can be ascertained.

Example – eligibility to a Phase II trial – gemcitabine in nasopharyngeal carcinoma

Foo, Tan, Leong *et al.* (2002) specify that patients were to have histologically confirmed undifferentiated carcinoma arising from the nasopharynx, *bidimensionally measurable* disease not within any prior radiotherapy fields, be between 18 and 75 years, with an Eastern Cooperative Oncology Group (ECOG) performance status (PS) < 2. In addition there were seven clinical chemistry limits that had to be satisfied before inclusion was possible. All patients were to receive $1250\,mg/m^2$ gemcitabine on days 1 and 8 of a 21-day cycle.

In contrast to pharmacokinetic, Phase I and II trials, in a Phase III trial in which a prospective new therapy is under test, the eligibility should reflect if possible the (wider) patient pool in which it is to be eventually used should it prove effective. Thus the emphasis now is to define simple and minimal eligibility criteria that allow all types of patients into the trial in whom benefit from the therapy may be expected. Essentially these include all the patient types for which the comparator in the trial is the current standard. If the eligibility criteria are too narrow, then, however good the test treatment, the clinical implications will affect only small groups.

Example – eligibility to a Phase III trial – burn wound management

Ang, Lee, Gan *et al.* (2001), in a randomised trial to compare Moist Exposed Burns Ointment (MEBO) with conventional dressing, specified that eligible patients were all patients with partial-thickness burns. The exceptions were those of very young age and very old patients (< 6 and > 80 years), and those with chemical or electrical burns. Patients with severe burns are by their very nature emergency admissions, so minimal time must be spent in assessing eligibility as protocol treatment must commence immediately.

There are at least two further aspects of the eligibility requirements that are important. The first is that the patient indeed has the condition in question and satisfies all the other requirements. There must be no specific reasons why the patient should not be included. For example, in some circumstances pregnant or lactating women (otherwise eligible) may be excluded for fear of impacting adversely either on the foetus or the newborn child. The second is that all the therapeutic options for study in the Phase III trial are equally appropriate for the particular patient. Only if both these aspects are satisfied should the patient be invited to consent to participate in the trial.

There will be circumstances in which a patient may be eligible for the trial but the attending physician feels (for whatever reason) that one of the trial options is 'best' for the patient. In which case the patient should receive that option, no consent for the trial is then required and the randomisation would not take place. In such circumstances, the clinician should not randomise the patient in the hope that the patient will receive the 'best' option. To withdraw the patient from the trial if the alternative option is allocated may seriously bias the trial conclusions.

7.4   INFORMED CONSENT

The ideal is that each patient or volunteer give fully informed and written consent. However, departures from this may be appropriate. For example, such departures may concern patients who may be unconscious at admission, patients with hand burns that are so severe that they affect their ability to sign the form, very young children or those with dementia. In these cases a proxy is required to consent for them.

PHARMACOKINETIC, PHASE I AND PHASE II TRIALS

In general, pharmacokinetic and Phase I trials are not comparative, so only details of the procedures that are to be involved and any potential side effects and risks need to be explained. For those involving patients, it would be important to explain that little therapeutic benefit could be expected.

Since most Phase II trials are not comparative also, only details of the procedures that are to be involved and any potential side effects and risks need to be explained. It would be important to explain to the patient that any therapeutic benefit hoped for, such as tumour shrinkage, may or may not transfer into benefit for the patient with respect to (say) increased survival or improved HRQoL. In the case of randomised Phase II trials, then considerations similar to those of Phase III would apply.

PHASE III TRIALS

Individually Randomised

In a comparative trial, all the options should be explained in detail to the patients concerned. This explanation must be provided before the randomisation is effected as

NMRC
National Medical Research Council
Singapore

Head & Neck
Cancer Group

CONSENT FORM

**Surgery And Adjuvant Radiotherapy Versus Concurrent Chemo-Radiotherapy
For Resectable [Non-Metastatic] Stage III / IV Head And Neck
Squamous Cell Cancer**

1. I have read the patient information sheet and understand its content.

2. I have had opportunity to discuss this study and have my questions answered by the investigators.

3. I have received satisfactory answers to all my questions.

4. I have received enough information about the study.

5. I confirm that I am not pregnant and have no intention of becoming pregnant during this study.

6. I understand that my participation is voluntary.

7. I understand that I am free to withdraw from the study:

    - at any time

    - without having to give reasons

    - without affecting my future medical care

8. Sections of my medical records relating to my participation in the study will be inspected by responsible individuals from a medical audit committee. All personal details will be treated as strictly confidential. I give my permission for these individuals to have access to my records.

9. I have had sufficient time to come to my decision.

10. I agree to participate in this study.

Patient :

....	....	....	....
Signature	Name	NRIC No.	Date

Witness :

....	....	....	....
Signature	Name	NRIC No.	Date

Investigator :

....	....	....	....
Signature	Name	NRIC No.	Date

Figure 7.2   Consent form utilised in a trial of head and neck cancer conducted by the National Cancer Centre, Singapore (and reproduced with their permission)

knowledge of the assignment may influence the way in which an investigator explains the alternatives. Otherwise greater stress or detail on the option selected by the randomisation procedure may be given. A key feature of the consent process is to explain the randomisation procedure.

An example of a consent form used in a randomised trial in patients with head and neck cancer is shown in Figure 7.2. This form satisfied the local regulations and was used concurrently with a patient information sheet explaining more about the trial and emphasising that participation was completely voluntary.

Randomised Consent Designs

In view of difficulties associated with obtaining informed patient consent to join a trial, various options have been proposed to minimise these difficulties. One suggestion is a Zelen (1992) design in which eligible patients are randomised to one of the two treatment groups before they are specifically contacted about the details of the trial. Once randomised, then those who are allocated to the standard treatment are all treated with it and no consent to take part in the trial is sought. The ethical argument is that this is the treatment they would have received in the absence of the trial, so no permission is needed. On the other hand, those who are randomised to the experimental treatment are asked for their consent; if they agree they are treated with the experimental treatment; if they disagree they are treated with the standard treatment. Huibers, Bleijenberg, Beurkens *et al.* (2004) describe a modification of the Zelen design in which patients are randomised before being approached but consent is then sought from both arms. However, neither arm is told of the existence of the alternative therapy.

The chief difficulty is that these designs each involve some deception and, although carried out with the best of intent, this is difficult to square with an ethical approach. Also most trials require additional measurements to be made on patients, even those in the control group and so consent is required for this and an explanation given of why the measurements are being made. This process clearly nullifies the advantage of a Zelen approach.

Cluster-randomised

Cluster-randomised trials, in which patients are randomised in clusters, are described in more detail in Chapter 9. For cluster-randomised trials there are two levels of consent. For example, the health care professionals consent to take part in the study, and then, after randomisation, the patients are informed that randomisation has occurred and that they are part of a study. However, for public heath promotion trials no consent by those receiving the intervention may be possible.

An ethical dilemma can occur when the health provider has been trained, in the context of a cluster design trial, to give a particular treatment in a certain way. Then, if an individual patient presents for a consultation, the individual does not have any choice as to how the treatment is given. In this context, in trials that compare a new approach with 'usual care', it would seem unnecessary to inform the patients in the 'usual care' group about the trial since their treatment is unchanged. Thus Donner,

Piaggio, Villar *et al.* (1998) used a Zelen design in a large multinational antenatal care trial.

In cluster designs there is an additional problem when blindness is an issue. For example, for many treatment trials validity is improved if the subject is unaware of what treatment they are receiving. Thus it would reduce bias if both groups of patients were aware that a trial was being carried out, but were not told specifically what treatment they would receive. In the 'patient-centred' trial of Kinmonth, Woodcock, Griffin *et al.* (1998) patients were asked afterwards if they felt their doctor was using a 'patient-centred' approach and a greater number thought so in the active group than in the control group. As a consequence, there is some concern with respect to the size of the potential bias in the final comparisons made.

7.5 THERAPEUTIC OPTIONS

The 'therapeutic' options should be well described within the trial protocol and details of what to do if treatment requires modification or stopping for an individual patient should be given. Stopping may arise either when patients merely refuse to take further part in the trial or from safety concerns with a therapy under test.

EQUIPOISE AND UNCERTAINTY

The randomised trial is the standard against which other trial designs may be compared. By the very term 'randomised', this design implies that the particular treatment given is chosen neither by the patient nor by the doctor, but by a randomisation device. In addition there must be genuine uncertainty as to which of the options is best for the patient. It is this uncertainty which provides the necessary equipoise to justify random allocation to treatment after due consent is given. When a trial is planned, it is therefore clear that there must be considerable 'uncertainty' with respect to the relative efficacy of the 'therapeutic' options. Without this uncertainty, the trial should not commence. On the other hand, once the trial is completed, one hopes that much of the initial uncertainty will be removed and that a recommendation with respect to one or other (or even both) of the options can be made. The very basis of planning the study size is that only when the trial has completed recruitment and follow-up, will one have sufficient information to reduce the uncertainty of the planning stage to a level that permits one option (say) to be recommended for future clinical use. At this stage the original 'equipoise' should no longer be in place.

STANDARD OR CONTROL THERAPY

At some stage in the development of a new therapy it is important to compare this with the current standard for the disease in question. In certain circumstances, the new therapy may be compared against a 'no-treatment' or placebo control.

> **Example** – *placebo-controlled trial – advanced hepatocellular carcinoma*
>
> In the randomised controlled trial conducted by Chow, Tai, Tan *et al.* (2002) in advanced liver cancer, patients were randomised to receive either placebo or tamoxifen. In this trial, both patients and the attending physicians were blind to the actual treatment that was given. Such a 'double-blind' or 'double-masked' trial is a design that reduces any potential bias to a minimum.

Placebo controls and 'no-treatment' controls are not possible in many circumstances. In this case, the 'control' will be the current best practice against which the new treatment will be compared and is usually termed the 'comparison' group. For example, in patients receiving surgery for the primary treatment of head and neck cancer followed by best supportive care, the randomised controlled trial may be assessing the value of adding post-operative chemotherapy to this 'standard' approach. In this case the comparison group are those who receive the current standard of no adjuvant treatment, whilst the 'test' group receive chemotherapy in addition.

TEST THERAPY

It is self-evident, that if there are only minor differences in the treatments included in a randomised trial, then only a very large-scale trial would detect any differences in efficacy, even if they were truly present. Thus it is best (within the realms of practicability and safety considerations) if the treatment options are as different as possible. For example, if a randomised trial is planned to test against placebo (dose $d=0$) a drug (at dose d), then d should be taken as high as possible. If in such a trial no effect is demonstrated, then one may be reasonably confident that the drug is not efficacious. On the other hand, if a lower dose $d/2$ (say) had been chosen to compare with placebo, then a negative outcome may be a result of the dose chosen being too low rather than the drug being truly inactive.

LARGE SIMPLE TRIALS

There are circumstances where small therapeutic advantages may be worthwhile demonstrating, particularly in the fields of cardiovascular disease and cancer. In terms of trial size, the smaller the potential benefit, essentially the effect size, then the larger the trial must be in order to be reasonably confident that the small benefit envisaged really exists at all.

Trials of this type, often involving many thousands of patients, are a major undertaking. To be practicable, they must be in common diseases in order to recruit the required numbers of patients in a reasonable time frame. They must be testing a treatment that has wide applicability and can be easily administered by the clinicians responsible or the patients themselves. The treatments must be relatively non-toxic, otherwise the small benefit will be outweighed by the side effects. The trials must be simple in structure and restricted as to the number of variables recorded, so that the recruiting clinicians are not overburdened by the workload attached to large numbers of trial patients going through the clinic. They also need to be simple in this respect for the responsible statistical centre to cope with the large amounts of patient data collected.

Example – *large simple trial* – *early breast cancer*

The ATAC (Arimidex, Tamoxifen Alone or in Combination) Trialists' Group (2002), as the group name suggests, was designed to test the combination of tamoxifen and anastrozole (arimidex) as adjuvant treatment for postmeno-pausal women with early breast cancer. The design had three arms of a 2×2 factorial design but omitted the double-placebo combination. The trial involved a relatively common disease and used very simple (and low-cost) treatments taken as tablets with very few anticipated side effects. In the event the trial recruited 9366 women and the preliminary results indicate that anastrozole is an effective and well-tolerated endocrine option for these patients.

INFLUENCING CLINICAL PRACTICE

Although we will talk specifically about trial size in the context of Phase I, II and III trials in the following chapters, there are general issues to consider. For example, when designing a new trial, the size (and of course design) should be chosen so that there is a reasonable expectation that the key question(s) posed will be answered. For Phase III trials, this implies that a realistic assessment of the potential benefit (the anticipated effect size) of the proposed test therapy must be made at the onset. The history of clinical trials research suggests that, in many circumstances, rather over-optimistic views of potential benefit have been claimed at their design stages. This has led to many inconclusive trials because of an inadequate number of patients. Such trials often reporting estimates of relative efficacy, had they been reliably established, of a clinically important magnitude. Thus the small trial conducted by Lau, Leung, Ho *et al.* (1999) indicated a large benefit for the use of adjuvant intra-arterial iodine-131-labelled lipiodol in resectable hepatocellular carcinoma but the alleged benefit was questioned as 'too-good-to-be-true' by Pocock and White (1999). Further reporting this small trial also compromised the possibility of confirmatory trials as the level of activity indicated, but certainly non-proven, impacted on the necessary 'equipoise' to justify randomisation in any subsequent trials.

Thus an important consideration at the design stage is to whether, should the new treatment prove effective, the trial will be reliable enough in itself to convince clinical teams not associated with the trial of the findings. Importantly, if a benefit is established, will this be quickly adopted in clinical practice? Experience has suggested that trials that will be adopted in practice are likely to be large, conducted by a respected group and have wide multicentre involvement. Thus there are considerations, in some sense outside the strict confines of the design, which investigators should heed if their findings are to have the desired impact.

7.6   PRACTICALITIES

INTENTION-TO-TREAT (ITT)

Once patients have been randomised to a clinical trial, treatment as specified in the protocol should start as soon as it is practicably possible. For the severely burnt patients either MEBO or conventional dressings can be immediately applied. On the other hand if patients, once randomised, have then to be scheduled for surgery, there may be considerable delay before surgery takes place. This delay may provide a period in which the patients change their mind about consent or, indeed, in those with life-threatening illness, some may die before the scheduled date of surgery. Thus, the number of patients actually starting the protocol treatment allocated may be less than the number randomised to receive it.

The 'intention-to-treat' (ITT) principle is that once randomised the patient is retained in that group for analysis whatever occurs, even in situations where a patient after consent is randomised to (say) *A* but then refuses and even insists on being treated by option *B*. The effect of such a patient is to dilute the estimate of the true difference between *A* and *B*. However, if such a patient was analysed as if allocated to treatment *B*, then the trial is no longer properly randomised and the resulting comparison may be seriously biased. The ITT principle ensures that for a trial set up to test differences, any estimate of treatment effect is, if anything, biased towards the null, whereas the difficulty with analysing a trial by the treatment patients actually received is that we do not know the direction of the bias.

One procedure that used to be in widespread use was to review the trial in detail once the protocol treatment and follow-up were complete and all the trial-specific information collected. This review would, for example, check that the patient eligibility criteria were satisfied and that there had been no important protocol deviations while on treatment. The problem is this tends to selectively exclude patients with the more severe disease. Usually, this review would not be blind to the treatment received. In fact even if the trial were double-blind, there might still be clues, once the data are examined in this way, as to which treatment is which.

Evidence for selective exclusion following such reviews is provided by Machin, Stenning, Parmar *et al.* (1997) who examined some of the first UK Medical Research Council randomised trials in patients with cancer. They showed that the earlier publications systematically reported on fewer patients in the more aggressive treatment arm despite a 1:1 randomisation. Thus, for example, any patient who had difficulties with this treatment, perhaps the more sick patients, were not included in the assessment of its efficacy and this systematic exclusion would tend to bias the results in its favour.

PER PROTOCOL

In general, the application of ITT to a superiority trial is conservative in the sense that it will tend to dilute between observed randomised treatment group differences and so reduce the chance of demonstrating efficacy. However, Piaggio and Pinol (2001) point out that for 'equivalence' (see section 9.3) trials the dilution caused by ITT will not be conservative as it will tend to favour the equivalence hypothesis. Too many patients failing to adhere to their allocated treatment, for whatever reason, will clearly dilute the respective treatments to such an extent that each becomes like the other and hence falsely 'equivalent'.

Thus in certain circumstances, a 'per protocol' summary may be more relevant. In such an analysis, the comparison is made only in those patients who comply (which has to be carefully defined in advance) with the treatment allocated. Lewis and Machin (1993) point out, as one example of a per protocol analysis, that if the toxicity and/or side-effects profile of a new agent are to be summarised, any analysis including those patients who were randomised to the drug but then did not receive it (for whatever reason) could seriously underestimate the true levels. If this is indeed appropriate for such endpoints, then the trial protocol should state that such an analysis is intended from the onset.

A clear statement of what distinguishes an ITT from a per protocol analysis is made by ICH (1999).

HEALTH RELATED QUALITY OF LIFE

Most Phase III trials are intended primarily to address questions of efficacy, although frequently there are important secondary objectives. Of these HRQoL may be particularly important. Indeed, it may be the endpoint of prime importance in patients with chronic conditions or in those who are terminally ill or psychologically impaired. However, the measurement process is now made by means of one or more HRQoL instruments. These instruments are developed according to a very strict series of procedures and, in general, cannot be quickly developed just for the trial in hand.

The HRQoL domains measured by these instruments may then be used as the definitive endpoints for clinical trials. If a single aspect of the HRQoL instrument, measured at one time point, is to be used for treatment comparison purposes then no new principles are required, either for trial design purposes or for analysis. On the other hand, and more usually, there may be several aspects of the QoL instrument that may need to be compared between treatment groups and these features will usually be assessed over time. This is further complicated by often-unequal numbers of assessments available from each patient, caused by missing assessments in the series for a variety of reasons related, perhaps in terminal patients once close to death, or unrelated to the health status of the patient concerned.

Although design principles may not change to a large degree, logistical problems are magnified. These range from determining the schedule for when the HRQoL assessments are to be made and by whom – the patient or the carer (although this may be instrument specific) – to checking that all questions are completed, to dealing with the large quantity of data at the analytical and reporting stages. Fayers and Machin (2000) and Fairclough (2002) discuss these and other features of HRQoL data in some detail.

ECONOMIC EVALUATION

As with HRQoL, there may be circumstances where an economic evaluation of the relative merits of two treatments is required. This may be particularly important if non-inferiority is to be demonstrated or if the relative costs associated with particular modalities are difficult to quantify. If we were to design a trial primarily to compare costs associated with different treatments we would follow the basic ideas of blinding and randomisation and then record subsequent costs incurred by the patient and the health provider. A very careful protocol would be necessary to define which costs are being considered so that this is measured consistently for all patients.

However, most trials are aimed primarily at assessing efficacy and a limitation of investigating costs in a clinical trial is that the schedule of, and frequency of, visits by the patient to the physician may be very different to what it would be in routine clinical practice. Typically patients are monitored more frequently and more intensely in a trial setting than in routine clinical practice. The costs recorded, therefore, in a clinical trial may well be different (probably greater) than in clinical practice.

The same limitation does, of course, apply to efficacy evaluations as the overall level of efficacy seen in clinical trials is often not realised in clinical practice. However, in a clinical trial, since it is the *relative* efficacy of one treatment over another that is determined then this limitation, whilst still important, can be considered less of an overall objection.

Recommendations of how trials incorporating health economics assessment should be conducted have been given by Drummond and McGuire (2002), while Neymark, Kiebert, Torfs *et al.* (1998) discuss some of the methodological issues as they relate to cancer trials.

7.7   TRIAL CONDUCT

REGISTERING CLINICAL TRIALS

An important criticism made by the teams conducting systematic reviews of clinical trials is that the relevant trial results are not always published. This may be because the trial was never completed or it turned out to give equivocal or negative results, or perhaps was due to mere indolence on the part of the investigating team. As a consequence, systematic overviews seek out those trials that are unpublished as well as those that are published in the medical literature. There has long been evidence that those unpublished trials may represent the more 'negative' of trials conducted so that if an overview is made without them the associated meta-analysis may provide an unduly optimistic view of the (new) therapy under test.

To overcome some of these difficulties, Dickersin and Rennie (2003) argue, as have many others, that an important first step in the trial development and conduct process would be to formally register trial protocols. This registration should be completed *before* a trial can even begin. They argue that each trial should be given a unique identifier so that there can be no ambiguity at a later date. This unique identifier would, for example, have to be quoted to the relevant journal editor when submitting the clinical results for publication. It would clearly allow those conducting systematic reviews to be sure that *all* relevant trials are included in their review. Some of the details that may be required for satisfactory registration purposes are listed in Figure 7.3.

Many of the items are obviously very easy to provide as they form part of the key information that will be included in all good clinical trial protocols. It is somewhat

Identifying Information	Name of organisation conducting the trial
	Name of trial sponsor
	Protocol number
Trial details	Purpose
	All interventions
	Title and acronym
	Disease or condition
	Eligibility criteria
	Design
	Planned trial size
	Locations where recruitment takes place
Funding	Full details of all funding with associated reference numbers
Contact	Lead principal investigator and other key personnel
Conduct	Date first patient entered
	Recruitment status
	Date of last patient entered

Figure 7.3 Suggested details necessary for trial registration purposes

more difficult to specify all the 'locations' where the trial may eventually take place. This tends to suggest that the registration will have to be updated as the trial progresses but provided the information required is not too extensive, this should not be too large a burden for a well-organised investigating team.

Although registration is certainly not mandatory or even possible at national level in most situations, it is goal that can be achieved by the funding bodies and, at least, the home institution of the leading investigators.

REGISTERING PATIENTS

Allied to the issue of registering the trial protocol, it is also very important to register the patient onto the trial so that ultimately the trial report concerns the outcome of all the registered patients. For randomised controlled trials, this registration will usually be an integral part of the randomisation process and it is customary for careful attention to be paid to this point. Indeed the reporting requirements of the clinical journals and the regulatory authorities for such trials, especially if the results are to be part of a product licence application, make it very explicit that this is required.

The magnitude of Phase III trials in terms of patient numbers forbids reporting of individual outcomes and in most cases this would not be sensible. However, for earlier phase studies anonymised patient specific data may be very valuable indeed as these trials are conducted at the more 'experimental' stages and such detail may provide interesting clues for other research teams. Sadly, the standard of reporting of Phase I and II studies does not often meet the high standards demanded of the Phase III randomised controlled trial. Indeed it is often difficult to know how many patients were actually included in some of these studies.

Example – *reporting a Phase I trial – pancreatic cancer*

An excellent example of the careful reporting of a Phase I trial is provided by Muler, McGinn, Normolle *et al.* (2004). They give patient-by-patient details of date 'on-study', the dose administered, the date 'off-study' and whether or not a dose-limiting toxicity (DLT) was observed. In this list was also included one patient (Patient 8) in whom DLT could not be assessed. This list, and other aspects of this report, allows the interested reader to obtain maximal information from their study.

DATA MONITORING

Once a clinical trial is under way, the responsible teams have much to do. Thus, in addition to recruiting and treating patients, often with a protocol which is more stringent than standard practice, and organising follow-up, they must monitor the accumulating data for safety (and efficacy). Although safety will be of paramount concern for the individual patients, collective concern over many patients may determine whether a regimen is safe enough for use and, if it is found unsafe (within the context of the trial), may justify premature closure of the study. It is also possible that the early trial data indicate a real advantage (or disadvantage) to the new therapy under test.

In general, it is best if an independent group monitors the trial progress, although the individual clinical and statistical teams should always be on the lookout for the untoward. It is usual that this Data Monitoring Committee (DMC) is constituted of clinical members and a medical statistician, cognisant of the issues concerned but not involved with the trial itself.

WHEN TO PUBLISH

The first rule after completing a clinical trial is to report the results – whether they are positive, negative or equivocal. Despite this mandate to publish, not least so that any benefits that may have been demonstrated may be passed to future patients as quickly as possible, some care has to taken in deciding the appropriate time for this. In circumstances where all patients have been recruited and complete efficacy details obtained from every patient as specified in the protocol, publication can be immediate. In contrast, if the trial involves long-term follow-up of patients, perhaps eventually recording their survival time from randomisation, then it may be a long time before all

Participants	Eligibility criteria for participants and the setting and locations where the data were collected
Interventions	Precise details of the interventions intended, and how and when they were actually administered
Objectives	Specific objectives and hypotheses
Outcomes	Clearly defined primary and secondary outcome measures
Sample size	How sample size was determined
Randomisation	Details of method used to generate the random allocation sequence – including details of strata and block size
	Method used to implement the random allocation – numbered containers, central telephone, or web based
Blinding	Description of the extent of the blinding in the trial – investigator, participant
Statistical methods	Statistical methods used for the primary outcome(s)
Participant flow	Flow of participants through each stage of the trial
Recruitment	Dates defining the periods of recruitment and follow-up
Follow-up	As many patients as possible to be followed up. Drop-outs should be reported by treatment group

Figure 7.4 Selected key items to be included in a clinical trial report (adapted and abbreviated from that recommended for a Phase III trial by Moher, Schultz and Altman, 2001)

patients have died. Such trials depend on the number of events observed and not just the numbers of subjects recruited. Thus an appropriate time to publish is once the number of events specified in the protocol has been observed. The time when this will occur can be estimated at the design stage, and refined as the trial progresses, so as this number approaches, steps can be taken for preparing the publication to minimise delays.

There will be circumstances where, for example, the new treatment in a Phase III trial may be much more efficacious than had been anticipated at the design stage. The temptation is then to stop the trial early or at least to publish the interim findings. However, seldom, if ever, will it be justifiable to publish interim results while the trial is still open, since it will certainly disturb the equipoise necessary for the randomisation and will affect the 'fully informed' consent process. However, any decision to stop a trial early, or to publish interim results, should not be made without prior consultation with the independent DMC who should be the only ones fully conversant with the full data. Once a randomised trial is stopped early, for whatever reason, it may not be possible to start again and the consequences of an inconclusive result thereby arising are of real concern.

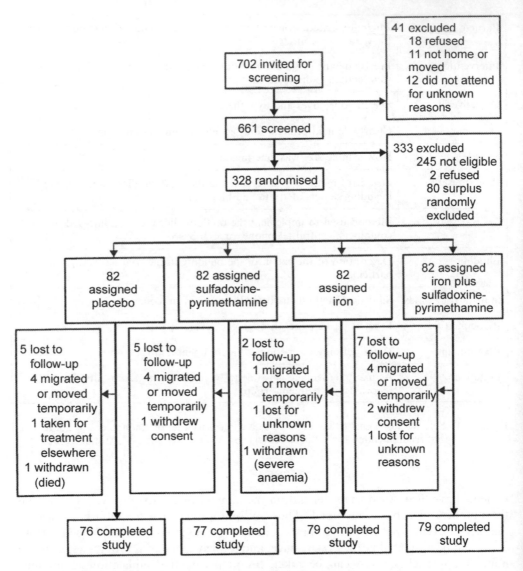

Figure 7.5   Trial profile following the CONSORT guidelines (from Verhoef, West, Nzyuko *et al.*, 2002; Reprinted with permission from Elsevier (The *Lancet*, 360, 908–914))

CONSORT

Considerable effort is required in order to conduct a clinical trial of whatever type and size and this effort justifies reporting of the subsequent trial results with careful detail. However, there is a wide variation in the quality of the standard of reporting of clinical trials. Some reports even omit key details such as the numbers randomised to each group in a Phase III trial. Nevertheless major strides in improving the quality have been made and pivotal to this has been the Consolidation of the Standards of Reporting Trials (CONSORT) statement described by Begg, Cho, Eastwood *et al.* (1996), amplified by Moher, Schultz and Altman (2001) and extended to cluster randomised trials by Campbell, Elbourne and Altman (2004). CONSORT describes the essential items that should be reported in a trial publication in order to give assurance that the trial has been conducted to a high standard. This is an internationally agreed recommendation, adopted by many of the leading medical journals, although there are still some who do not appear to insist that their authors comply with the requirements. Some of the key items from CONSORT are listed in Figure 7.4.

One particular feature of the CONSORT statement is that the outcomes of all participants randomised to a clinical trial are to be reported. Thus a full note has to be provided on those who post-randomisation, for example, then refuse the allocation and perhaps then insist on the competitor treatment. Figure 7.5 gives an example of the CONSORT style patient flow through the 2×2 factorial randomised trial conducted by Verhoef, West, Nzyuko et al. (2002) in anaemic children. The schema clearly shows the numbers randomised to each group, and the detailed reasons why 21 of the children, roughly equal numbers per randomised group, did not complete the study.

For those designing clinical trials it is clearly important to be aware of the demands that will be made at the reporting stage. Thus a careful investigating team will take due note of these requirements and modify the design as necessary and ensure as the trial progresses the necessary information is accumulated.

Design features

Consider the full range of design options

Careful definition of eligibility criteria

Careful definition of endpoints

Careful monitoring for safety

Consider the ethical aspects – approval, consent and patient information

Ensure all patients are registered

Use the CONSORT checklists – to verify the key requirements are met at the design stage

Have a target journal for publication in view

8 Early Clinical Trials

Summary

Once the activity of a compound has been established in the laboratory (usually by use of experimental animals) the next stage of development is to bring this forward to man in what are often termed early phase clinical trials. A pharmacokinetic study aims to establish an effective dosing regimen for the compound in order to reach concentrations within the therapeutic window as quickly as possible, and to stay within the desired range by suitable choice of maintenance dose and dosing interval. The usual aim of Phase I trials is to determine a maximal safe dose with which more rigorous investigation of activity in a Phase II trial can be conducted. The Phase II trial, if demonstrating activity that suggests efficacy, may be the precursor to a randomised Phase III trial comparing the agent with a standard treatment for the disease or condition in question. This chapter deals with issues related to the design of such early human studies.

8.1   INTRODUCTION

As we have indicated earlier, the design of any study is the key component for obtaining a satisfactory answer to the question posed. We shall see later in Chapter 9 that careful consideration is given to the design (and sample size) aspects when considering randomised controlled trials. However, an important factor when considering the design of these Phase III trials is the information provided from earlier stage studies and trials. Consequently since the development of, for example, new therapies or medical devices, tends to progress at the clinical stage through pharmacokinetic (PK), Phase I to Phase II then to Phase III trials as in Figure 7.1 the sequential nature of this structure implies that reliable information from one step is important for the next. Poor 'experimentation' at the relevant stage can clearly jeopardise the design of the next stage and, at best, results in a waste of resource and, at worst, may compromise patient safety. Unfortunately, the evidence provided by published reports of early stage trials suggests that these have often not been well designed or well reported.

PK studies attempt to characterise the fate of a drug in the body while a Phase I trial aims to determine (often from a pre-selected range of potential doses) the dose that can be utilised at the next stage of development and so focuses on selecting the highest practicable dose. The presumption is that the greater the dose the greater the

Design of Studies for Medical Research. D. Machin and M. J. Campbell
© 2005 John Wiley & Sons Ltd. ISBN 0 470 84495 7

anti-disease effect will be. However, safety considerations dictate that the dose chosen for the subsequent trials should have an acceptable toxicity profile. Early indications of activity against the disease may be noted at the Phase I stage, but this is often incidental to the main purpose of the trial.

The objective of a Phase II trial is to assess the activity of a new drug with a view to deciding whether or not the regimen has sufficient potential efficacy to warrant further study. Thus for patients with solid tumour cancers, patients are recruited to a Phase II trial and the proportion in whom there is complete or partial tumour shrinkage (these have to be carefully defined) is determined. If this proportion is sufficiently high a randomised Phase III trial comparing this (new) treatment with the current standard for the disease in question may be recommended as the next step in the development sequence.

The two primary outcomes of toxicity and sufficient activity can be considered simultaneously in certain Phase II designs. Although in most instances Phase II trials are single-arm studies, there may be several compounds available to study as potentials for a future Phase III trial in which case a randomised comparative design may be appropriate.

Although in this chapter we use the development of a new compound as the principal example, the methods do have wider applicability, for example, testing two established compounds but combined together in a single regimen.

8.2   PHARMACOKINETIC STUDIES

AIMS

The aims of a PK study are to establish tolerability of a new compound and determine the dose to use, the appropriate route and the associated schedule. They are often extended to investigating potential interactions with other drugs likely to be used in the target population and identification of patient characteristics, such as gender, weight, ethnic group or renal function, that exert an effect on the kinetics of the drug substantial enough to warrant dose adjustment.

THERAPEUTIC WINDOW

Underlying most dosage regimens is the idea of a 'therapeutic window', which is a range within which drug concentrations should be maintained to achieve clinical benefit. Concentrations that are too low may not achieve efficacy, whereas higher levels may result in undesirable side effects. For instance, most antibiotics require a certain minimum inhibitory concentration to be sustained to maintain efficacy against a particular target organism. An effective dosing regimen should aim to reach concentrations within the therapeutic window as quickly as possible, and to stay within the desired range by suitable choices of maintenance dose and dosing interval.

For some classes of agents, it may be unlikely that there is a common therapeutic window for all patients. Indeed subject-specific factors may alter the relationship between drug concentration and effect to such a degree that the desirable concentration range may differ substantially across patients.

Example – pharmacokinetic study – telithromycin for respiratory tract infection

Bhargava, Lenfant, Perret *et al.* (2002) state that in preliminary studies in humans telithromycin has been found to be well tolerated and to possess a pharmacokinetic profile supporting a once-daily 800 mg oral dose taken in the mornings with 240 ml water. They indicate that this dose has been selected for use in Phase III clinical trials against respiratory tract infections.

COMPARTMENTAL MODELS

Underlying all PK studies is the concept of a compartmental model. Essentially these represent the body as a system of compartments that communicate reversibly with each other. A compartment is not so much a particular anatomical or physiological region, but rather a tissue or tissues with similar blood flow and drug affinity. For example, the liver and kidneys, being highly perfused organs, are often considered as being in the same compartment as the circulation. The compartments are assumed well mixed with a uniform distribution of the administered drug throughout. Figure 8.1 shows a two-compartment model to describe drug kinetics following a single intravenous (IV) bolus injection of a drug in which, following essentially instantaneous absorption of the drug into the circulation, it is assumed to distribute into the two compartments. The central compartment (V_1) represents the blood, extracellular fluid and highly perfused organs and tissues. The second (peripheral) compartment (V_2) may be thought of as other, poorly perfused, tissues. For the model of Figure 8.1, elimination of the drug is assumed to occur from the central (plasma) compartment only. The rate constants, $k_{1,0}$, $k_{1,2}$ and $k_{2,1}$, govern the kinetic transfers into and out of the relevant compartments.

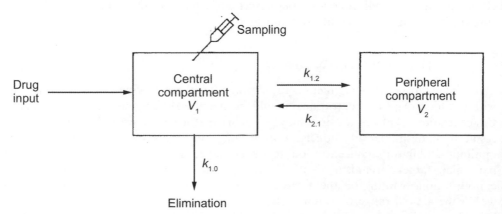

Figure 8.1 Two-compartment model to describe drug kinetics following a single intravenous bolus injection (from Mant and Allen, 2001. Early phase studies, pharmacokinetics and adverse drug interactions. In I Di Giovanna and G Hayes, *Principles of Clinical Research*. Wrightson Biomedical Publishing, Petersfield, pp 117–160. [8])

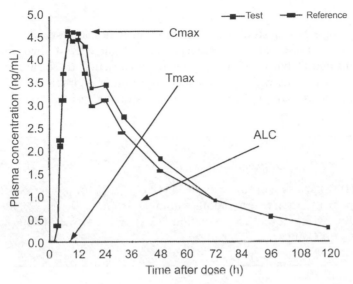

Figure 8.2 Pharmacokinetic profiles for a test and reference formulation (from Julious, 2004, Figure 4; reproduced by permission of John Wiley & Sons Ltd)

Sampling Design

A full population PK sampling design requires that blood samples should be drawn from subjects at various times (typically one to six time-points) following drug administration. The objective is to obtain multiple drug levels per patient at different times to describe the individual PK profiles. These are then averaged over all subjects studied. The number of repeated measures taken, and their location in time, will depend on the shape of the PK profile and this will depend on the type of drug under investigation.

The basic features of a PK profile are given in Figure 8.2, which plots the concentration of the drug in the plasma against the time from the dose being given. The area under this concentration/time curve, AUC, serves to measure the extent of absorption, whereas, in the case of fast-releasing formulations, the maximum concentration, C_{Maximum}, and the time of occurrence, t_{Maximum}, characterise the rate of absorption.

Example – repeated measures design – telithromycin for respiratory tract infections

Venous blood samples were taken by Bhargava, Lenfant, Perret *et al.* (2002) for telithromycin plasma level determination immediately before and at 0.5, 1, 1.5, 2, 2.5, 3, 3.5, 4, 5, 6, 8, 12, 24, 34, 48 and 58 h after medication. In this example, measures extended over a 2.5-day period but were most frequent in Day 1. Clearly the early observation points will focus on estimating C_{Maximum} and t_{Maximum}, while the later observations are crucial to establish the AUC.

Study Size

Since in these single-group studies each subject provides an estimate of $C_{Maximum}$, $t_{Maximum}$, and AUC, these can be averaged over all subjects studied for summary purposes. Julious and Debarnot (2000) state categorically that these summaries should be on the logarithmic scale, which is equivalent to quoting their geometric rather than arithmetic mean values. Sample sizes can then be estimated using equation (3.3).

***Example** – sample size – mean log $C_{Maximum}$*

Wooding (1994) gives an example of mean log $C_{Maximum}$ for a drug as 3.36 and, on the same scale, the corresponding within-subject as $SD_{Within}=0.40$. For a 95% CI of width $\omega=0.25$, equation (3.3) gives, $N = 4[0.40^2/0.25^2]\times 1.96^2 = 39.4 \approx 40$ subjects.

BIOEQUIVALENCE

In certain situations, one may wish to compare the PK profiles of different formulations of the same compound or the same compound used in different circumstances, perhaps in a paediatric as opposed to an adult population. In either case the studies may be seeking equivalence rather than superiority. Bioequivalence of different formulations of the same drug is usually taken to mean equivalence with respect to rate and extent of drug absorption. For many drug substances, a large between-subject variation is known to exist and so crossover designs are recommended for bioequivalence studies. It is usual to employ a balanced two-period design. In such a crossover trial, if a test (T) formulation is to be compared with the reference (R) formulation, then the subjects will usually be randomised equally between the sequences TR and RT.

***Example** – crossover bioequivalence study – absorption of telithromycin in healthy volunteers*

Bhargava, Lenfant, Perret et al. (2002) describe a two-period design in which 18 healthy volunteers took a single dose, 800 mg in two tablets, of telithromycin on one occasion following fasting (F) and on another occasion following a meal (M). Their summary results at each observation time are given in Figure 8.3. The object of the study was to determine whether or not the rate and extent of absorption of this antibacterial remained unaffected by food intake. Each period comprised 58 hours of post-drug observation requiring venous blood samples at 16 different time points. The wash-out period was between 6 and 8 days.

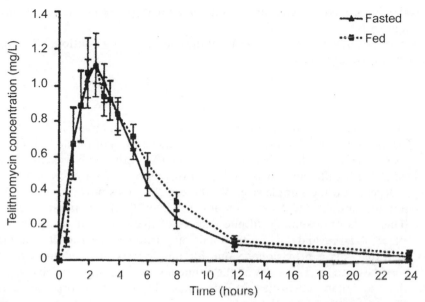

Figure 8.3 Group results from a randomised two-treatment, two-period crossover trial of the effect of food on the bioavailablity of telithromycin (from Bhargava, Lenfant, Perret *et al.*, 2002; reproduced by permission of Taylor & Francis)

Ratio of Means

As we have indicated, measures of drug absorption are plausibly log-Normally distributed and studies should focus on the ratio of the two means, $\theta = \mu_{\text{Test}}/\mu_{\text{Reference}}$, with corresponding null hypothesis H_0: $\theta = 1$, rather than their difference. Thus lower and upper bounds of bioequivalence are expressed as above and below the null hypothesis ratio of unity. Commonly used values for these are $\theta_L = 0.8$ and $\theta_U = 1.25$. On a logarithmic scale these are equidistant from log $1 = 0$, since log $0.8 = -0.22$ and log $1.25 = +0.22$. Bioequivalence is conceded if the two-sided $100(1 - 2\alpha)\%$ CI for the ratio $\mu_{\text{Test}}/\mu_{\text{Reference}}$ is completely contained within the interval (θ_L, θ_U).

Although many bioequivalence studies continue to be planned and reported with respect to a difference between means rather than by a ratio, Julious and Debarnot (2000) do not advocate this approach and so it is omitted here.

Study Size

Since bioequivalence studies are usually small, the sample-size equations require that (essentially) the Normal distribution values $z_{1-\alpha}$ and $z_{1-\beta/2}$ are replaced by those of the Student's t-distribution $t_{f, 1-\alpha}$ and $t_{f, 1-\beta/2}$ respectively, where f is the number of degrees of freedom.

Thus adapting equation (3.22) for the equivalence of two means for larger sample sizes and specifying equal group sizes, that is $\lambda = 1$, the required number of subjects, half to receive the sequence TR and half RT, is

$$N_{\text{Bioequivalence}} = \frac{2\sigma^2(t_{f,1-\alpha} + t_{f,1-\beta/2})^2}{\varepsilon^2}. \tag{8.1}$$

Here, ε is the limit for equivalence and it is assumed that $\mu_{\text{Test}} = \mu_{\text{Reference}} = \mu$ hence their ratio is equal to 1.

Equation (8.1) can be expressed in terms of the coefficient of variation, $CV = \sigma/\mu$, and if we also define $\Omega = \varepsilon/\mu$, then

$$N = \frac{2CV^2(t_{f,1-\alpha} + t_{f,1-\beta/2})^2}{\Omega^2}. \tag{8.2}$$

Now, for example, $t_{f,1-\alpha}$ besides depending on α also depends on the number of degrees of freedom, f, utilised to estimate σ in the final analysis of the design. For a two-period crossover design in which there is no period effect, if the analysis is by means of a paired t-test of the N differences observed, then there are $f = N-1$ degrees of freedom. Thus $t_{f,1-\alpha}$ depends on the sample size, N, whereas $z_{1-\alpha}$ does not.

To obtain the sample size from equation (8.1), or (8.2), an iterative process is required. This starts by assuming infinite degrees of freedom, that is, using $z_{1-\alpha}$ and $z_{1-\beta/2}$ in place of $t_{f,1-\alpha}$ and $t_{f,1-\beta/2}$ to obtain a starting value for the sample size, denoted N_{I}. From this a provisional value for the degrees of freedom is $f_{\text{I}} = N_{\text{I}} - 1$. This can then be used in Table T9 of the Student's t-distribution to give $t_{f_{\text{I}},1-\alpha}$ and $t_{f_{\text{I}},1-\beta/2}$, which are then substituted in equation (8.1). This then provides a revised estimate of the sample size, N_{II} and so $f_{\text{II}} = N_{\text{II}} - 1$. The whole process is then repeated as often as necessary until convergence.

***Example** – sample size – ratio of two means*

Wooding (1994) gives an example of defining bioequivalence on a ratio scale and gives the planning mean log C_{Maximum} as $\mu_{\text{Plan}} = 3.45$ and within-subject SD, $\sigma_{\text{Plan}} = 0.40$. Then with $\alpha = 0.1$, $\beta = 0.1$ and if we assume $\varepsilon = 0.22$, Table T1 and equation (8.1) gives

$$N_1 = \frac{2 \times 0.12^2(1.6449 + 0.8416)^2}{0.2^2} = 4.45 \approx 5.$$

From this $f_1 = 5 - 1 = 4$ and from Table T9 of Student's t-distribution, $t_{4,0.95} = 2.132$ and $t_{4,0.8} = 0.941$. Substituting these in equation (8.1) gives

$$N_{\text{II}} = \frac{2 \times 0.12^2(2.132 + 0.941)^2}{0.2^2} = 6.8 \approx 8$$

when rounded up to the next even integer. Now for $f_{\text{II}} = 8 - 1 = 7$, Table T9 gives $t_{7,0.95} = 1.895$ and $t_{7,0.8} = 0.896$. Substituting these in equation (8.1) gives

$$N_{\text{III}} = \frac{2 \times 0.12^2(1.895 + 0.896)^2}{0.2^2} = 5.6 \approx 6.$$

Repeating this process once more finally gives $N_{\text{Bioequivalence}} = 8$. This implies that $m = 4$ subjects will be randomised to one sequence and 4 to the other in the planned crossover trial.

> **Design features – PK studies**
>
> *Identify the type of subjects or patients required*
>
> *Decide on the summary characteristics of the PK profile required – C_{Maximum}, t_{Maximum}, AUC*
>
> *Consider carefully, the number and location of observations in time*
>
> *Ensure balance between experimental rigour and subject discomfort*
>
> *For bioequivalence – choose the value for equivalence on the ratio scale*
>
> *Anticipate the action to take if the full profile is not obtained in some subjects*

8.3 PHASE I TRIALS

In broad terms the aim of a Phase I trial is to establish the maximum tolerated dose (MTD) of a particular compound or treatment modality that can then be used in a subsequent Phase II trial to assess the corresponding activity. In some circumstances, the treatment under test may prove to be too toxic and so no MTD is established. In this case a Phase II trial would not be initiated for subsequent further testing. Underestimation of the MTD may lead to an apparent lack of efficacy at the later stages. Overestimation may lead to unacceptable toxicity (even death) in some patients. In either situation, a potentially useful compound may be shelved and opportunities for a therapeutic advance stalled.

THE MAXIMUM TOLERATED DOSE

For patients with a specific disease, one objective of treatment may be to reduce (or eradicate) the disease burden. However, it is recognised that any attack on the disease itself by a chemotherapeutic or other agent may bring collateral damage to normal tissue and vital organs. The usual strategy is to attempt to balance the two by establishing the concept of dose-limiting toxicity (DLT) by means of a Phase I trial. Such trials establish the dose at which DLT occurs and then step down from this dose by one step to define the MTD. The purpose is to establish the dose for use in any subsequent Phase II trial.

The level and type of DLT may be very specific to the clinical situation under investigation but should be defined before the Phase I trial commences. Once so determined, the presence or absence of such toxicity is recorded carefully when a patient receives the compound under study. However, this presumes that a first dose (say d_{Start}) has been identified for the design and that this has been given to the first patient.

Example – DLT and MTD – paediatric cancers

Shepherd, Burkes, Cormier *et al.* (1996) define the DLT as an absolute neutrophil count less than $0.5 \times 10^9/L$, or a platelet count less than $25 \times 10^9/L$, or any grade 3 non-haematological toxicity on the WHO scale. Following their Phase I trial, Estlin, Pinkerton, Lewis *et al.* (2001) recommended a MTD of $640\,mg/m^2/day$ following DLT at $768\,mg/m^2/day$ for nolatrexed dihydrochloride in children with advanced cancer.

ASSESSING TOXICITY

Since the assessment of toxicity is the key measure in these designs this must be defined very carefully indeed. This may be defined in general terms, for example, any WHO grade 3 toxicity of whatever type, or may very specific. It is very important that standard criteria are used to define the corresponding grades of toxicity. In oncology, a frequently adopted standard is set by the Common Terminology Criteria for Adverse Events (CTCAE) of the National Cancer Institute (2003).

CHOOSING THE DOSES TO INVESTIGATE

In advance of the first patient being recruited in a Phase I trial, the investigators first identify the range of doses to use and all the specific dose levels to test. Thus d_{START} will be one of these options and the ultimately identified MTD will also be one of these predefined doses. There are some difficulties with such an approach, since one is likely to start at low dose and then proceed dose-step by dose-step to successively higher doses. The choice of doses to investigate in humans will often depend on what has been observed in animal studies. These animal studies may have determined, for example, the MTD for a certain species of animal and experience has suggested that a reasonable starting dose for human studies may be one-tenth of this value. Caution (for safety reasons) may then dictate an even lower dose should be considered, but then there is concern that such low doses may be entirely innocuous and so could never be of benefit. The chances therefore of treating patients at potentially ineffective doses are clearly high. So, even with Phase I trials, there is concern that too low a dose may bring no potential benefit to the patient yet expose them to some (possibly high) risk.

Example – initial dose – cancer studies

Smith, Lee, Kantarjian *et al.* (1996) describe examples of initial doses for Phase I studies in patients with cancer as: 1/50 safe dose in mouse, 1/3 low-toxic dose in dog, 1/20 lethal dose (LD) in rat and less than 1/10 LD in mouse. It is clear that the design and conduct of the experiments leading to these recommendations are crucial.

Table 8.1 Dose-escalation methods based on the Fibonacci series and that used for a Phase I study of nolatrexed dihydrochloride conducted by Estlin, Pinkerton, Lewis *et al.* (2001). A phase I study of nolatrexed dihydrochloride in children with advanced cancer. A United Kingdom Children's Cancer Study Group Investigation. *British Journal of Cancer*, **84**, 11–18. [8]

Dose	Fibonacci ratio		Nolatrexed dihydrochloride	
	Full	'Modified'	Escalation	Dose (mg/m²/day)
d_1	1	1	1	600
d_2	2	2	**1.33**	800
d_3	1.50	1.67	1.20	960
d_4	1.67	1.50	1.17	1120
d_5	1.60	1.40	1.07	1200
d_6	1.63	1.33	1.20	1440
d_7	1.62	1.33	1.11	1600
...	...	...		
d_∞	**1.33**	**1.33**		

Once the minimum dose to investigate, d_{MINIMUM}, is determined, then attention naturally turns to establishing what might be considered the therapeutic range and the setting of the maximum dose, d_{MAXIMUM}, for the study. Once these are established then the remaing doses to study will then also be determined.

For convenience we label the k doses finally chosen as $d_1 = d_{\text{MINIMUM}}$, d_2, d_3, ..., $d_k = d_{\text{MAXIMUM}}$. However, we still need to choose k and the specific values for each of the intermediate doses between the minimum and maximum values already defined. Statistical design considerations may suggest that these should be chosen equally spaced between d_{MINIMUM} and d_{MAXIMUM} on either a linear or a logarithmic scale. The doses may depend on how the drug is 'packaged' – perhaps in tablet form or vial of a certain volume where dose choice may be limited, or in a powder or liquid more easily constituted into any dose.

However, practice has often recognised that as the dose increases in equal steps it may become sequentially more and more toxic and hence possibly dangerous for the wellbeing of the patient. This caution has then led many investigators to decrease the step sizes as the dose increases. One method uses the Fibonacci series. Fibonacci (*c.* 1180 to *c.* 1250) was an Italian mathematician who first studied the following mathematical series: $a_0 = a_1 = 1$, then from a_2 onwards $a_{n+1} = a_n + a_{n-1}$. This gives the series: 1, 1, 2, 3, 5, 8, 13, 21, 34, etc. The corresponding Fibonacci ratios of successive terms are: $1/1 = 1$, $2/1 = 2$, $3/2 = 1.5$, $5/3 = 1.667$, $8/5 = 1.600$, $13/8 = 1.625$, $21/13 = 1.615$, $34/21 = 1.619$, ..., and eventually as n gets larger and larger this approaches $1.33 = 2/(\sqrt{5} - 1)$. These ratios are shown in Table 8.1 and, for relatively small n appropriate to the number of dose levels in a Phase I study, the ratio oscillates up and down. In mathematical terminology the series of ratios is not monotonically decreasing and so in fact does not provide successively decreasing step sizes. There is no theoretical reason why this or any other mathematical series should be chosen – they are merely empirical devices.

Nevertheless, it is usually regarded as desirable that successive doses are a decreasing multiplier of the preceding dose and thus (often without a clear explanation provided) 'modified' Fibonacci multipliers like those of Table 8.1 are substituted in practice. However, it is usually pragmatic considerations that determine the modifications and no systematic rationale underlies the changes.

***Example** – Phase I trial design – nolatrexed dihydrochloride in advanced paediatric cancer*

In the Phase I study of nolatrexed dihydrochloride in children with advanced cancers conducted by Estlin, Pinkerton, Lewis *et al.* (2001) the corresponding protocol states: 'The study is designed to incorporate a minimal number of patients in order to achieve the primary aim of a Phase I study, i.e. estimation of the MTD (Korn, Midthune, Chen *et al.*, 1994). At most dose levels, three to a maximum of six patients are to be included, so formal statistical analysis is not planned'.

In fact the doses actually recommended in this protocol, which are given in Table 8.1, are not entirely uniformly decreasing in terms of the ratio of successive doses, and only the first escalation corresponds to the limiting Fibonacci ratio of 1.33. No reason for the sequence chosen is explicit in the protocol itself.

C33D

A common, sequential, design is to choose a 'low' starting dose, perhaps with $d_{START} = d_{MINIMUM}$, and a fixed number of replicates (often 3). The choice of the next dose, d_{NEXT}, then depends on the number of patients (0, 1, 2 or 3) experiencing DLT. Clearly if no patients experience DLT then the subsequent dose to investigate will be higher than that just tested. This process continues until either the stopping level of DLT is attained in the successive groups of three patients or $d_{MAXIMUM}$ has been tested.

Commencing with the lowest dose:

(a) if zero of three experience DLT, then escalate to the next higher dose level.

(b) if one of three patients experience DLT, then add three more patients at that dose level:

  (i) if zero of these three patients experience DLT (i.e. only one of six patients at the dose level), then escalate to the next higher dose level.

  (ii) if one (or more) of these three patients experience DLT, then the MTD has been exceeded; three more are then added at the previous dose level (if only three patients had been treated previously at the prior level).

Figure 8.4 Establishing the MTD in a C33D for a Phase I trial (after Smith, Bernstein, Bleyer *et al.*, 1998. Conduct of phase I trials in children with cancer. *Journal of Clinical Oncology*, **16**, 966–978. [8]

In circumstances where the first two patients both experience DLT at a particular dose, it is not usual to give the third patient this same dose but to change the dose chosen to a lower one from the pre-specified dose range. Using this type of strategy Smith, Bernstein, Bleyer *et al.* (1998) state that the MTD from a Phase I design is established by adding cohorts of three patients at each dose level, and using the rules of Figure 8.4 to determine whether dose escalation should occur. This is known as a Cumulative '3+3' Dose (C33D) approach and is one that is used by the cancer chemotherapy programme of the USA National Cancer Institute.

Although this process will (in general) establish the MTD it is only a pragmatic consideration that dictates that the Phase I trial should have tested at least six patients at d_{MTD}. This usually implies (as indicated in Figure 8.4) that once first identified, extra patients are then recruited and tested at this provisional d_{MTD} until six patients in total have experienced this dose.

Example – *DLT and MTD – nolatrexed dehydrochloride in childhood cancer*

Estlin, Pinkerton, Lewis *et al.* (2001) report on the Phase I study conducted in children with advanced cancer the design of which was described earlier in Table 8.1. The three doses actually tested are given in Table 8.2 and were not those specified in the design. At the conclusion of this study, Estlin, Pinkerton, Lewis *et al.* (2001) recommended a MTD of 640 mg/m^2/day of nolatrexed dihydrochloride. However, it is clear from their report that DLT was observed with a dose of 768 mg/m^2/day, although only four rather than six patients required of the C33D design were accumulated at the recommended MTD of 640 mg/m^2/day.

However, practical (and ethical) issues usually constrain the size of Phase I trials and a maximum size in the region of 24 (8 × 3) is often chosen. This multiple of 3 arises from the use of the C33D design. This implies that if predetermined doses are to be used, and the final dose chosen will have three extra patients tested, then $k=7$ dose options are the maximum that can be chosen for the design as $(k \times 3)+3=24$ patients.

Table 8.2 Results of Phase I study of nolatrexed dihydrochloride in childhood cancer (adapted from Estlin, Pinkerton, Lewis *et al.*, 2001. A phase I study of nolatrexed dihydrochloride in children with advanced cancer. A United Kingdom Children's Cancer Study Group Investigation. *British Journal of Cancer*, **84**, 11–18. [8])

Patient	Dose (mg/m^2/day)	Dose escalation	DLT (0=No, 1=Yes)
1, 2, 3	480		0/3
4, 5, 6, 7	640	1.33	0/4
8, 9, 10, 113	768	1.20	3/4

Storer Design

Storer (2001) describes what is essentially a modification to the C33D design by adding a stage before that design is implemented. The strategy is essentially to start the C33D process at a more informative dose than $d_{MINIMUM}$. This adjunct design suggests recruiting single individuals (rather than three) to successive doses and moving up and down the dose escalation scale according to whether or not a DLT is observed. The design moves into C33D once the current patient has not experienced a DLT *and* one previous patient has experienced DLT *and* one has not.

Limitations

The C33D design, with or without the Storer (2001) modification, has no real statistical basis, and more efficient alternatives have been sought. Efficiency here can be thought of as achieving the right MTD and with as few patients as possible. However, the design is easy to implement and requires little (statistical) manipulation – only keeping a count of the number of patients experiencing DLT at each dose tested. However, published studies appear to suggest that many variations from the basic C33D occur in practice. Indeed, Smith, Lee, Kantarjian *et al.* (1996) comment, following a review of Phase I studies conducted at the MD Anderson Cancer Center, Houston, USA, that: 'investigators sometimes entered cohorts of patients at a dose intermediate between two previously tested levels'. This clearly makes designing Phase I trials somewhat problematic but perhaps unavoidable since critically ill patients are often involved. Nevertheless, such difficulties imply that the results need to be interpreted with due caution and carefully reviewed before taking the next step in the development process.

CONTINUAL REASSESSMENT METHOD

O'Quigley, Pepe and Fisher (1990) and O'Quigley (2001) have proposed the continual reassessment method (CRM) as an alternative to C33D. This design recruits the first patient to a dose closer to the centre of the range of pre-specified doses than the $d_{MINIMUM}$ of C33D. Essentially, if DLT is observed in this first patient then the next patient (Patient 2) is given the dose below d_{START}, whereas if no DLT is observed he or she receives the dose above d_{START}. Once this second patient receives the corresponding dose, and presence or absence of DLT is observed, the subsequent dose to utilise (which may be below, at or above the dose last used) is determined. However, at any stage of this process, the results from all individual patients so far recruited are utilised to provide the basis for the choice of the dose to be tested in the next patient recruited.

Selecting the Doses

The same process of selecting the range and actual dose in the C33D design is necessary for the CRM design. In addition, however, to implement CRM it is necessary to attach to each of these doses (based on investigator opinion) the probability of patients experiencing DLT at that dose. We label these probabilities $\theta_1, \theta_2, \theta_3, \ldots, \theta_k$. This *prior* elicitation of investigator opinion about toxicity leads to CRM being termed a Bayesian design.

It is implicit in the method of selecting these probabilities that, once they are assigned, then a 'reasonable' starting dose, d_{START}, would correspond to the dose that gives a value of θ_{START} close to some 'acceptable' value. This probability is often chosen as less than 0.3 – the 0.3 arising as a less than 1 in 3 chance, the '3' coming from history associated with the use of C33D. The chosen d_{START} would not usually correspond to the extremes $d_{MINIMUM}$ or $d_{MAXIMUM}$ of the dose range cited.

Example – *selecting the doses for CRM – non-Hodgkin's lymphoma*

In the Phase I study of Flinn, Goodman, Post *et al.* (2000) summarised in Table 8.3, a dose-escalation strategy was utilised with decreasing multiples of the previous dose used. They defined minimum, $d_{MINIMUM}=40$, and maximum, $d_{MAXIMUM}=100$, doses with six $10\,mg/m^2$ steps. A CRM-based design was used and the investigator prior probabilities attached to each dose are given in Table 8.3. As might be expected, as the dose is increased the anticipated probability of DLT increases, so that with dose $40\,mg/m^2$, θ is only 0.05 (or anticipated to be seen in 1 in every 20 patients with this dose), whereas at dose $100\,mg/m^2$ θ is 0.8 (four in every five patients).

Table 8.3 DLT observed in patients with advanced non-Hodgkin's lymphoma treated with liposomal daunorubicin with constant doses of CVP (after Flinn, Goodman, Post *et al.*, 2000. A dose-finding study of liposomal daunorubicin with CVP (COP-X) in advanced NHL. *Annals of Oncology*, **13**, 11, 691–695. Oxford University Press)

Liposomal daunorubicin (mg/m²)	Dose escalation	Prior probability of DLT, θ	Number of patients recruited	Number of patients with DLT
40	—	0.05	—	—
50 (start)	1.25	0.10	4	0
60	1.20	0.20	4	1
70	1.17	0.30	3	0
80	1.14	0.50	7	2
90	1.13	0.65	2	2
100	1.11	0.80	—	—

The $d_{START}=50\,mg/m^2$ chosen corresponding to the prior probability of toxicity θ close to 0.1 and not the 0.3 we indicated as a common value to be used. A total of 20 patients were eventually included in total. Their final conclusion was that in patients with advanced non-Hodgkin's lymphoma (NHL) the MTD for liposomal daunorubicin was 70–80 mg/m².

Implementation

Although the CRM method is more efficient than the C33D design it is considerably more difficult to implement, as the (statistical) manipulation required to determine the

C33D	CRM
Requires establishing the specific doses to be used at the design stage	Requires establishing the specific doses to be used at the design stage
	Requires clinical opinion of the associated probability of toxicity at each of the chosen doses
For each patient, requires the presence of DLT to be determined	For each patient, requires presence of DLT to be determined
Dose for the next patient easily established	Requires clinical opinion of the associated probability of toxicity at each of the chosen doses
	Dose for the next patient requires detailed calculation
	Dose for the next patient uses information on all those so far included in the study
	Usually requires fewer patients
Easy to explain	Difficult to explain
Requires no specialist statistical software	Requires specialist statistical software

Figure 8.5   Basic features of the C33D and CRM designs

next dose to use is technically complex and requires specialist computer statistical software such as that of Vernier, Brown and Thall (1999). The design reduces the number of patients receiving the (very) low dose options and thereby avoids patients receiving doses at which there is little prospect of them deriving benefit. Nevertheless, the design has been criticised by Korn, Midthune, Chen *et al.* (1994) for exposing patients to the risk of receiving potentially very toxic doses. However, modifications to the original design have been proposed to overcome both these difficulties (too low or too high) by Goodman, Zahurak and Piantadosi (1995) who suggest assigning more than one patient to each dose level chosen, and only allowing escalation/de-escalation by one dose level at a time.

PRACTICALITIES

C33D or CRM

The comparative features of the C33D and CRM designs are summarised in Figure 8.5.

Small Size

It has to be recognised that Phase I trials, however carefully designed, will include relatively few patients and so the corresponding level of uncertainty with respect to the true MTD will be high. It is also recognised that the designs do not (in one sense) estimate the MTD but rather choose one of the options presented by the investigators. This implies that very careful consideration needs to be given to the dose options available within the design. Further patients are not randomised to the doses chosen for investigation.

Phase I – design and conduct issues

Clearly define patient eligibility

Clearly define the DLT

Establish the dose levels to be investigated

Choose the design, C33D or CRM

Consider the Storer option

If CRM, elicit the prior probabilities of DLT for each dose

Ensure that all patients are registered

Ensure all evaluations are made

Ensure the final report details information on all patients

8.4   PHASE II TRIALS

In contrast to Phase I trials, there are a relatively large number of alternative designs for Phase II trials. These include single-stage designs, in which a predetermined number of patients are recruited and two-stage designs, in which patients are recruited in two stages and the move to Stage 2 is consequential on the results observed in Stage 1. Multi-stage designs have been proposed, but the practicalities of having several decision points have limited their use because of the inherent further delays involved with each extra stage. Most Phase II trials are of a single-arm, non-comparative design. However, randomised Phase II selection designs, in which the objective is to select only one, the 'best', of several agents tested simultaneously, are strongly recommended in some situations.

Since most Phase II trials are single-arm experiments, Estey and Thall (2003) point out difficulties if the results are used for comparative purposes. Thus when different treatments are studied in separate single-arm trials, actual differences between response rates associated with the treatments (*treatment effects*) are confounded, as there is no randomisation to treatment, with differences between the trials (*trial effects*). Consequently an apparent treatment effect may in reality only be a trial effect.

In considering the design of a Phase II trial of a new drug, the investigators will usually have some knowledge of the activity of other drugs for the same disease. The anticipated response to the new drug is therefore compared, at the planning stage, with the observed responses to other therapies. This may lead to the investigators pre-specifying a response probability that, if the new drug does not achieve it, results in no further investigation. They might also have some idea of a response probability that, if achieved or exceeded, would certainly imply that the new drug has activity worthy of further investigation, perhaps in a Phase III randomised trial to determine efficacy.

As with Phase I designs, if a Phase II trial either fails to identify efficacy or overestimates the potential efficacy, there will be adverse consequences for the next stage of the development process.

ASSESSING RESPONSE

For a Phase I trial, the key endpoint measure is DLT as determined by pre-specified levels of toxicity and so an integral part of the design process is to define these precisely and, during the course of the trial, to carefully record their presence or absence. For Phase II studies, the endpoint is usually some measure of anti-disease activity and this translates into a measure of response. However, it is first essential to define what is meant exactly by response.

SINGLE-STAGE DESIGN

Fleming–A'Hern

Fleming (1982) proposed a single-stage procedure for Phase II trials in which a predetermined number of patients are recruited to the study and a decision about activity obtained from the number of responses observed amongst these patients alone.

In constructing the design, the investigators are asked to determine the largest response proportion as π_0 which, if true, would clearly imply that the treatment does not warrant further investigation. For example, for a new anti-tumour drug this may be set at 0.1 because the investigators are aware of 'many' alternative agents for the same tumour that have at least that level of efficacy. The investigators are then asked to judge what is the smallest response proportion, π_{New}, that would, if demonstrated, imply the treatment warrants further investigation. For a new anti-tumour drug this may be set at 0.2, but will vary from circumstance to circumstance. This choice implies that, should the response rate turn out to be larger than this, then the agent under test would be worthy of future investigation, perhaps in a Phase III comparative trial. Obviously, between these limits, one is left in a position of not knowing quite how to proceed.

Study Size

The structure implied by defining π_0 and π_{New}, means that, in the Phase II trial itself, two, *one-sided* hypotheses, are to be tested. These are that the true response rate π is either $\leqslant \pi_0$ or $\geqslant \pi_{New}$. It is then necessary to specify α, the probability of rejecting the hypothesis $\pi \leqslant \pi_0$ when it is, in fact, true. Further, one specifies β, the probability of rejecting the hypothesis $\pi \geqslant \pi_{New}$ when that is true.

For this design, Fleming (1982) gives an approximation to the sample size required but A'Hern (2001) has used more exact methods for the calculation and his table of sample sizes should be used in all circumstances.

Example – *sample size using Fleming–A'Hern Phase II design* – *whole body hyperthermia*

To illustrate the differences in Phase II trial size for the Fleming design, A'Hern (2001) uses the study of Van der Zee, van Rhoon, Wike-Hooley *et al.* (1983) as an example. This describes a Phase II trial of whole-body hyperthermia in 27 patients with various cancers. He supposed a further Phase II trial is planned but only in patients with lung adenocarcinoma in which two of the three patients with this disease had complete remission in this trial. The investigators set the lowest response probability of interest to be $\pi_0 = 0.15$ and the treatment would be developed further only if the response was greater than $\pi_{New} = 0.50$. They also require a (one-sided) test size $\alpha = 0.01$ and a power $1 - \beta = 0.9$.

Using these values in A'Hern (2001, Table 1) gives $N_{A'Hern} = 21$ with $r_{A'Hern} \geqslant 8$ responses for acceptance that the higher rate is more plausible. The approximations given by Fleming (1982) give $N_{Fleming} = 18$ and $r_{Fleming} \geqslant 7$ which suggest three fewer patients and one fewer response required. Such differences are clearly important for the design process.

TWO-STAGE DESIGN

In a single-stage design, all the patients are recruited before the response rate is calculated and the decision on level of efficacy made. Should the final response rate turn out to be low, then in a sense, the patients have been exposed to an ineffective regimen. Of course, we do not know this at the commencement of the trial but as the trial progresses interim information on activity does become available. The strategy of a two-stage design is to review this accumulating data (but not too often) so as to keep to a minimum the number of patients treated with the drug should it be ineffective. The implication, at the commencement of Stage 2, is that there is sufficient indication in Stage 1 that there is an acceptable minimum response rate that would enable (ethically) the continued use of this drug. The requirement is that a suffcient number of patients recruited to Stage 2 will be expected to obtain some benefit.

Gehan Design

In the approach suggested by Gehan (1961), a minimum requirement of efficacy π_0 is set, as with Fleming's design, but patients are recruited in two stages, that is, n_{G1} in Stage 1 and a further n_{G2} ($\geqslant 0$) in Stage 2.

Study Size

In these circumstances the probability of n_{G1} successive patients failing on the drug in Stage 1, if its efficacy is exactly that of the minimum efficacy π_0, is

$$\beta = (1 - \pi_0)^{n_{G1}}. \tag{8.3}$$

If the value of β is specified by the design, then equation (8.3) can be rearranged to give

$$n_{G1} = \frac{\log\beta}{\log(1 - \pi_0)}, \qquad (8.4)$$

as the Stage 1 sample size.

If no responses ($r_{G1}=0$) are observed in Stage 1, no patients are recruited to Stage 2. In these circumstances the estimate of π is $p_{G1}=0/n_{G1}$ or 0%. This estimate of π then has a 95% CI ranging from 0% to $[100 \times 1.96^2/(n_{G1} + 1.96^2)]\% \approx [400/(n_{G1}+4)]\%$ using the methods described by Newcombe and Altman (2000). For example, if $n_{G1}=14$ and $r_{G1}=0$, then the upper limit of the 95% CI is from 0% to 22%, implying a great deal of uncertainty with respect to the true value of π at this stage.

On the other hand, if $r_{G1} \geqslant 1$ responses are observed, then the size of the recruitment to Stage 2 depends on their actual number. Assuming that once Stage 1 is complete, r_{G1} ($\geqslant 1$) responses are observed, then the estimated response rate is $p_{G1}=r_{G1}/n_{G1}$ and a further n_{G2} patients are recruited to Stage 2. This gives a total of $N_{Gehan}=n_{G1}+n_{G2}$ patients in all. The value of n_{G2} is chosen to give a required value of the standard error, $SE(p)$ for the final estimate, p, of the true activity π, that is,

$$SE(p) = \sqrt{\frac{p(1 - p)}{n_{G1} + n_{G2}}} = \varepsilon, \qquad (8.5)$$

where ε is set by the investigating team. Rearranging equation (8.5), the required number of patients for the second stage is

$$n_{G2} = \frac{p(1 - p)}{\varepsilon^2} - n_{G1}. \qquad (8.6)$$

However, at the end of Stage 1, we do not know the final estimate p, only $p_{G1}=r_{G1}/n_{G1}$, the proportion of successes in the first stage. Thus, to estimate n_{G2} from equation (8.6), we must use p_{G1} rather than p. However, n_{G1} is usually so small that the resulting p_{G1} will be very imprecise. As a consequence, rather than using p_{G1} to replace p in equation (8.6), Gehan used π_{UL} the one-sided upper (arbitrarily chosen) 75% confidence limit for π obtained at the end of Stage 1. This gives the estimate for the Stage 2 sample size.

$$n_{G2} = \frac{\pi_{UL}(1 - \pi_{UL})}{\varepsilon^2} - n_{G1}. \qquad (8.7)$$

This depends rather critically on the number of successes r_{G1} observed in Stage 1 of the trial.

If there are r_{G2} responses in Stage 2, then $p=(r_{G1}+r_{G2})/(n_{G1}+n_{G2})$ is the final estimate of the activity of the drug based on N_{Gehan} patients.

***Example** – sample size using Gehan Phase II design – non-responsive breast cancer*

Lehnert, Mross, Schueller *et al.* (1998) used the Gehan design for a Phase II trial of the combination dexverapamil and epirubicin in patients with breast cancer. For Stage 1 they set $\pi_0=0.2$ and $\beta=0.05$, obtaining $n_{G1}=14$. Of these

14 patients, $r_{G1}=3$ responses were observed, then their requirement of $\varepsilon=0.1$ implies a further $n_{G2}=9$ patients were to be recruited. Finally a total of four (17.4%) reponses was observed from the $N_{Gehan}=n_{GI}+n_{G2}=23$ patients, the result giving a 95% CI for π from 7 to 37%.

Simon – Optimal and Mini-max Designs

As is clear, from the chosen upper limit of a 75% CI used by Gehan (1961) to determine the number of patients to enter Stage 2 of his design, rather arbitrary assumptions are made when developing statistical designs for Phase II trials. Thus Simon (1989) describes two, two-stage designs with somewhat different properties from those of Gehan. He describes a Phase II design that is 'optimal' for Stage 1, in that the sample size is minimised for that stage if the regimen has low activity. The second, or 'mini-max', design aims to minimise the maximum total (Stage 1 plus Stage 2) sample size, N.

As with the Fleming design, these designs specify the parameters π_0 and π_{New}, where again α is the probability of rejecting the hypothesis $\pi \leqslant \pi_0$ when it is in fact true and β the probability of rejecting the hypothesis $\pi \geqslant \pi_{New}$ when that is true. Simon establishes his designs by checking for every total sample size N, each possible division into two stages, those that satisfy these conditions. From these he then chooses for the 'optimal' design that which has the smallest Stage 1 sample size, and for the 'mini-max' that with the minimal total sample size. For each of these designs, the corresponding sample size for each stage is given together with the minimum number of responses required to trigger the start of Stage 2 and the total number of responses required to suggest activity.

Example – Simon's optimal design – advanced non-small-cell lung cancer

Baldini, Tibaldi, Ardizzoni *et al.* (1998) used a Simon's optimal two-stage design so as to minimise the expected number of patients to be accrued in the case of low activity, in which case, only Stage 1 would be implemented. The use of 'expected (total) number' refers to the statistical properties of the design as one does not know while planning the study if Stage 2 will, or will not, be implemented. They state, with some notational changes, in the statistical methods section of their paper: 'Sample size was calculated on the following assumptions: $\alpha=0.05$, $\beta=0.1$; π_0 (clinically uninteresting true response rate) and π_{New} (sufficiently promising true response rate), defined according to Simon, were set at 10% and 30% respectively'.

This design implied recruiting 18 patients to Stage 1 and if two or fewer responses were observed, the accrual had to be stopped. Otherwise, 17 more patients were to be accrued in Stage 2. The drug combination was considered of interest if seven or more responses were observed out of 35 evaluable patients.

Example – *Simon's mini-max design* – *metastatic nasopharyngeal cancer*

Foo, Tan, Leong *et al.* (2002) used the mini-max design of Simon (1989) for two Phase II trials that were to be conducted in parallel. In one study chemonaive patients with metastatic nasopharyngeal cancer were recruited and, in the other, those who had received previous chemotherapy for their disease. The investigators determined the design parameters, π_0 and π_{New} for each trial separately as summarised in Table 8.4, and for both studies set $\alpha = 0.05$ and $\beta = 0.2$.

Table 8.4 Simon mini-max designs utilised, and results obtained, by Foo, Tan, Leong *et al.* (2002) in patients with metastatic nasopharyngeal cancer

Previous chemo-therapy	π_0	π_{New}	n_{S1}	r_{S1}	r	n_{S2}	N_{Simon}	r_S	R (%)	95% CI for π
				Response			Total		Response rate	
No	0.1	0.3	15	2	3	10	25	6	7 (28.0)	15.9 to 44.4
Yes	0.05	0.2	13	1	7	14	27	4	13 (48.1)	33.2 to 63.4

The Stage 1 results of Table 8.4 allowed both studies to proceed to Stage 2 since $r > r_{S1}$ in both cases. However, at the close of Stage 2 for the chemonaive patients, efficacy was just claimed with a total of $R = 7$ responses observed against the requirement of $r_S = 6$. In contrast, for the previously treated group, efficacy was clearly established with $R = 13$ responses observed against the requirement of $r_S = 4$.

When deciding on which of the two Simon (1989) designs to use for a study, the design team need to balance two consequences: (1) the undesirable prospect of giving too many patients what turns out to be an ineffective drug against (2) minimising the total number of patients necessary to complete the Phase II design. Clearly, if no effective drug is available for the disease under consideration then one may not be so concerned with the first of these and would prefer to keep the overall study size to a minimum.

Tan–Machin Single- and Dual-threshold Designs

In the Phase II designs discussed, the final response rate is estimated by R/N, where R is the total number of responses from the total number of patients recruited N (whether obtained from a single- or two-stage design). This response rate, together with the corresponding 95% CI, provides the basic information for the investigators to decide if a subsequent Phase III trial is warranted. However, even after the trial is completed, as in the examples of Table 8.4, there often remains considerable uncertainty about the true value of π. Thus even for the high response rate of 48.1% observed in Table 8.4 the corresponding 95% CI is consistent with a true response rate as small as 33% and one as high as 63%, an almost twofold difference. Thus we would not be confident for the chemonaive patients that $\pi > \pi_{\text{New}} = 0.3$. Although for the previously treated patient we may be reasonably confident that $\pi > \pi_{\text{New}} = 0.2$.

One consequence of this type of uncertainty led Tan and Machin (2002) to argue that what is of key relevance to the decision as to whether to proceed to a Phase III trial, is the knowledge of the probability that the response rate, π, is greater than, for example, π_{New}. Thus in their two-stage single-threshold design (STD) the investigator first sets the target reponse rate π_{New}, (which they denote as R_U) and π_{Prior}, the anticipated value of the drug being tested. However, in place of α and β, λ_1 the required threshold probability following Stage 1 that $\pi > \pi_{\text{New}}$ and λ_2 the required threshold probability after completion of Stage 2 that $\pi > \pi_{\text{New}}$ are specified. Further, once the first stage of the trial is completed, the estimated value of λ_1, that is l_1, can be computed and, should the trial continue to Stage 2, then, on trial completion, l_2 can be computed.

Example – Tan–Machin Phase II STD design – gemcitabine in metastatic nasopharyngeal cancer

Tan, Machin, Tai *et al.* (2002) re-analysed the Phase II trial of Foo, Tan, Leong *et al.* (2002) for previously treated patients as if they had been designed by the methodology of Tan and Machin (2002). First they back-calculated from the two-stage Simon mini-max design utilised, that this choice implied for their STD values of $\lambda_1 = 0.728$ and $\lambda_2 = 0.774$ respectively. Using the actual trial data, they then compute $l_1 = 0.997$ (which is clearly greater than $\lambda_1 = 0.728$) and $l_2 = 0.999$ (which is clearly greater than $\lambda_2 = 0.774$). So had the STD been used this re-analysis suggests that, at the end of Stage 1 continuation to Stage 2 would have been appropriate. Further information at the end of Stage 2 recommended that gemcitabine was considered to have sufficient activity for Phase III evaluation.

In the two-stage dual-threshold design (DTD) of Tan and Machin (2002) the investigator first sets the target reponse rates of π_0 and π_{New} (which they denote as R_L and R_U) as with the Fleming design. They then set $\pi_{\text{Prior}} = (\pi_0 + \pi_{\text{New}})/2$ as the anticipated value of the drug being tested. Again, in place of α and β, λ_1 is now set as the required threshold probability following Stage 1 that $\pi < \pi_0$, while λ_2 remains the required threshold probability after completion of Stage 2 that $\pi > \pi_{\text{New}}$. Again, once the first stage of the trial is completed, the estimated value of λ_1, that is l_1, can be computed and should the trial continue to Stage 2 then, on its completion trial, l_2 can be computed. The latter is then used to help make the decision whether or not a Phase III trial is suggested.

Example – *Tan–Machin Phase II DTD design* – *gemcitabine in metastatic nasopharyngeal cancer*

For the chemonaive study of Foo, Tan, Leong *et al.* (2002), the actual trial data gives $l_1 = 0.01$ and $l_2 = 0.37$. These can be equivalently expressed by the probability that $\pi > \pi_0$ is $1 - l_1 = 0.99$ (1%) but the probability of being greater then π_{New} is 0.37 (37%). These together imply that the response rate is truly in the region of uncertainty, $\pi_0 \leqslant \pi \leqslant \pi_{New}$, has a high probability of 62%.

Tan and Machin (2002) suggest planning values for (λ_1, λ_2) as (0.6, 0.7), (0.6, 0.8) or (0.7, 0.8). These imply, for this trial, that Stage 2 should commence since $(l_1 = 0.99 > 0.6)$, as was indeed the case, but gemcitabine should not be recommended for a Phase III trial on the basis of the final evidence available since $l_2 = 0.37 < 0.7$.

Bryant and Day – Toxicity and Response Design

Bryant and Day (1995) point out that a common situation when considering Phase I and Phase II trials is that although the former primarily focuses on toxicity and the latter on efficacy, each in fact considers both. This provides the rationale for their Phase II design which incorporates toxicity and activity considerations. Essentially they combine the optimal two-stage Simon design for activity with a similar design for toxicity where one is looking for *acceptable* toxicity but *high* activity.

Their design implies the same, two, *one-sided* hypotheses, are to be tested as for the Fleming and Simon designs which are that the true rates π are either $\leqslant \pi_0$ or $\geqslant \pi_{New}$. But now, these values have to be set for both response and toxicity. It is then necessary to specify α_R the probability of rejecting the hypothesis $\pi_R \leqslant \pi_{R0}$ and similarly α_T for the hypothesis $\pi_T \leqslant \pi_{T0}$ when they are, in fact, true and β is set as the probability of failing to recommend a treatment that is acceptable with respect to activity and toxicity. Since both toxicity and response are assessed in the same patient, the distributions of response and toxicity are not independent, and these two are linked by means of

$$\phi = \frac{\eta_{00}\eta_{11}}{\eta_{01}\eta_{10}}. \qquad (8.8)$$

Here η_{00} is the true proportion of patients who both fail to respond and also experience unacceptable toxicity, η_{01} is the proportion of patients who fail but have acceptable toxicity, η_{10} is the proportion of patients who respond but who have unacceptable toxicity, and finally η_{11} is the proportion of patients who respond and also have acceptable toxicity. Fortunately the designs suggested by Bryant and Day (1995) turn out to be little affected by the magnitude of ϕ, and so in Table T10 levels of toxicity and activity are assumed independent, in which case $\phi = 1$. For pragmatic reasons, when selecting the designs, Bryant and Day (1995) restrict their choice to those for which the size of Stage 2 is $n_2 \leqslant 1.25\, n_1$.

Example – *Bryant–Day toxicity and response Phase II design* – *ifosfamide and vinorelbine in ovarian cancer*

González-Martín, Crespo, García-López *et al.* (2002) used the Bryant and Day two-stage design with a cutoff point for the response rate of 10% and for severe toxicity, 25%. Severe toxicity was defined as grade 3–4 non-haematological toxicity, neutropenic fever or grade 4 thrombocytopenia. They do not provide full details of how the sample size was determined but their choice of design specified a Stage 1 of 14 patients and Stage 2 a further 20 patients. In the event, in these advanced platinum-resistant ovarian cancer patients, the combination of ifosfamide and vinorelbine was evidently very toxic. Hence the trial was closed after 12 patients with an observed toxicity level above the 25% contemplated.

RANDOMISED 'SELECTION' DESIGNS

In situations where there is more than one agent available for Phase II testing and all (or at least several) of them prove to be potentially worthwhile there is a difficulty in proceeding to the Phase III stage. This is because with many options it may not be possible to test all of them against the current standard treatment for the disease in a definitive Phase III trial as the sample size then required for a multi-arm trial would be unacceptably large. Thus an alternative strategy is to first screen the new therapies in a Phase II trial, but in a design setting the aim of which is to select only one to test in Phase III. In this screen of two or more agents, patients are assigned at random to the alternatives in the Phase II trial. Such 'selection' designs have been proposed by Simon, Wittes and Ellenberg (1985), but their use is really confined to agents or combinations of agents that indicate real promise from earlier studies. This approach chooses the observed best treatment for the Phase III trial, however small the advantage over the others. The trial size is determined in such a way that if a treatment exists for which the underlying efficacy is superior to the others by a specified amount, then it will be selected with a high probability.

Trial Size

Table T11 gives the sample size requirements for randomised Phase II selection designs with binary outcomes with $g=2$, 3 and 4 groups. The improvement in response rate in one group (labelled group g for convenience) is anticipated to be at least $\delta=0.15$ or 0.20 over the remainder (termed the baseline).

Except in extreme cases, when π_i is small or large, Table T11 indicates the sample size is relatively insensitive to these baseline response rates, that is, the response rates of groups 1 through to $g-1$. Since precise knowledge of these may not be available, a conservative approach to trial design is to always use the largest sample size for each g. For example, with $\delta=0.15$ (which may result from many possibilities for the components of $\pi_{New} - \pi_i$ but all leading to the same value of δ) use the row of Table T11 giving the largest number of patients. This is the row with $\pi_i = 0.45$, $\pi_{New} = 0.60$ giving **37, 55** and **67** patients per group for $g = 2$, 3 and 4, respectively. Similarly with $\delta = 0.20$ use the row with $\pi_i = 0.40$, $\pi_{New} = 0.60$ giving **21, 31** and **38** patients per group. When randomisation is conducted, the g groups form a natural block size. For example, if four compounds are to be compared the experimental design may be configured in a way similar to Figure 4.3. In this case there would be $b = 38$ balanced blocks of size four each containing the $t = 4$ different treatments (compounds), or alternatively $b = 19$ balanced blocks of size 8, with $r = 2$ patients receiving each of the $t = 4$ treatments.

Unfortunately, with $g \geqslant 4$ groups these designs lead to relatively large randomised trials and this may limit their usefulness.

Example – *randomised Phase II design* – *non-Hodgkin's lymphoma*

Itoh, Ohtsu, Fukuda *et al.* (2002) describe a randomised two-group Phase II trial comparing dose-escalated (DE) with biweekly (dose-intensified) CHOP (DI) in newly diagnosed patients with advanced-stage aggressive non-Hodgkin's lymphoma. Their design anticipated at least a 65% complete response rate (CR) in both groups. To achieve a 90% probability of selecting the better arm when the CR rate is 15% higher in one arm than the other, at least 30 patients would be required in each arm. [The more detailed tabulations of Table T11 give 29 as opposed to 30.]

In the event, they recruited 35 patients to each arm and observed response rates with DE and DI of 51% and 60% respectively. The follow-on study, a randomised Phase III trial, compares DI CHOP with the standard CHOP regimen.

WHICH DESIGN TO USE

With such a plethora of different options for Phase II designs, it is clearly important that the investigators choose that which is best for their purpose. In some cases the choice will be reasonably clear, for example, if one has several compounds to test at the same time then the randomised selection design will be preferred to (say) a series of parallel single-arm studies. In other circumstances, the patient pool may be very limited and a key consideration will be the maximum numbers of patients that might have to be recruited. Features to guide investigators in their choice are summarised in Figure 8.6.

The essential difference beween the Tan–Machin designs and the others is that in the former the statistical design parameters are set through λ_1 and λ_2 rather than α and β.

Single-stage	No stopping rules	
Fleming–A'Hern	Sample size fixed	Size determined at the design stage
Randomised	Sample size fixed	Size determined at the design stage and depends on the number of compounds under test

Two-stage	Allow early termination	
Gehan	Maximum sample size unknown	Final sample size depends on the number of responses in Stage 1
Simon – Optimal	Maximum sample size fixed	Stage 1 sample size chosen to ensure inactive compound does not go to Stage 2
Simon – Mini-max	Maximum sample size fixed	Designed for maximum sample size to be a minimum
Tan–Machin – STD	Maximum sample size fixed	Stage 1 sample size chosen to ensure inactive compound does not go to Stage 2
Tan–Machin – DTD	Maximum sample size fixed	Designed for maximum sample size to be a minimum

Two-stage	Allow early termination	Dual endpoint
Bryant–Day – Optimal	Maximum sample size fixed	Stage 1 sample size chosen to ensure inactive or too toxic compound does not go to Stage 2

Figure 8.6   Comparative properties of alternative Phase II designs

---

Phase II – design and conduct issues

Clearly define patient eligibility

Clearly define the measures of response (and toxicity)

Choose a single- or two-stage design

Consider the importance of not proceeding to Stage 2 if activity low

Consider whether a CI or threshold probability approach is to be used for interpretation

Consider the possibility of a randomised selection design

Ensure that all patients are registered

Ensure all evaluations are made

Ensure the final report details information on all patients

8.5   PRACTICALITIES

Although PK, Phase I and Phase II studies are often of modest or even small size, the temptation to conduct these studies without due attention to detail should be resisted. In fact, these studies (imprecise though they may be) provide key information for the drug development process. It is therefore essential that they are carefully designed, painstakingly conducted and meticulously reported in full.

Although we have discussed design, care must also be taken to prepare for the unexpected to occur. Perhaps a level or type of toxicity not anticipated may occur and one should think of ways in which the basic design may have to be modified in such an eventuality.

It is also important that all patients are registered for the trial (and hence are in the trial database) and that the final report includes information on all these patients. This is particularly important if a review process of, for example, each objective response in a Phase II trial reveals that certain patients admitted to the trial either were not truly eligible, or had not received the full treatment as specified by the protocol or could not be evaluated for the endpoint. Perhaps it is unclear whether or not they had sufficient tumour shrinkage for a satisfactory response. It must be clear in the study protocol itself, and in the subsequent report of the study results, whether these 'ineligible', 'non-compliant' and 'non-evaluable' patients are or are not included in the reported response rates. This equally applies for any assessment of toxicity, whether or not toxicity is a formal endpoint for the design as it is in Phase I studies and the Bryant–Day design of Phase II.

Recruitment

One difficulty with some Phase I designs is that the results from each patient must be known before the dose for the next patient can be determined. This almost certainly implies inbuilt delays in the recruitment process and hence studies of lengthy duration. For the same reason, there may be delay between Stage 1 and Stage 2 of a two-stage Phase II design. However, continuous monitoring of the patient responses may trigger Stage 2 before the formal recruitment to Stage 1 is complete, if there are already sufficient responses. However, this may be difficult in a multicentre setting and so a formal review, once Stage 1 is complete, may be justified before embarking on Stage 2.

For both Phase I and II trials of any design, in most circumstances patient numbers, and often response rates, are quite low; so investigators should always use exact confidence interval methods when reporting their results.

8.6   TECHNICAL DETAILS

THE BINOMIAL DISTRIBUTION

In Phase II trials, the underlying reponse rate is assumed to be constant and to have probability π. If N patients are recruited to a study then $r = 0, 1, \ldots, N$ responses may be observed. The probability of r responses from N patients is given by the binomial distribution as

$$P(r) = \frac{N!}{r!(N-r)!} \pi^r (1-\pi)^{N-r}, \tag{T8.1}$$

where $r! = 1 \times 2 \times 3 \times \ldots \times (r-1) \times r$ and if $r=0$, then $r! = 0! = 1$. This distribution has mean $\mu = N\pi$ and standard deviation $\sigma = \sqrt{[N\pi(1-\pi)]}$.

In circumstances when N is reasonably large, and π is not close to 0 or to 1, this can be approximated to by a Normal distribution with the same mean, μ, and standard deviation, σ. This was the approximation used by Fleming (1982). However, in Phase II trials N may not be large and small values of π may be anticipated so A'Hern (2001) used the exact binomial probabilities themselves when tabulating the designs.

CONFIDENCE INTERVALS

If a Phase II study is conducted in N subjects and r patients respond, then the estimate of the true proportion of responses π, is given by $p = r/N$ and this has a standard error (SE) estimated by

$$SE(p) = \sqrt{\frac{p(1-p)}{N}}. \tag{T8.2}$$

The use of the Normal distribution leads to the following approximate $100(1-\alpha)\%$ CI for the true probability π as

$$p - z_{1-\alpha/2}\sqrt{\frac{p(1-p)}{N}} \quad \text{to} \quad p + z_{1-\alpha/2}\sqrt{\frac{p(1-p)}{N}}. \tag{T8.3}$$

However, as we have pointed out, when N is small, as will often be the case, and particularly if π is small (as it may be in Phase II trials), Newcombe and Altman (2000) provide exact CIs and these should replace equation (T8.3) in all circumstances.

9 Phase III Trials

Summary

This chapter deals with the main design features of randomised Phase III trials. These include the two-treatment–two-period crossover trial, parallel designs of two or more groups, and factorial designs. Contrasts are made between trials designed to detect superiority and those to demonstrate equivalence and non-inferiority. We also describe cluster trials in which the randomisation to the intervention is not made on an individual subject basis. Methods of estimating the appropriate numbers of subjects to be recruited are indicated.

9.1 INTRODUCTION

We have described how randomised Phase III trials may emerge as one consequence of a sequence of preclinical studies, Phase I and Phase II trials. Their objective is to test if the 'new' compound (or intervention) is as at least as effective as the current standard for the 'disease' in question. Alternatively, Phase III trials may evolve from questions arising in clinical practice and not from a specific development process. Thus one may wish to compare different approaches to treatment in which no drugs are involved, for example, the contrast of an entirely surgical approach to cancer treatment with a combined modality involving radiotherapy. Key components in the design of Phase III trials of whatever type are randomisation, an appropriate degree of blinding and the numbers of patients to be recruited.

Many Phase III trials have one characteristic in common and that is that the unit that is randomised (usually a patient) is the same as the unit that is analysed. However, another type of trial is one in which subjects are randomised to the alternative interventions in groups which are then termed clusters. In a two-group cluster randomised trial several (usually half) of the groups will receive one intervention and the remainder the other intervention. Thus a whole group, consisting of a number of individuals depending on the context, is assigned en bloc. Nevertheless, just as for the individually randomised situation, the outcome is measured on each individual.

9.2 CROSSOVER TRIALS

BEFORE-AND-AFTER DESIGN

The simple 'before-and-after' study is not suitable for evaluation of alternative therapies. To illustrate this, suppose a trial is planned to compare the current standard

---

Design of Studies for Medical Research. D. Machin and M. J. Campbell
© 2005 John Wiley & Sons Ltd. ISBN 0 470 84495 7

therapy (S) against a test therapy (T). Patients in Period I of the design are first recruited to S, then when a new therapy comes along all subsequent patients are switched to T during Period II of the design. Unfortunately, although the differences between the before-and-after observations may measure the effect of the intervention, any observed changes (or their apparent absence) may also be attributed to changes that are temporal in nature. Such changes may be outside the control of the investigator, so that the true benefit of the intervention cannot be estimated.

In addition, to use this kind of approach, the clinical team is unlikely to design such a trial completely prospectively. That is they are unlikely to decide at the planning stage to first recruit m patients to S then, once recruitment is complete, switch to T and recruit a further m patients. It is more likely that they will begin T with new patients and then look back in the medical records to see how patients they had treated with S had fared. Essentially the efficacy of T is then assessed by comparison with historical data on S. In these circumstances seldom can one guarantee that the eligibility criteria applied at the time the patients of this retrospective review were recruited would be the same as for the prospective component. Perhaps no consent procedures were involved for S, since it was the standard therapy and treatment was not part of a clinical trial, whereas consent would have to be obtained for T. This consent process may remove certain types of patients from the 'after' group biasing the eventual comparison in an uncertain way. It is also often the case that the follow-up data arising from the historical patient record may not be of sufficient quality of completeness, and methods of clinical assessment perhaps not as rigorous as would be demanded in a prospective clinical trial context.

TWO-TREATMENT–TWO-PERIOD DESIGN

Nevertheless, the 'before-and-after' type of approach can be adapted to form a 'crossover' trial. An example is a two-treatment–two-period trial in which the patient first receives one of the treatments, say A, then following that the other, say B. In this case, although each patient receives both of the two treatments, half receive these in the order A followed by B (AB) and half in the reverse order (BA). This eliminates, or more correctly takes account of, the temporal changes when the analysis is made.

In a two-treatment–two-period crossover trial, the randomisation is between the sequences AB and BA. In which case, the randomisation will be constrained to ensure m subjects are randomised to the sequence AB and m to BA. If the 1:1 ratio is not achieved, then the statistical properties of the crossover design are compromised.

Example – *crossover trial* – *red ginseng and erectile dysfunction*

Hong, Ji, Hong et al. (2002) describe a randomised placebo (P) controlled, two-period crossover trial of Korean red ginseng (G) in patients with erectile dysfunction. During the course of the trial, the erectile function of the men was assessed using the International Index of Erectile Function score. The trial participants and investigators were blinded to the order in which the trial medication was administered. The trial design is summarised in Figure 9.1.

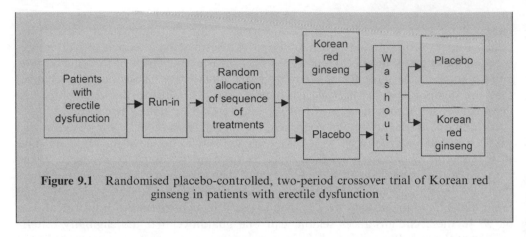

Figure 9.1 Randomised placebo-controlled, two-period crossover trial of Korean red ginseng in patients with erectile dysfunction

Typically in a two-period crossover trial, there is 'run-in' stage in which the subject receives neither treatment, followed by randomisation to one of the two sequences. Then the Period I treatment stage commences, followed in turn by a washout in which no treatment is given, then Period II starts with the second treatment of the sequence. So in the trial of Hong, Ji, Hong *et al.* (2002) there was a run-in period of 1 week, an 8-week treatment period, followed by a washout of 2 weeks' duration, and then a final 8 weeks on the other treatment.

The run-in establishes a baseline measure of erectile function, and the washout period is included to enable the level of erectile dysfunction experienced by the men to return to the same or similar levels to that experienced during the run-in period. Thus there is an implication that the patient returns to essentially the same state at the beginning of Period II as he was at the start of Period I. If this is achieved then there is no 'carry-over' effect of the treatment received in Period I into that given in Period II. That is, if the sequence *GP* is given, then any effect of *G* given in Period I will not be present in Period II when the man receives *P*. Similarly, the same principles apply to the reverse sequence *PG*.

Should the treatment that is given in Period I have a long-term effect on the condition, then this will carry over into Period II and hence affect the final comparison of *G* with *P*. As an extreme example, should the treatment of Period I cure the erectile dysfunction, then Period II treatment becomes inappropriate and the crossover design cannot be completed. At the analysis stage, a check on whether or not there is a Period effect can be made. This is done by comparing the mean of all the observations made in Period I (half made on *G* and half on *P*) with the same mean for Period II (half made on *P* and half on *G*). It is important to ensure that the between-treatment comparison (*G* v *P*) within the patient remains unaffected by anything other than the change in treatment itself and random variation.

Although verification at the analysis stage is always important, the design team should try to ensure that 'carry-over' is unlikely to be a problem in the proposed trial. Thus they should ensure a suitable washout period. If this period is too short, then carry-over is a distinct possibility; if it is too long, then the trial duration is clearly extended unnecessarily. For a drug the choice of washout interval will entail knowledge of its pharmacokinetics. In a drug trial of two active compounds, one could either have a period in which neither compound is given, which, of course would be apparent to the subject, or a period in which a placebo treatment is given. In this latter case, the subject may be blind to the start of washout and the start of Period II. In non-blind situations, one may not wish to take measurements during the washout. For any intervention, one should have some idea of how long it will take for the outcome measure to return to its baseline values. Crossover trials can be tricky to design in cases where the non-active control is a placebo. Clearly one would not expect any carry-over effect from this treatment. However, one should still have a washout period, even when this is given as the initial treatment of the sequence, in order to mimic the washout design when the active treatment is the first.

Drop-out is a major problem in crossover trials, because they require considerable cooperation from the subjects. A subject who misses the second period effectively nullifies their contribution in the first period. One way of reducing drop-out rates is to ensure the trial is as short as possible and so a balance has to be struck between this and extending the washout to ensure that Period II is free of carry-over. This also requires some knowledge of how quickly the treatments under test will affect the outcome measures as this will determine the length of each period.

The characteristics of this design, for example, the run-in and the washout periods, imply that only certain types of patients for whom active treatment can be withheld in this way are suitable for recruitment. These include chronic diseases that are relatively stable such as arthritis or asthma. In essence the associated therapies may be for symptom relief, so that when they are removed the symptoms return to baseline. Similarly the design can be used to compare medications for migraine, although in this situation the time between Period I and Period II may have to vary according to the frequency of attacks in the individual patient.

THREE OR MORE PERIODS AND/OR TREATMENTS

With some treatments there is a real possibility that one treatment will work differently when taken as a first-line treatment (Period I), compared to when being taken as a second-line (Period II) treatment. This change in efficacy is termed a 'treatment-by-period' interaction. With a two-period–two-treatment crossover trial this interaction is confounded with any carry-over effect, and so cannot be estimated separately from it. As discussed by Senn (2002), one solution is to extend the trial to three periods, using the treatment sequences AAB and BBA, so that one can estimate the carry-over for A twice (A into A, then A into B) in one sequence and B twice in the other. However, this makes strong assumptions about the size of the carry-over, in that it only extends into the next period and not beyond. In this design it is possible to test for carry-over and if it is found, then there is a problem with the interpretation. As we have indicated, it is important to understand the pharmacokinetics of the treatments involved and thereby ensure a design with no carry-over.

If there are three or more treatments to compare, then it is required to extend the numbers of periods also. Use can be made of the Latin squares of Table T4 to generate the alternative sequences.

Trial Size

For the paired design of a crossover trial one has to specify an anticipated effect size so, if the variable being measured is continuous and can be assumed to have a Normal distribution, we define this in the familiar form of $\Delta = \delta/\sigma_{\text{Within}}$. Here δ remains the anticipated difference in mean outcomes when the patients receive options A and B. However, because the design is paired, the SD rather than representing variation *between*-patients (more fully denoted σ_{Between}) is now the *within*-patient SD, σ_{Within}.

Example *– crossover trial size – red ginseng and erectile dysfunction*

The results given by Hong, Ji, Hong *et al.* (2002) allow one to back-calculate the within-subject SD of the differences between placebo and red ginseng with respect to the score for orgasmic function. This turned out to be $\sigma_{\text{Within}} \approx 3$ units. Suppose we wished to replicate this trial and choose orgasmic function as the endpoint of interest. Further it was also thought that the observed difference in this trial of $d = 5.61 - 4.92 = 0.69$ score units would be a clinically important benefit if it could be reliably established. As a consequence we set $\delta_{\text{Plan}} = 0.69$, $\sigma_{\text{Plan}} = 3$, giving a standardised effect size of $\Delta_{\text{Plan}} = \delta_{\text{Plan}}/\sigma_{\text{Plan}} = 0.69/3 \approx 0.25$. For test size $\alpha = 0.05$ and power $1 - \beta = 0.8$, equation (5.2) leads to $N_{\text{Units}} = 128$. That is, 128 men would be randomised, 64 to the sequence GP and 64 to PG.

Design features of crossover trials

Patients act as their own controls

Can be more efficient than a parallel group design – the within-patient SD is often less than the between-patient SD

Careful choice of suitable patients

Assumes symptoms return to pre-treatment values when treatment stops

Only suitable for chronic conditions such as arthritis or asthma, where treatment is palliative, not curative

Consider the length of the run-in period

Consider the length of the treatment period. This should be sufficiently long that treatment has had a chance to work, but not so long as to extend the trial duration too much

Consider the length of the washout period. This should be sufficient for the effect of treatment in the first period to wear off

Consider the extent of blinding

Randomisation is between sequences, not treatments

The within-subject *SD* quantifies the anticipated variation among measurements on the same individual, irrespective of the treatment received. It is a compound of true variation in the individual and any measurement error. The between-subject *SD* quantifies the anticipated variation between subjects.

One pragmatic way to obtain the within-subject *SD* for planning purposes is to postulate the range of values the difference within the units is likely to take, and divide this range by four. Alternatively, if an anticipated value of the between-subject *SD*, σ_{Between}, is available, then it is known that the within-subject *SD* is given by $\sigma_{\text{Within}} = \sigma_{\text{Between}} \times \sqrt{1 - \rho}$, where ρ is the autocorrelation coefficient between the values of the outcome measure on two occasions. Experience suggests that these correlations are often between 0.60 and 0.75.

The number of patients required for the crossover design is estimated by equation (5.2) but in this situation, $\lambda = 1$ is the only possible value as the 'unit', or the 'pair', is the patient observed on two occasions, once when receiving *A* and once when receiving *B*.

9.3   PARALLEL GROUPS

TWO GROUPS

The most common design for a Phase III trial is a simple two-group comparison. This design will often compare a test therapy with a standard (or control) therapy. Most often too, the patients will be assigned at random to the options on a 1:1 basis. If randomisation is not possible, then a very clear justification for this is required.

***Example** – two-group parallel design – open versus laparoscopically assisted colectomy*

Tang, Eu, Tai *et al.* (2001) describe a randomised trial of the effect of open (*O*) versus laparoscopically assisted (*L*) colectomy on systemic immunity in patients with colorectal cancer. The basic structure of their trial is given in Figure 9.2.

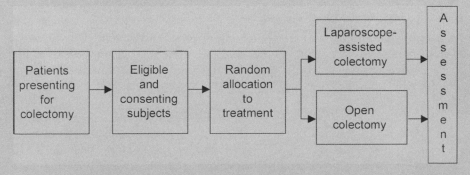

Figure 9.2   Randomised clinical trial of the effect of open versus laparoscopically assisted colectomy on systemic immunity in patients with colorectal cancer

Eligible patients were those with a clinical diagnosis of colorectal cancer based on colonoscopy or barium enema following histological confirmation, were at least 18 years of age, and were suitable for elective surgical resection by left hemicolectomy, sigmoid colectomy, anterior or abdominoperineal resection. In addition, there were several specific exclusion criteria.

A 1:1 randomised allocation was made through a central randomisation office to L or O after eligibility had been confirmed and informed consent obtained. Alternating randomised blocks of size $b=4$ and 6 were used to ensure treatment balance between the two arms after each 10 successive patients. The precise details of this were not revealed to the clinical team until after the trial was closed to patient entry.

In certain situations, there may be gain in recruiting a larger number of patients to one group than the other. For example, there may be a restricted supply of the new or test treatment, whereas the standard is more readily available. In this case, the number of patients for which the test can be given is fixed (perhaps at a relatively small number), but recruiting more than this number to the control group can increase the statistical efficiency of the design.

Trial Size

If the variable being measured is continuous and can be assumed to have a Normal distribution, then the number of subjects, m, for one group, when there are λm in the other, of an independent (non-paired) two-group trial can be estimated by equation (3.14). On the other hand, if the final endpoint is binary or a survival time, then equation (3.15) or (3.20) respectively will be used.

Example – *trial size* – *open versus laparoscopically assisted colectomy*

For the trial of Figure 9.2, Tang, Eu, Tai *et al.* (2001) state: 'It was anticipated that the T-cell number in patients having open surgery would be reduced to approximately 25 per cent of the baseline value. It was hoped that the laparoscopic approach would result in the third post-operative day T-cell counts being maintained at baseline levels or, at most, being reduced by 10 per cent'.

On this basis, for $\alpha=0.05$, power $1-\beta=0.8$, and anticipated difference in mean percentage reduction of $\delta=0.15$ (15%), assuming $SD=0.40$ and $\lambda=1$, equation (3.14) leads to $m=113$ and so $N=2m=226$ or approximately 250 patients. Were the power set to 90% then a larger trial of $N=300$ patients would be required.

In fact the trial was designed as one component of an international multicentre trial with a survival endpoint and the target of 200 patients was set from both a resource limitation point of view, and a prespecified width of the 95% CI for the secondary endpoint of reduction in T-cell counts between the treatment groups. Thus Tang, Eu, Tai *et al.* (2001) state: 'The difference in percentage reduction of 15 per cent would have a 95 per cent confidence interval (CI) of approximately 5 to 35 per cent based on a trial of 200 patients'.

Example *– trial size – chronic heart failure*

The CHARM-Added trial of McMurray, Östergren, Swedberg *et al.* (2003) randomised patients with chronic heart failure (CHF) who were being treated with ACE inhibitors to placebo or candesartan. The primary outcome was a composite event of the first of: unplanned admission to hospital for the management of worsening CHF or time to cardiovascular death. The authors state: 'The planned sample size of 2300 patients was designed to provide around 80% power to detect a 16% relative reduction in the primary outcome, assuming an annual placebo event rate of 18%'.

In the event 2548 patients were enrolled, 1272 to placebo and 1276 to candesartan. However, the report of the trial was based on 538 and 483 events respectively – far fewer than the number of patients randomised.

The above disparity is typical of trials with survival time endpoints, as the number to recruit derived from equation (3.20) is effectively the number needed to recruit 'in order to observe the required number of events'. If we can anticipate the rate at which events are likely to occur, then we can determine in advance the likely duration of the recruitment period, and the subsequent follow-up period required.

MORE THAN TWO GROUPS

Although there are many examples of clinical trials conducted on three or more groups, they do pose difficulties at the design stage in relation to trial size as more than one hypothesis is often under test. The approach to trial design will depend on the types of interventions involved and the precise comparisons intended.

Several Comparisons with Placebo

In certain situations there may be several potentially active treatments under consideration each of which it would be desirable to test against a placebo. The treatments considered may be entirely different formulations and one is merely trying to determine which, if any, are active relative to placebo rather than to make a comparison between them. In such cases a common minimum effect size to be demonstrated may be set by the clinical team for all the comparisons. Any treatment that demonstrates this minimum level would then be considered as 'efficacious' and perhaps then evaluated further in subsequent trials.

The conventional parallel group design would be to randomise these treatments and placebo (g options) equally, perhaps in blocks of size, $b=g$ or $2g$. However, Fleiss (1986, pp. 95–96) has shown that in this situation it is statistically more efficient to have a larger number of patients receiving placebo than each of the other interventions. This is because every one of the $g-1$ comparisons is made against placebo so that its effect needs to be well established. The placebo group should have $\sqrt{(g-1)}$ patients for every one patient of the other treatment options. For example, if $g=5$, then $\sqrt{(g-1)}=\sqrt{4}=2$, thus the recommended randomisation is 2:1:1:1:1 which can be conducted in blocks of size $b=6$ or 12. However, if $g=6$ for example, then $\sqrt{6}=2.45$ which is not an integer but with convenient rounding this leads to a randomisation ratio of 2.5:1:1:1:1:1 or equivalently 5:2:2:2:2:2. The options can then be randomised in blocks of size, $b=15$ or 30.

Example – *comparisons with placebo – prophylaxis following myocardial infarction*

Wallentin, Wilcox, Weaver *et al.* (2003) include in a randomised trial placebo and four doses of ximelagatran to test for its possible use for secondary prophylaxis after myocardial infarction. In this case, the aim of the trial is to establish the lowest dose which has sufficient activity of clinical relevance. Patients were randomly allocated to placebo or 24, 36, 48 and 60 mg twice daily of ximelagatran for 6 months on a 2:1:1:1:1 basis. The authors give no indication of the block size used in their trial.

Trial Size

If the variable being measured is continuous and can be assumed to have a Normal distribution then the number of subjects m, for the non-placebo treatment groups can be calculated by suitably modifying equation (3.14) by setting $\lambda=\sqrt{(g-1)}$ to give

$$m = \left(1+\frac{1}{\sqrt{g-1}}\right)\left[\frac{(z_{1-\alpha/2}+z_{1-\beta})^2}{\Delta_{\text{Plan}}^2}+\frac{z_{1-\alpha/2}^2}{8}\right], g>1. \qquad (9.1)$$

This leads to a total trial size of $N=(g-1)\times m+\sqrt{(g-1)}\times m=m[(g-1)+\sqrt{(g-1)}]$ patients.

If the endpoints are binary or are a survival time, then corresponding adjustments to equations (3.15) or (3.20) would have to be made.

Example

Suppose $g=5$, and the minimal standardised effect size of clinical interest has been set at $\Delta_{\text{Plan}}=0.5$, then with test size $\alpha=0.05$ and power, $1-\beta=0.8$, equation (9.1) gives $m=48$. This implies $\sqrt{(5-1)}\times 48=96$ would receive placebo. The total trial size of $N=(5-1)\times 48+\sqrt{4}\times 48=288$ or approximately 300 patients. This trial could then be conducted in $r=50$ replicate randomised blocks of size $b=6$ patients or with $r=25$ and $b=12$.

Dose Response

The example of comparing four doses of a single drug with placebo to determine which doses provide a minimally important clinical difference can be recast into examining a full dose-response situation. However, for Phase III trials there will be few occasions when this will be required as the doses to be used will often have been determined in an early phase of the development process.

Trial Size

If a sample size is required for a dose-response Phase III trial then, assuming the dose response is linear on some scale and the endpoint of interest is a continuous measure, equation (5.8) and the nomogram of Figure 5.2 can be utilised for this purpose.

However, sample-size calculations are often calculated from a rather pragmatic standpoint as the following example illustrates.

Example – *dose response* – *tamoxifen in inoperable hepatocellular carcinoma*

Chow, Tai, Tan *et al.* (2002) describe a randomised double-blind trial of the use of tamoxifen (TMX) in patients with inoperable hepatocellular carcinoma. The doses of TMX compared were 0 (placebo), 60 and 120 mg/d and patients were randomised to these in a double-blind manner. The outcome variable was the survival time as measured from the date of randomisation. The authors state:

> The trial was designed to compare placebo (P) with tamoxifen 120 mg/d (TMX120). To assess a possible dose response, an intermediate group of tamoxifen 60 mg/d (TMX60) was included and patients were randomized into one of 3 groups (P, TMX60, TMX120) in a ratio of 2:1:2. It was assumed that the 6-month survival rate with P would be 40% and that the minimum clinical important difference to detect with the TMX120 group was 20% greater than this value. For a 2-sided test of 5% and a power of 80%, this gave approximately 200 patients. The 3-arm trial comparing P, TMX60, and TMX120 in the ratio 2:1:2 would test the possibility of a dose response with survival and would require 250 patients. This was increased to 300 (120, 60, and 120 patients respectively) to account for a possible attrition rate.

Thus the authors gave no formal justification for the sample size for the TMX60 group but rather a pragmatic explanation. However, the intermediate dose in this design gives the potential to test for departures from linearity at the analysis stage.

In fact this trial provides a cautionary tale for those designing studies. The results are given in Figure 9.3 and were the opposite of what was anticipated! Thus at 6 months survival with TMX120 was about 20% *worse* than with placebo. Additionally, the evidence from the intermediate outcome with TMX60 suggested that the adverse outcome was not merely due to tamoxifen having an adverse effect at high doses but a possibly beneficial one at more moderate dose levels.

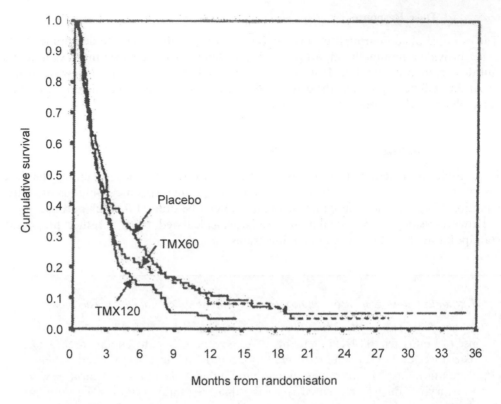

Figure 9.3 Survival in patients with inoperable hepatocellular carcinoma treated with oral tamoxifen (TMX) at 0, 60 or 120 mg per day (from Chow, Tai, Tan *et al.*, 2002. No role for high-dose tamoxifen in the treatment of inoperable hepatocellular carcinoma: an Asia-Pacific double-blind randomised controlled trial. *Hepatology*, **36**, 1221–1226. [1, 4, 7, 9, 11])

In contrast to the CHARM-Added trial conducted by McMurray, Östergren, Swedberg *et al.* (2003) in CHF, where 2300 patients were planned for in order to observe 1000 cardiovascular events in a reasonable time frame, inoperable hepatocellular carcinoma is usually fatal within a relatively short time. It was anticipated that the majority of the patients recruited would have died (median survival is only 3 months) at the time of analysis. This was indeed the case as 296 (91%) had died of the 324 patients recruited. Remarkably only three patients (less than 1%) were lost to clinical follow-up in this multinational trial.

Factorial Designs

The basic structure of factorial designs, and sample-size calculations, have been described earlier and indicate that, for example, the 2 × 2 design allows two questions to be posed simultaneously. The advantage is that the number of subjects thereby required may be as little as half the number that would be required if the two questions had been addressed in two entirely separate trials. The design may be particularly useful in circumstances where, say, factor *A* addresses a major therapeutic question, while factor *B* poses a more secondary one. For example, *A* might be the addition of a further drug to an established combination chemotherapy for a cancer while *B* may the choice of anti-emetic delivered with the drugs. However, the concern over the estimation of any interaction between the two factors remains, although its very presence could not be detected if the two questions were not posed simultaneously.

Example – 2^3 *factorial design – prevention of falls in the elderly*

Day, Fildes, Gordon *et al.* (2002) describe a 2^3 design in a trial of falls prevention in the elderly. For this trial, one factor was concerned with improving strength and balance (*S*), one with reducing home hazards (*H*) and one with assisting vision (*V*). This led to the eight combinations (**1**), (*s*), (*h*), (*v*), (*sh*), (*hv*), (*vs*) and (*vhs*). The endpoint was the time from randomisation to the time to a participant's first fall. Their results are summarised by factor in Figure 9.4.

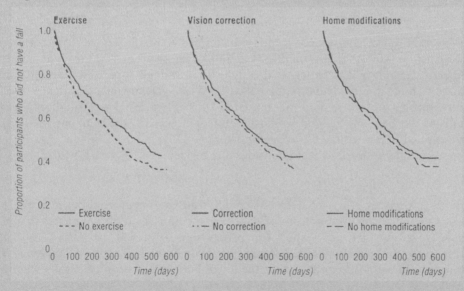

Figure 9.4   Kaplan–Meier plots showing the probability of remaining fall-free for each of three interventions separately amongst older people living in their own homes (from Day, Fildes, Gordon *et al.*, 2002. Randomised factorial trial of falls prevention among older people living in their own homes. *British Medical Journal*, **325**, 128–131. [9])

The authors concluded that although all factors contributed to the reduction in the risk of a fall, it was improving strength and balance, *S*, that was the most potent intervention tested.

Piantadosi (1997, p. 397) gives a list of some important trials that have used factorial designs of one kind or another.

EQUIVALENCE AND NON-INFERIORITY TRIALS

Equivalence

As we indicated in Chapter 3, in certain situations, a new therapy may bring certain advantages over the current standard, possibly in a reduced side-effects profile, in easier administration or in lower cost, but may not be anticipated to be better with respect to the primary efficacy variable. For example, if the treatments to compare are for an acute (but not serious) condition, then perhaps a cheaper but not so efficacious (within quite wide limits) alternative to the standard may be acceptable. However, if the condition is life-threatening then the limits of 'equivalence' would be narrow as any advantages of the new approach must not be offset by an unacceptable increase in, say, death rate.

In these circumstances, to design a trial, a level of 'therapeutic equivalence' should be defined.

Non-inferiority

One special form of equivalence trial is that termed a 'non-inferiority' trial. Here we only wish to be sure that one treatment is 'not worse than' or is 'at least as good as' another treatment; if it is better, that is fine (even though superiority would not be required to bring it into common use). All we need is to get convincing evidence that the new treatment is not worse than the standard. Thus in Figure 3.3 we would only set the boundary $-\varepsilon$, but not $+\varepsilon$, and would be quite concerned if the outcome of the trial were reflected by one of the CIs: F, G or H.

These considerations lead us to consider a one-sided $100(1-\alpha)\%$ CI for δ as

$$[Difference - z_{1-\alpha}.SE(Difference)] \text{ to } UL, \qquad (9.2)$$

where $z_{1-\alpha}$ replaces $z_{1-\alpha/2}$ of a two-sided CI, and the upper confidence limit, UL, depends on the context but not on the data. For a comparison of two means in a non-inferiority setting, $UL=\infty$, while for proportions it would be $UL=+1$. These correspond to the largest possible difference that can occur between two outcomes. The requirement for non-inferiority is that the lower limit of equation (9.2) falls wholly to the right of $-\varepsilon$.

Example – *adjuvant treatment of postmenopausal women with early breast cancer*

The ATAC Trialists' Group (2002) conducted a three-group randomised trial of anastrozole (arimidex) (***a***), tamoxifen (***t***) and the combination (***at***) in postmenopausal women with early breast cancer. The trial was designed to test

> two hypotheses. One was that that the combination (*at*) was superior to tamoxifen alone (*t*) and the second that anastrozole (*a*) was either non-inferior or superior to tamoxifen alone (*t*). This latter comparison comprises the 'equivalence' component to the trial.
> The trial report quotes:
>
> > 'Disease-free survival at 3 years was 89.4% on anastrozole and 87.4% on tamoxifen (hazard ratio 0.83 [95% CI 0.71–0.96] $p=0.8$)'. Thus with a better disease-free survival (DFS) at 3 years there was no evidence of inferiority with anastrozole as compared to tamoxifen. One can be confident of non-inferiority but this does not imply a conclusion of superiority even though the 3-year DFS rate is higher by 2.0%.

Jones, Jarvis, Lewis and Ebbutt (1996) suggest that a per protocol as well as an ITT analysis should be conducted in any equivalence trial, and a one-sided CI used in the situation when non-inferiority is to be established. Neither of these approaches appears to have been adopted by the authors.

Practicalities

As explained by Simon (2000), trials to show that two (or more) treatments are 'equivalent' to each other pose special problems in design, management and analysis. 'Proving the null hypothesis' in a significance-testing scenario is never possible. The strict interpretation when a statistically significant difference has *not* been found is that 'there is insufficient evidence to demonstrate a difference'. Small trials typically fail to detect differences between treatment groups, but this is not necessarily because no actual difference exists. Indeed it is unlikely that two different treatments will ever exert truly identical effects.

Although analysis and interpretation can be quite straightforward, the design and management of equivalence trials is often much more complex. In general, careless or inaccurate measurement, poor follow-up of patients, poor compliance with study procedures and medication all tend to bias results towards no difference between treatment groups. This implies that an ITT analysis is not likely to be appropriate since we are trying to offer evidence of equivalence; poor study design and logistical procedures may therefore actually help to hide treatment differences. In general, therefore, the quality of equivalence trials needs especially high compliance of the patients with respect to the treatment protocol.

Trial Size

Continuous Outcome

For a two-sided CI approach, the sample size per group required to demonstrate the equivalence of two means in a 1:1 randomised design based on an anticipated common mean, μ, with *SD*, σ, and level of equivalence set as $\pm\varepsilon$, is given by equation (3.22) which we repeat here for convenience. Thus

$$m_{\text{Equivalence}} = \frac{2(z_{1-\alpha} + z_{1-\beta/2})^2}{\Delta^2}, \tag{9.3}$$

where $\Delta = \varepsilon/\sigma$ is the relevant effect size.

For a non-inferiority trial, since a one-sided CI is appropriate for analysis, $\beta/2$ is replaced by β in the above equation.

Example – *home or institutional care in the elderly*

Regidor, Barrio, de la Feunte *et al.* (1999) anticipated that elderly patients following a period in hospital are likely to have a mean social functioning (SF) of about 65, with $SD \approx 25$, if assessed by the SF-36 health questionnaire. Suppose that such patients, with no potential family support, can either be discharged to their *own* home with additional home-help provided, or to institutional care. Home-care is considered the best option, and there is concern that HRQoL may be compromised in those referred for institutional care.

If the clinical team regard the two approaches to be essentially equivalent if SF-36 in the institutional care group is no more than five points below those who are discharged home, what size of non-inferiority trial is needed?

The non-inferiority value is set at $\varepsilon = 5$, $\sigma_{\text{Plan}} = 25$ and these give $\Delta_{\text{Plan}} = 5/25 = 0.2$. We then use equation (9.3) but with β replacing $\beta/2$. Thus we have from Table T1 for $\alpha = 0.1$, $z_{1-\alpha} = z_{0.9} = 1.2816$ and $\beta = 0.2$, $z_{1-\beta} = z_{0.8} = 0.8416$ also. These imply

$$m_{\text{Non-inferiority}} = \frac{2(1.2816 + 0.8416)^2}{0.2^2} = 225.4$$

or approximately 230 giving a total of $N_{\text{Non-inferiority}} = 2 \times 230 = 460$. To allow for drop-outs perhaps we would recruit 500 in all. In the trial, elderly patients would then be randomised, half to be discharged home with additional support, and half to institutional care.

Binary Outcome

The total sample size required for a trial to test for equivalence of proportions from two groups of equal size and anticipated to have the same proportion of responses, π, is

$$N_{\text{Equivalence}} = \frac{4\pi(1 - \pi)(z_{1-\alpha} + z_{1-\beta/2})^2}{\varepsilon^2}. \tag{9.4}$$

Once again for a non-inferiority trial $\beta/2$ is replaced by β in the above equation.

> **Design features of equivalence trials**
>
> *Decide on whether equivalence or non-inferiority is required*
>
> *Decide the limits for equivalence or non-inferiority*
>
> *Ensure very careful attention to detail in trial conduct especially patient compliance*
>
> *Plan for a per protocol analysis*

9.4   CLUSTER TRIALS

In certain situations, the method of delivery of the intervention prevents it being given on an individual subject basis; it can only be delivered to blocks or clusters of individuals. For example, if a public health campaign conducted via the local media is to be tested, it may be possible to randomise locations to either receive or not the planned campaign. It would not be possible, however, to randomise individuals to receive or not the subsequent public health intervention.

A further situation where cluster designs are useful is where there is a possibility of 'contamination' in the delivery of the intervention itself. For example, in a trial to investigate if training in 'patient-centred' consultation procedures is useful, half the primary care physicians participating might receive the 'training', T, whereas the other half would not. Instead they would rely on their standard practice, S. Clearly, if instead patients were randomised to receive either S or T consultations from their own doctor all doctors would have to be trained. It would then be very difficult for the doctor to switch 'on and off' between patients, as the randomisation would demand, and so contamination would occur. Any differences in the effect of the two interventions would then become diluted. Thus a cluster design, where the doctor provides only one of T or S, ensures that the trial is free of this contamination.

> *Example* – *cluster design* – *treatment of menorrhagia*
>
> Fender, Prentice, Gorst *et al.* (1999) use a cross-sectional design in the Anglia Menorrhagia Education Study (AMES) trial in which 348 doctors from 100 practices in primary care were recruited and 54 randomised to intervention, 46 to control. The intervention, an educational package describing the appropriate treatment of menorrhagia, was designed with the objective to reduce the number of referrals to hospital. The package was given to small practice-based groups. In the year post randomisation, the number of patients referred by the intervention group was 20% compared to 29% in the control group suggesting the desired effect of the package.

In these trials, observations made on the individual subjects are used to assess the effectiveness of an intervention although the intervention itself is aimed at health care professionals. Here the interventions only indirectly affect the patients.

INTRA-CLASS CORRELATION

Despite the lack of individualised randomisation, and the receipt of a more group-based intervention, the assessment of the effect is made at the individual subject level. As a consequence of the clustering, an important feature of cluster-randomised trials is that variables measured on the patients within a cluster are not completely independent. Thus patients treated by one health care professional tend to be more similar amongst themselves than those treated by a different health care professional. So, if we know which doctor is treating a patient, we can predict, by reference to experience with other patients, slightly better than by chance, the outcome for the patient concerned. Consequently the patient outcomes for one doctor are positively correlated and so are not completely independent of each other. Due note of the magnitude of this correlation is required in the design process.

The strength of the dependence amongst observations made within a particular cluster is measured by the intra-cluster correlation (ICC) which we define in Section 9.5.

Example – ICC – primary care practices in England

Campbell (2000) quotes the ICCs from the Health Check Study in which nine primary care practices were chosen in the north and nine in the south of England. The values of the within-region ICC given in Table 9.1 are small, although somewhat increased when adjusted for smoking levels in the practices, suggesting that patients of the clusters are relatively homogeneous. However, once calculated across all 18 practices in the two regions, the ICC is more than doubled.

In general, the more heterogeneity there is between the clusters, the greater the ICC as this inflates the between clusters SD, $\sigma_{Between}$ (see equation T9.2) leading to the higher value.

Table 9.1 Intra-class correlations (ICC) calculated from primary care practices in the north and in the south of England (after Campbell, 2000; reproduced by permission of Hodder Arnold)

Adjusted for smoking levels	England		All
	North	South	
Number of clusters	9	9	18
No	0.004	0.008	0.021
Yes	0.008	0.025	0.011

Ukoumunne, Gulliford, Chinn *et al.* (1999) have shown that a common value of an ICC is around 0.05 although this value is somewhat larger than those of Table 9.1. One method of reducing the effect of between cluster variation is to have a design with pair-matched clusters chosen on the basis of their characteristics before randomisation. In the above example, that may involve pairing each primary care practice from an urban setting with another from a similar setting, and each rural practice with another.

In general, cluster trials will compare $g=2$ or more interventions and will involve c clusters, a fraction of which, often $1/g$, will receive one of the interventions, each cluster comprising k subjects. Design options include the choice of c and k, both of which may include non-statistical considerations in their choice, perhaps determined by the number of clusters willing to participate, and the practical limitations for the number of subjects recruited per cluster.

RANDOMISATION

In carrying out randomisation, the clusters are decided in advance and then randomised before the intervention is applied. However, the subjects from these clusters who are eventually involved may be patients, for example, incident cases of diabetes or depression who are not themselves identified at the time of randomisation. Thus one cannot rely on randomisation to balance, in the alternative intervention groups, the known and unknown factors associated with prognosis as one would if the patients had been individually randomised to the intervention options. Thus the purpose of randomisation in cluster trials is to try and balance confounding factors associated with the *cluster*. Since the number of clusters is inevitably limited, the scope for randomisation to achieve balance is also limited. Of course as the number of clusters increases we would expect cluster unit characteristics, on average, to balance, and so patient characteristics should also balance as a consequence. Thompson, Pyke and Hardy (1997) used a pair-matched design for the Family Heart Study in which primary care practices were matched, before randomisation, to improve balance of prognostic factors.

PRACTICAL ISSUES

Optimising Delivery

Many cluster design trials involve behaviour change amongst patients, which can be very difficult to achieve. Unfortunately, the educational packages used in such trials often lack modern psychological insight into facilitating change. Indeed many education-type trials in primary care go straight into Phase III with a package that is not extensively tested beforehand to try and optimise its delivery. This contrasts with conventional pharmaceutical trials that go through a number of early phases; only after extensive testing does a company embark on Phase III trial to make a direct comparison with current practice. Advice on the design of trials to evaluate complex interventions has been given by the Medical Research Council (2002).

Baseline Data

Although baseline measures are usually to be recommended, in intervention trials it is likely that measuring or assessing people at baseline may change their future response as the act of measuring at baseline may prime subjects to be more receptive of the intervention that follows. In this way, the baseline measurement becomes part of the intervention package. If, after the trial is completed and the intervention is shown to be effective, it is then used omitting the baseline measurements as would be the usual case, it may become less effective than had been anticipated. Thus in planning studies, the improvement in efficiency gained by baseline variables should be weighed against the associated increased cost and their potential effect on the interventions planned.

Motivation

If a training intervention is planned which affects the health care professionals, there can be severe problems in recruiting and maintaining enthusiasm amongst the control groups. After all, they are health care professionals who were recruited because of their interest in the particular disease or condition and in obtaining training. Therefore if they are then told, following randomisation, that they are not to get the intervention, they may either seek training elsewhere and/or drop out from participation in the trial. In these circumstances, a useful stratagem is to offer the intervention to the control group once the trial itself is complete. Thus Thompson, Kinmonth, Stevens et al. (2000), as part of the Hampshire Depression Project, offered training to the general practitioners allocated the control arm but one year later than in those of the intervention arm. In this case, it was felt that a one-year trial would be sufficient time to measure the intervention effect.

Cluster Size

For practical reasons, a cluster-randomised trial will often have a preset duration and so the numbers of subjects per cluster cannot be fixed in advance. Consequently there can be considerable differences in the number of subjects recruited per cluster. This leads to problems at the analysis stage. If the condition under study is relatively rare, and some clusters are small, there is a real possibility that in some clusters no patients will be recruited. This possibility needs to be considered at the design stage, since it can adversely affect the ability of the trial to detect differences between the interventions involved.

Trial Size

With cluster trials there are two further sample-size issues. One is how many clusters should be involved and the other is, for each cluster, how many patients should be recruited. The sample-size calculation process begins by assuming the trial is to be an *individually* randomised trial for a given effect size, significance level and power. Thus, depending on the type of endpoint, continuous, binary or survival, the number of subjects required per intervention group, $m_{Individual}$, is obtained from equations (3.14), (3.15) or (3.20).

However, the sample size, $m_{Individual}$, is then inflated to give that appropriate for the *cluster* design. The inflation required to the individual-based sample-size calculation is termed the design effect (*DE*). This is given by

$$DE = 1 + (k - 1)\rho_{Cluster}, \qquad (9.5)$$

where k is the anticipated number of subjects per cluster and $\rho_{Cluster}$ the ICC.

From this the total number of patients required in each intervention group, comprising c clusters of size k subjects, of the trial is

$$m_{Cluster} = m_{Individual} \times DE \qquad (9.6)$$

If for a g-group trial, the total number of clusters, c, is fixed, Campbell (2000) shows that the number of patients per cluster, k, for a cluster-randomised trial with ICC$=\rho_{Cluster}$ is given by

$$k = \frac{m_{Individual}(1 - \rho_{Cluster})}{(c/g) - m_{Individual}\rho_{Cluster}}. \qquad (9.7)$$

The number of patients per cluster increases rapidly as $m_{Individual}\rho_{Cluster}$ approaches c/g, although Donner and Klar (2000) noted that it is seldom worth having more than about $k=60$ individuals per cluster.

Example   trial size – cholesterol levels

The Family Heart Study Group (1994) give the intra-primary care practice correlation for serum cholesterol as about 0.02. Suppose an investigator wishes to design a cluster-randomised trial involving 50 practices and wishes to detect a relatively modest reduction in mean serum cholesterol equivalent to a standardised effect size of 0.3 by an intervention based on an educational package.

Assuming a two-sided test size $\alpha=0.05$ and power $1-\beta=0.8$, then equation (3.12) gives $m_{Individual}=176$. Assuming a 1:1 randomisation of 'intervention' or 'no intervention' to practices, then with $c/g=50/2=25$ practices involved per group and $\rho_{Cluster}=0.02$,

$$k = \frac{176(1 - 0.02)}{[25 - (0.02 \times 176)]} = 8.02$$

or eight subjects per practice. This compares with $m_{Individual}/25=176/25=7.04$ or seven subjects. Thus the number of subjects involved with the cluster-randomised design will be $N_{Cluster}=c \times k=50 \times 8=400$, compared to the somewhat fewer $N_{Individual}=50 \times 7=350$.

In reality, it might be that $k=8$ is the planned *average* number of subjects per cluster. If there is likely to be considerable variation around this figure, then the sample size may need to be adjusted upwards to account for this heterogeneity. A cautious approach may then recommend this is further increased by 10% to give an average of nine subjects per practice.

> **Design features of cluster trials**
>
> *Randomise clusters, not individual patients*
>
> *Need to choose the number of clusters as well as number of patients per cluster*
>
> *Consider the potential variation in the number of subjects per cluster that may be recruited*
>
> *Often all clusters are available at the start of the trial and randomisation is carried out only once*
>
> *Stratifying by cluster size is important*
>
> *Interventions are often complex, and should be thoroughly developed before the trial starts*

9.5   TECHNICAL DETAIL

INTRA-CLASS CORRELATION

In the model for a cluster design comparing two interventions, equation (1.1) has to be modified in several ways to take note of the different clusters involved. The model for a subject in cluster i is

$$y_i = \beta_0 + \beta_1 \tau + \alpha_i + \varepsilon. \tag{T9.1}$$

The coefficients β_0 and β_1 have the same interpretation as in equation (1.1) and $\tau=0$ for one intervention, and $\tau=1$ for the other. In addition, α_i is the effect for cluster i and is assumed random with the *between*-clusters *SD* of σ_{Between}. This is similar to the situation described in discussing compound symmetry in equation (T5.1). The error term ε is assumed to be random with mean 0, but with a *within*-clusters *SD*, σ_{Within}.

The strength of the dependence amongst observations made within a particular cluster is measured by the intra-cluster correlation (ICC). This is given by

$$\rho_{\text{Cluster}} = \frac{\sigma^2_{\text{Between}}}{\sigma^2_{\text{Within}} + \sigma^2_{\text{Between}}}. \tag{T9.2}$$

This equation has similar form to that of equation (T5.2). In general as σ_{Between} increases ρ_{Cluster} increases.

10 Diagnosis

Summary

An important part of the process of examining a patient is to check clinical measures taken from the patient against a 'normal' or 'reference' range of values. Evidence of the measure lying outside these values may be taken as indicative of a particular diagnosis. In this chapter we describe the methods for establishing reference intervals and a related problem for receiver operating curves in distinguishing diseased from non-diseased subjects. We also describe the design of agreement studies, with respect to the degree of self-reproducibility of a single observer, and the strength of two-observer or more, agreement.

10.1 INTRODUCTION

When a physician is in the process of establishing a diagnosis in a patient who presents with particular symptoms, the patient may be subjected to a series of tests, the results from which may then suggest an appropriate course of action. For example, a patient complaining of not feeling well may be tested for the presence of a bacterium in their urine. On the basis of the reading obtained the patient may then be classified as infected. It is this infection that is then presumed to be the cause of 'not feeling well'. The object of treatment will then be to remove this infection in the expectation that this will then alleviate the presenting symptoms.

In other circumstances a patient may be referred to a specialist centre for further examination and diagnosis. Thus in patients suspected of liver cancer it is routine to take blood samples from which their α-fetoprotein (AFP) levels are determined. A high level is indicative of liver cancer although further and more detailed examination may be required to confirm the eventual diagnosis. The judgement as to whether or not a particular patient has a high AFP is made by comparison with individuals whose AFP has also been measured but are known to be free of the disease in question. In most circumstances, the range of values of AFP in patients who do indeed have liver cancer will overlap with healthy subjects who are free of the disease. In view of this overlap, and to help distinguish the diseased from the non-diseased, receiver operating curves (ROC) are constructed to help determine the best cut-point value for diagnosis.

In many situations, once a specimen is collected from a patient for diagnosis, an assessment is made as to whether or not this indicates the presence of the disease in

---

Design of Studies for Medical Research. D. Machin and M. J. Campbell
© 2005 John Wiley & Sons Ltd. ISBN 0 470 84495 7

question. This process may involve some subjectivity on the assessor's part, so after appropriate training perhaps, one may wish to measure the assessor's reproducibility. In much the same scenario there may be more than one assessor responsible for reviewing patient material, in which case one would like to be sure that they are in broad agreement in their decisions. Thus for the same specimen, readers may not agree, and there remains a possibility that if each reviewed the material again that their decisions may not be the same. In both instances, if there were substantial disagreement, then this would raise concern with respect to the diagnostic processes involved.

10.2   REFERENCE INTERVALS

The objective of a study to establish a normal range or reference interval (RI) is to define the interval for a particular clinical measurement within which the majority of values, often 95%, of a defined population will lie. Individuals subsequently found to be outside these limits may be thought to require medical intervention in some way.

CHOOSING THE SUBJECTS

Samples are taken from populations to provide estimates of population parameters; in our situation the cut-point(s) of the RI. The purpose of summarising the behaviour of a particular group is usually to draw some inference about a wider population of which the group is a sample. Thus, although a group of volunteers are investigated, the object is to represent the RI of the general population as a whole, which will include the healthy and those who are not. As a consequence, it is clearly important that the 'volunteers' are chosen carefully so that they do indeed reflect the population as a whole and not a particular subset of that population. If the 'volunteers' are selected at random from the population of interest then the calculated RI will be an estimate of the true RI of the population. If they are not, then it is no longer clear what the RI represents and at worst it may not be appropriate for clinical use.

NORMAL DISTRIBUTION

If the variable that has been measured has a Normal distribution form, then the data x_1, $x_2, \ldots, x_N$ from the N subjects can be summarised by the sample mean, $\bar{x}$, and sample SD, s. These provide estimates of the associated population mean, μ, and SD, σ, respectively.

In this situation, the $100(1-\alpha)\%$ RI is estimated by

$$\bar{x} - z_{1-\alpha/2}s \qquad \text{to} \qquad \bar{x} + z_{1-\alpha/2}s. \tag{10.1}$$

Often a 95% RI is required, in which case $\alpha=0.05$ and from Table T1, $z_{1-\alpha/2} = z_{0.975} = 1.9600$.

If we denote the cut-points of the lower and upper limits of this RI as R_{Lower} and R_{Upper}, then its width is

$$W_{\text{Reference}} = R_{\text{Upper}} - R_{\text{Lower}} = 2z_{1-\alpha/2}s. \tag{10.2}$$

Example – reference interval – myocardial iron deposition

Anderson, Holden, Davis *et al.* (2001) established normal ranges for T2-star (T2*) values in the heart. T2* is a magnetic resonance technique which can quantify myocardial iron deposition, the levels of which indicate the need for ventricular dysfunction treatment. They quote a 95% normal range for T2* as 36 to 68 ms obtained from 15 healthy volunteers (9 males, 6 females, aged 26–39).

They also quote RIs given by Li, Dhawale, Rubin *et al.* (1996) as 26.5 to 39.5 ms based on 13 normal subjects; Wacker, Bock, Hartlep *et al.* (1999) as 39 to 57 ms from six patients with coronary disease; and by Reeder, Faranesh, Boxerman *et al.* (1998) as 32 to 44 ms in the mid-septum in five volunteers. These RIs are determined from very few subjects and are very variable in the range of T2* values they cover and in their location, as well as in their width.

Study Size

A key property of any RI is the precision with which the cut-points are estimated. Thus of particular relevance to design are the width of the CIs for the estimated cut-points R_{Lower} and R_{Upper}. Harris and Boyd (1995) state that if the sample is large ($N > 100$) then the standard error (SE) of these cut-points is

$$SE(R_{Lower} = SE(R_{Upper} = \sigma\sqrt{(3/N)} = 1.7321\sigma/\sqrt{N}. \tag{10.3}$$

Thus the approximate $100(1-\gamma)\%$ CI for the true R_{Lower} is

$$R_{Lower} - z_{1-\gamma/2} \times \frac{1.7321s}{\sqrt{N}} \quad \text{to} \quad R_{Lower} + z_{1-\gamma/2} \times \frac{1.7321s}{\sqrt{N}}, \tag{10.4}$$

and there is a similar expression for R_{Upper}. The width of these CIs is

$$W_{Cut} = 2 \times z_{1-\gamma/2} \times \frac{1.7321s}{\sqrt{N}}. \tag{10.5}$$

One design criterion for determining an appropriate study size to establish an RI is to fix a value for the ratio of W_{Cut} to $W_{Reference}$. The design therefore sets $\rho = W_{Cut}/W_{Reference}$ to some pre-specified value. In this case it follows, from dividing equation (10.5) by (10.2) and rearranging, that the sample size is estimated by

$$N = 3 \left[\frac{z_{1-\gamma/2}}{\rho z_{1-\alpha/2}} \right]^2. \tag{10.6}$$

For the particular case when we choose α and γ to have the same value, equation (10.6) simplifies to

$$N = 3/\rho^2. \tag{10.7}$$

Practical values for ρ suggested by Linnet (1987) range from 0.1 to 0.3. Table T12 gives N for different α, γ and ρ. From both equation (10.7) and the table one can see that as ρ

decreases from 0.3 to 0.1 the corresponding value of N increases quite dramatically, so that a relatively large study is required.

Example – *sample size* – *myocardial iron deposition*

We presume that we are planning to estimate the 95% RI for myocardial T2* and we have the study of Anderson, Holden, Davis *et al.* (2001) available. From their study, $W_{Reference} = 68 - 36 = 32$ ms and we intend to quote a 90% CI for the cut-point(s) so determined. With $\alpha = 0.05$, $\gamma = 0.10$ Table T1 gives $z_{0.975} = 1.9600$ and $z_{0.95} = 1.6449$; then use of equation (10.6) with $\rho_{Plan} = 0.1$ giving $N = 3 \times [1.6449/(0.1 \times 1.9600)]^2 \approx 210$. Direct entry into T12 with $\alpha = 0.05$, $\gamma = 0.10$ and $\rho_{Plan} = 0.1$ gives $N = 211$ subjects. Had $\rho_{Plan} = 0.2$ been chosen, then $N \approx 53$ subjects are required.

These estimates of study size contrast markedly with the 15 volunteers used by Anderson, Holden, Davis *et al.* (2001). In terms of the design criteria we have introduced here, their study corresponds to the use of $\rho_{Plan} \approx 0.4$, which is outside the range recommended by Linnet (1987).

NON-NORMAL SITUATION

If the data do not have a Normal distribution then in some circumstances an algebraic transformation of the data may have to be made. The only sensible transformation is a logarithmic one. In which case, the RI for $y = \log x$ will take the form of equation (10.1) but with y replacing x in the calculation of the mean and *SD*. Further the sample size can still be estimated by equations (10.6) and (10.7). However, the corresponding RI on the x-scale is then obtained from the antilogarithms of the lower and upper limits of this range. That is the reference range for x is

$$\exp(\bar{y} - z_{1-\alpha/2}s_y) \qquad \text{to} \qquad \exp(\bar{y} + z_{1-\alpha/2}s_y). \tag{10.8}$$

If the data cannot be transformed to the Normal distribution form, then an RI can still be calculated. In this case, the data $x_1, x_2, \ldots, x_N$ are first ranked from largest to smallest. These are labelled $x_{(1)}, x_{(2)}, \ldots, x_{(j)}, \ldots, x_{(N)}$. The lower limit of the $100(1 - \alpha)\%$ reference range is then $x_{(j)}$, where $j = N\alpha/2$ (interpolating between adjacent observations if $N\alpha/2$ is not an integer). Similarly the upper limit is the observation corresponding to $j = N(1 - \alpha/2)$. These limits provide what is often known as the *empirical* normal range.

Campbell and Gardner (2000) define the ranks of the lower and upper limits of a $100(1 - \gamma)\%$ CI for any quantile q, as

$$r_q = Nq - [z_{1-\gamma/2} \times \sqrt{Nq(1 - q)}]$$

and   (10.9)

$$s_q = 1 + Nq + [z_{1-\gamma/2} \times \sqrt{Nq(1 - q)}].$$

These values are then rounded to the nearest integer. These integers provide the r_qth and s_qth observations in this ranking and hence the relevant lower and upper confidence limits. To determine those for R_{Lower}, one sets $q = \alpha/2$ in equation (10.9) and for R_{Upper}, $q = 1 - (\alpha/2)$ is used.

However, these are the *ranks* of the observed values corresponding to R_{Lower} and R_{Upper}, not the values themselves. Hence there is no equivalent algebraic form to W_{Cut} of equation (10.5) in this case. However, we can obtain an approximation to their *SE*. This is provided for by the *SE* which is appropriate for quantiles estimated using ranks *but* assuming these ranks had arisen from data having a Normal distribution form. This gives, in place of equation (10.3),

$$SE(R_{\text{Lower}}) = SE(R_{\text{Upper}}) = \frac{\sigma}{\sqrt{N}} \sqrt{\frac{(\gamma/2)[1 - (\gamma/2)]}{\phi_{1-\gamma/2}^2}} = \eta \frac{\sigma}{\sqrt{N}}. \tag{10.10}$$

Here

$$\phi_{1-\gamma/2} = \frac{1}{\sqrt{2\pi}} \exp\left(-\frac{z_{1-\gamma/2}^2}{2}\right)$$

is the height of the Normal distribution at $z_{1-\gamma/2}$. Values of η, for different values of γ, are given in Table T13. For example, when $\gamma = 0.05$, $z_{0.975} = 1.9600$, then direct calculation or use of Table T13 gives $\eta = 2.6713$. This multiplier, 2.6713, is larger than that, $\sqrt{3} = 1.7321$, of equation (10.3).

Thus an approximation to the $100(1-\gamma)\%$ CI for the true R_{Lower} of the $100(1-\alpha)\%$ RI is

$$R_{\text{Lower}} - z_{1-\gamma/2} \times \eta \frac{\sigma}{\sqrt{N}} \quad \text{to} \quad R_{\text{Lower}} + z_{1-\gamma/2} \times \eta \frac{\sigma}{\sqrt{N}}. \tag{10.11}$$

This CI has width

$$W_{\text{CI}} = 2 \times \eta \times z_{1-\gamma/2} \times \frac{\sigma}{\sqrt{N}}. \tag{10.12}$$

Study Size

One method to determine the sample size would be first to use equation (10.6) to give N_{Initial} and then inflate this by use of η to obtain $N_{\text{Final}} = \eta\, N_{\text{Initial}}/\sqrt{3}$. This will lead to a larger study size to establish an RI than those given in Table T12 for the Normal distribution case by a factor of $\eta/\sqrt{3} \geq 1$. This illustrates why, if at all possible, transforming the scale of measurement to one that is approximately Normal in distribution is very desirable.

Example – *sample size for an empirical normal range – myocardial iron deposition*

Suppose we presume in estimating the numbers of subjects required for a 95% RI for myocardial T2* we did not have a Normal distribution. The earlier calculations using Table T12 with $\alpha=0.05$, $\gamma=0.10$, $\rho_{Plan}=0.1$ gave $N_{Initial}=211$. Then with $\gamma=0.10$ the last column of Table T13 gives $\eta\sqrt{3}=1.22$. The planned study size for the RI determination is $N_{Final}=1.22\times211=258$ or approximately 260 individuals.

Design features – reference intervals

Careful selection of volunteers

Are measures used on volunteers the same as those to be used on patients and made in the same manner?

Are strata required: male–female; young–old?

10.3   RECEIVER OPERATING CURVES

In the process of making a diagnosis for a particular patient, a clinician establishes a set of diagnostic alternatives or hypotheses. The clinician then attempts to reduce these by progressively ruling out specific diseases and in the process initiates tests both to exclude certain diagnoses and to confirm the presence of the disease which is indeed present. For a particular diagnosis, a good diagnostic test should indicate clearly either that the disease is very unlikely or that it is very probable.

REFERENCE TEST

There clearly has to be a process by which patients who present with a particular set of symptoms become ultimately, and ideally unambiguously, diagnosed or deemed free of the disease in question. Thus, for example, a patient may be suspected to have a particular type of cancer, but only once surgery is undertaken and the tumour removed can one unequivocally say that it is a cancer of a particular type. In this case the reference test is the combined surgical and post-surgical processes in coming to this final diagnosis.

The reference test is usually the currently accepted best available and feasible diagnostic test to determine the presence or absence of the disease in question.

Clearly when evaluating the potential of a new diagnostic test, the person who performs the reference test should be 'blind' to the results of the diagnostic test and vice versa. This is especially so if the tests involve some degree of subjectivity in their interpretation. This is often the case with a pathological specimen, although seemingly objective laboratory measures may not be free of all subjectivity as might often be claimed.

DESIGN OPTIONS

Cases (Diseased) and Controls (Healthy)

One design to establish a diagnostic test takes values of the measurement of interest from subjects (controls) who are known to be free of the disease and in patients known to have the disease in question. However, this design does not reflect the clinical situation in which tests will be applied. Essentially this process takes two groups, one from each end of the disease spectrum, and omits the intermediate when making comparisons. This creates an artificial gap in test values between those categorised as healthy and those diseased and so exaggerates the value of the diagnostic test. Thus this design is not recommended.

Consecutive Patients

As de Vet, van der Weijden, Muris *et al.* (2001) point out, in clinical practice diagnostic tests are never used in healthy persons but only in groups for which the diagnostic test is indicated, including patients with the disease present in various levels of severity. So the best approach to evaluate the diagnostic accuracy of a test is to use a sample of consecutive patients for whom the test is indicated. A careful description of the eligibility characteristics of this group needs to be provided. These patients will undergo the new diagnostic test and also those for the reference test by which they will be categorised as non-diseased or diseased. Thus for every patient one has the test result and the ultimate decision.

SINGLE MARKER

When a diagnostic test produces a continuous measurement, then a diagnostic cut-point is selected. This is then used ultimately to divide future subjects into those who are suspected to have the disease and those who are not.

This diagnostic cut-point is determined by first calculating the sensitivity and specificity at each potential cut-point. The sensitivity of a test is the proportion of those *with* the disease who also have a positive diagnostic result, that is, they are above the cut-point. On the other hand, the specificity of a test is the proportion of those *without* the disease who also have a negative result, that is, they are below the cut-point. The sensitivity on the y-axis (vertical) against ($1-$specificity) on the x-axis (horizontal) obtained for each possible cut-point is then plotted. The final (diagnostic) cut-point, C, is usually chosen at a point which provides sensible balance between sensitivity and specificity. For a particular test this requires an assessment of the relative medical consequences and costs of making a false diagnosis of disease (false positive, FP) or of not diagnosing disease that is present (false negative, FN).

Example – *ROC curves* – *primary angle-closure glaucoma*

Devereux, Foster, Baasanhu *et al.* (2000) made anterior chamber depth measurement of the eye to detect occludable angles by means of optical

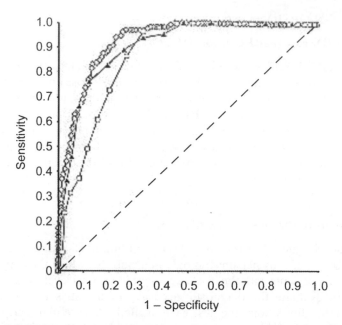

Figure 10.1 ROCs for detecting occludable angles for three different methods on the same subjects (from Devereux, Foster, Baasanhu *et al.*, 2000. Anterior chamber depth measurement as a screening tool for primary angle-closure glaucoma in an East Asian population. *Archives of Ophthalmology*, **118**, 257–263. [6, 10]

pachymetry, O, slit-lamp mounted, S, and hand-held, H, ultrasound tests in individuals. The corresponding ROCs are summarised in Figure 10.1 and the corresponding areas beneath the curves were 0.93, 0.90 and 0.86 for the respective methods. The optical method gave a sensitivity of 85% and specificity of 84% at a screening cut-off of $C < 2.22$ mm for detecting occludable angles.

A perfect diagnostic test would be one with no FP or FN results and would be represented by a line that started at the origin and went up the y-axis to a sensitivity of 1, and then across to a false positive rate of $(1 - \text{specificity}) = 0$. A test that produces false positive results at the same rate as true positive results would produce a ROC on the diagonal line $y = x$.

Study Size

If the objective is to estimate the area, AUC, under an ROC, then sample size can be determined using an expression similar to equation (3.2) from which the width, ω, of this CI can be calculated. The study size is then

$$m_{\text{Diseased}} = 4 \left[\frac{\sigma^2}{\omega^2} \right] z_{1-\alpha/2}^2. \tag{10.13}$$

The right-hand side of this equation is identical in form to equation (3.4). However, because evaluation of a diagnostic test determined through the ROC requires two subject groups, the diseased and non-diseased, the method of estimating σ has to take this into account. In fact Obuchowski and McClish (1997) show that it is a complex function of the ratio of non-diseased subjects to diseased subjects, R, in the study and the required sensitivity and specificity. The latter requirements are equivalent to setting the test size α and the power $1 - \beta$. Specifically,

$$\sigma = \frac{\exp(-\theta^2/4)}{2\sqrt{\pi}} \sqrt{\left(1 + \frac{1}{R} + \frac{5\theta^2}{8} + \frac{\theta^2}{8R}\right)}, \tag{10.14}$$

where $\theta = z_{1-FPR} - z_{1-TPR}$, FPR and TPR are the false positive and true positive rates respectively, and $R \geqslant 1$.

From this $m_{Non\text{-}diseased} = R \times m_{Diseased}$, so that the final estimated study size is $N = m_{Diseased} + m_{Non\text{-}diseased}$.

Values of the total sample size required (diseased plus non-diseased) are given for $R = 1$ and 1.5 in Table T14 for a range of FPR, TPR and widths, w, of the corresponding 95% CI for the AUC.

Example – *sample size for ROC curves – cartilage abnormalities*

Obuchowski and McClish (1997) consider the planning of a study to estimate the accuracy of magnetic resonance imaging (MRI) for detecting cartilage abnormalities in patients with symptomatic knees. Patients in the study were to undergo MRI for arthroscopy, which is considered the gold standard for determining the presence/absence of abnormalities. Following a five-point scoring, it is anticipated that 40% of patients will have a cartilage abnormality, so $R = 60/40 = 1.5$. Assuming the FPR $= 0.1$, TPR $= 0.5$, then for width $w = 0.10$, Table T14 gives the total sample size required as $N = 283$ or approximately 300, of which $0.4 \times 300 = 120$ would be anticipated to be diseased and 180 non-diseased.

SEVERAL MARKERS

In situations where more than one test is available for the same diagnostic problem one might compare the respective ROC curves and choose that which is closest to a perfect diagnostic test. The area under this perfect ROC curve is then the total area of the panel; that is, $AUC = 1 \times 1 = 1$. In the example of Figure 10.1, the three tests are not 'perfect' but one can see that the AUC is greater for one of the tests than the others. Thus the AUC is a measure of the performance of a diagnostic test against the ideal and may also be used to compare different diagnostic tests. Thus Obuchowski and McClish (1997) refer to the AUC as the accuracy of the test.

***Example** – several markers – primary angle-closure glaucoma*

In the case of Devereux, Foster, Baasanhu *et al.* (2000), the design involved the three screening tests, *O*, *S* and *H*. In such circumstances, if a single observer is involved, then it is a good idea to randomise the order in which these assessments are used in the individual patients. This can be done by means of a series of 3 × 3 Latin squares. For example, the first 36 patients, and examinations, could be allocated by first replacing *A*, *B* and *C* by *O*, *S*, *H* respectively. The order in which the corresponding 12 Latin squares of Table T4 are used is then randomised. Assume that we use the first two digits of the first column of Table T3 for this purpose, then the first four squares are chosen using the remainders after dividing by 12 of 75, 80, 94 and 67. These are 3, 8, 10 and 7; then the first 12 subjects would be examined as in Figure 10.2.

	Subject											
	1	2	3	4	5	6	7	8	9	10	11	12
Examination 1	*O*	*S*	*H*	*S*	*O*	*H*	*H*	*S*	*O*	*S*	*H*	*O*
Examination 2	*H*	*O*	*S*	*O*	*H*	*S*	*O*	*H*	*S*	*O*	*S*	*H*
Examination 3	*S*	*A*	*O*	*H*	*S*	*O*	*S*	*O*	*H*	*H*	*O*	*S*

Figure 10.2 First four of a random sequence of 3 × 3 Latin squares for a single observer study using three diagnostic methods on each of successive subjects

Study Size

Although methods of estimating study size for both independent and paired or matched designs to compare the *AUC* of two diagnostic tests have been given by Obuchowski and McClish (1997), they require specialist computer programs for their evaluation.

REPORTING

Bossuyt, Reitsma, Brund *et al.* (2003), with many simultaneous publications of the same article in many leading journals, provide the elements necessary for complete and accurate reporting of studies of diagnostic accuracy. This publication was part of the Standards for Reporting of Diagnostic Accuracy (STARD) initiative and has been widely adopted. The list of items in Figure 10.3 provides a suitable checklist of some important elements to consider when designing a study investigating a diagnostic test.

Methodological criteria
1. Was the study relevant with respect to the purpose of the test?
Study population
2. Were individuals with and without disease included in the evaluation?
3. Was the study population appropriate for evaluating the proposed use of the diagnostic test?
4. Were the inclusion and exclusion criteria that were used to select study patients described?
5. Were demographic and clinical characteristics of the study patients described?
6. Was the source of the study population described?
7. Was a wide spectrum of non-diseased and severity of diseased patients included?
8. Were patients with co-morbid conditions included in the case (diseased) group?
Diagnostic test and reference standard
9. Was an appropriate reference standard used?
10. Was the reference standard appropriately performed in a standard manner in all patients?
11. Were the interpretation of the reference standard and of the diagnostic test applied independently (blindly)?
12. Was the reproducibility of the test described?
13. Was a normal/abnormal reference ('gold') standard and normal/abnormal test result adequately defined?
Results
14. Were data presented in enough detail to calculate appropriate test characteristics?
15. Were uninterpretable results enumerated and described?
16. Was an appropriate sample size considered?

Figure 10.3 List of criteria assessing the quality of diagnostic studies (based on Kluwer Academic Publishers, de Vet, van der Weijden, Muris *et al.*, 2001, Table 1. Systematic reviews of diagnostic research. Considerations about assessment and incorporation of methodological quality. *European Journal of Epidemiology*, **17**, 301–306 [10] with kind permission of Springer Science and Business Media

---

Design features – ROC

Careful selection of consecutive patients

Careful selection of diseased patients

Estimate the ratio between the diseased and non-diseased from previous cohorts as determined by the reference

Double-blind assessment by new test and reference

Study size

Cross-check the design with the STARD requirements

10.4   AGREEMENT

Many measurements that are taken during any study require some degree of subjective judgement, whether assessing the results of diagnostic procedures or the effects of therapics. As a consequence, were the same observer to repeat, or different observers to measure, the same outcome, they may not give identical results. Observer agreement studies investigate the reproducibility of a single observer and the level of the consensus between different observers assessing the same unit, be it specimen, radiograph or pathology slide. Typically, in observer agreement studies, several observers make assessments on each of a series of experimental units and these assessments are compared. For example, to examine the variation in measurements of the volume of intracranial gliomas from computed tomography, different observers might evaluate scans from a series of patients. The values of tumour volume so recorded could then be compared. In other circumstances, the assessments may be of binary form such as a conclusion with respect to the presence or absence of metastases seen on liver scintigraphy. Clearly an ideal situation is one in which all the observers agree *and* the answer is correct. The correct answer can only be known if there is a 'gold' standard available.

To quantify the agreement between observers, studies will typically involve choosing the material to assess and defining the feature that one is trying to summarise. This requires definitions to work to, the number and choice of the specimens to review, the (random) order in which they should be reviewed and the number of observers required. In its simplest form such studies would involve two observers, each assessing all the specimens with no gold standard with which to compare.

SINGLE OBSERVER – REPRODUCIBILITY

Suppose a single observer makes a diagnostic decision after examining a patient (or perhaps a specimen taken from a patient), then how likely is the observer to draw the same conclusion were the specimen to be examined a second time? To assess this, we require the same assessments to be repeated by the same observer. For example, the same slide would need to be reviewed by the pathologist on two occasions. The second review would need to be undertaken 'blind' to the results of the first review and clearly some time later. A 'washout' period long enough to ensure that the pathologist did not 'recognise' the slide but not too much later if the period may cause deterioration of the specimen or after the observer (now more experienced) changes his/her methods in a systematic way.

For a single observer, the degree of reproducibility is quantified by the probability of making a chance error in diagnosis, ξ. This is the probability of ascribing either absent (coded 0) to a diagnosis when it should be present (coded 1), or a 1 to a diagnosis that should be 0. This review process generates for each of the specimens reviewed, one of the four possible binary pairs (0, 0), (1, 0), (0, 1) and (1, 1) as indicated in Table 10.1. The corresponding number of specimens, in each of these pairs, is represented by d_{00}, d_{10}, d_{01} and d_{11}.

Table 10.1   Possible outcomes for a single observer reviewing the same material on two occasions, or two observers reviewing the same material on two occasions

Second review(er)	First review(er)		Total
	Absent	Present	
Absent	d_{00}	d_{01}	
Present	d_{10}	d_{11}	
Total			m_{Repeat}

From Table 10.1, it is clear that the proportion of times the observer agrees with him- or herself is

$$p_{Agree} = \frac{d_{00} + d_{11}}{m_{Repeat}}. \tag{10.15}$$

while the proportion of disagreements is

$$p_{Dis} = \frac{d_{10} + d_{01}}{m_{Repeat}}. \tag{10.16}$$

Freedman, Parmar and Baker (1993) show that the degree of reproducibility of the reviewer is estimated by

$$\xi = \{1 - \sqrt{[2p_{Dis}]}\}/2. \tag{10.17}$$

This has a $100(1-\alpha)\%$ CI,

$$\xi - z_{1-\alpha/2} \times SE(\xi) \qquad \text{to} \qquad \xi + z_{1-\alpha/2} \times SE(\xi) \tag{10.18}$$

where

$$SE(\xi) = \sqrt{\frac{\xi(1-\xi)[1 - 2\xi(1-\xi)]}{2(1-2\xi)^2 m_{Repeat}}}. $$

Study Size

Sample-size calculations are based on the achievement of sufficient precision of the estimate of ξ which is governed primarily by the number of duplicate assessments, m_{Repeat}. For a given ξ, and desired width W_ξ, of the $100(1-\alpha)\%$ CI, the number of repeats necessary is given by

$$m_{Repeat} = \frac{2\xi(1-\xi)(1 - 2\xi + 2\xi^2)z_{1-\alpha/2}^2}{W_\xi^2(1-2\xi)^2}. \tag{10.19}$$

Example – *sample size* – *number of specimens*

Suppose that we anticipate that the probability of error by the observer is 5% and that we plan to estimate this probability with a 95% CI of width for the estimate of 10%. How many repeat observations should be made?

Here, $\xi = 0.05$, $W_\xi = 0.1$, and for $\alpha = 0.05$, Table T2.1 gives $z_{1-\alpha/2} = 1.9600$, then from equation (10.19),

$$m_{\text{Duplicate}} = \frac{2 \times 0.05 \times 0.95 \times [1 - (2 \times 0.05) + (2 \times 0.05^2)] \times 1.9600^2}{0.1^2[1 - (2 \times 0.05)]^2} = 40.77.$$

This implies that the observer should repeat his or her assessments on approximately 40 specimens.

TWO OBSERVERS – AGREEMENT

Disagreement

If agreement between observers is to be quantified then specimens will be assessed by each of two observers and each observer has to decide on a binary diagnosis (Absent or Present) for each specimen and scores these 0 or 1 respectively. This study then generates data also in the form of Table 10.1 but 'First review' and 'Second review' are now replaced by 'First reviewer' and 'Second reviewer'. The estimated probability of disagreement is now

$$p_{\text{Dis}} = \frac{d_{10} + d_{01}}{m_{\text{Two}}}. \tag{10.20}$$

Study Size

If the corresponding anticipated value for the probability of disagreement, π_{Dis}, is not too close to zero, and the sample size is reasonably large, then for a specified width, W_{Dis}, of the $100(1-\alpha)\%$ CI, the sample size is

$$m_{\text{Two}} = 4 \times \left(\frac{\pi_{\text{Dis}}(1 - \pi_{\text{Dis}})}{W_{\text{Dis}}^2} \right) z_{1-\alpha/2}^2. \tag{10.21}$$

This is an equivalent expression to equation (3.6) but, as we have warned previously, it may not be reliable if π_{Dis} is close to 0 or 1. Typical values of π_{Dis} range from 0.05 to 0.4. In most situations high disagreement values would not be anticipated but low values may be quite common. We therefore recommend the use of Table T1 in such situations.

Example – *two observers* – *disagreement*

It is anticipated that two observers will have a probability of disagreement of approximately 25% but it is desired to estimate this with a 95% CI of width 10%. How many observations should be made?

Here, $\pi_{\mathrm{Dis}}=0.25$, $W_{\mathrm{Dis}}=0.1$ and $\alpha=0.05$, hence equation (10.21) gives

$$m_{\mathrm{Two}} = 4 \times \left(\frac{0.25(1-0.25)}{0.1^2} \right) \times 1.96^2 = 288.$$

This agrees very closely with the more exact calculation of Table T1 which gives $N=286$. So for such a study, this implies that the two observers examine the same 300 specimens independently.

Cohen's Kappa, κ

Inter rater agreement is often measured by Cohen's κ, which takes the form

$$\kappa = \frac{p_{\mathrm{Agree}} - p_{\mathrm{Exp}}}{1 - p_{\mathrm{Exp}}} \qquad (10.22)$$

where p_{Agree} is the proportion of rater pairs exhibiting perfect agreement and p_{Exp} the proportion expected to show agreement by chance alone. From Table 10.1, as we have shown before, $p_{\mathrm{Agree}}=(d_{00} +d_{11})/m_{\mathrm{Repeat}}$. To get the expected agreement we use the row and column totals to estimate the expected numbers agreeing for each category. For negative agreement (Absent, Absent) the expected proportion is the product of $(d_{01}+d_{00})/m_{\mathrm{Repeat}}$ and $(d_{10}+d_{00})/m_{\mathrm{Repeat}}$, giving $(d_{00}+d_{01})(d_{00}+d_{10})/m_{\mathrm{Repeat}}^2$. Likewise for positive agreement the expected proportion is $(d_{10}+d_{11})(d_{01}+d_{11})/m_{\mathrm{Repeat}}^2$. The expected proportion of agreements for the whole table is the sum of these two terms, that is

$$p_{\mathrm{Exp}} = \frac{(d_{00} + d_{01})(d_{00} + d_{10})}{m_{\mathrm{Repeat}}^2} + \frac{(d_{10} + d_{11})(d_{01} + d_{11})}{m_{\mathrm{Repeat}}^2}. \qquad (10.23)$$

Study Size

Suppose the same $k=2$ raters rate each of a sample of m_{Repeat} subjects independently. If their ratings are binary in nature, and denoted as either a success (1) or a failure (0), then we can think of π as the underlying true proportion of successes. Then for an anticipated value of κ, Donner and Eliasziw (1992) quote the corresponding $SE(\kappa)$. If κ, is not too close to zero, and the sample size is reasonably large, then for a specified width W_κ of the $100(1-\alpha)\%$ CI, the sample size is

$$m_{\mathrm{Kappa}} = 4 \times \frac{(1-\kappa)}{W_\kappa^2} \left((1-\kappa)(1-2\kappa) + \frac{\kappa(2-\kappa)}{2\pi(1-\pi)} \right) z_{1-\alpha/2}^2. \qquad (10.24)$$

Example – sample size – Cohen's kappa

Suppose we believe that $\pi=0.3$, we anticipate $\kappa_{Plan}=0.4$ and we wish to determine this with $W_\kappa=0.2$ for a two-sided 95% CI. Then from equation (10.24)

$$m_{Kappa} = 4 \times \frac{(1-0.4)}{0.2^2}\left((1-0.4)[1-(2\times 0.4)] + \frac{0.4(2-0.4)}{2\times 0.3 \times 0.7}\right) \times 1.96^2.$$

This leads to $m_{Kappa}=378.9$ or about 400 subjects are needed.

The situation in which π is different for each of the two raters is discussed by Cantor (1996).

Cicchetti (2001) gives a useful general discussion of the problem of estimating a valid sample size in this area. He states, although this also applies in general, that sample size estimation '...involves much more than simply plugging numbers into confidence interval formulas, applying them to data from already published test manuals and then using them as a bench mark for sample size requirements'. Importantly he points out that clinically useful results can be obtained with relatively modest values of κ, and there is diminishing gain from increasing the sample size much above 100.

Intra-class Correlation Coefficient

The intra-class correlation (ICC) is the equivalent to κ when the k raters are asked to record on a continuous rather than on a binary scale. It was defined previously in equation (T9.2), but we repeat it here for convenience, as

$$\rho = \frac{\sigma^2_{Between}}{\sigma^2_{Within} + \sigma^2_{Between}}. \tag{10.25}$$

Study Size

To estimate the study size, typically one proposes a minimally acceptable level of inter-rater reliability as, say, ρ_0. In contrast, ρ_1 is then set as the value that we anticipate for our study. The design choice, is the combination $N_{Observations}=km_{Repeat}$, that is the optimum combination of numbers of raters (or observations) per subject, k, and numbers of subjects, $m_{Subjects}$.

Walter, Eliasziw and Donner (1998) suggest an effect size C_0 where

$$C_0 = \frac{1 + k\left[\dfrac{\rho_0}{1-\rho_0}\right]}{1 + k\left[\dfrac{\rho_1}{1-\rho_1}\right]}. \tag{10.26}$$

The number of subjects, m_{Subjects}, then required for two-sided significance α and power $1-\beta$ is given by

$$m_{\text{Subjects}} = 1 + \frac{2(z_{1-\alpha/2} + z_{1-\beta})^2 k}{(\log C_0)^2 (k-1)}. \tag{10.27}$$

Example – *sample size* – *intra-class correlation*

Walter, Eliasziw and Donner (1998) describe a study in which therapists are assessing children with Down's syndrome using the Gross Motor Functional Measure (GMFM). This has been validated for use in children with cerebral palsy and it was felt necessary to check its validity in children with a different disease.

The investigators were hoping for an inter-rater reliability of at least 0.85, and had determined that a reliability of 0.7 or higher would be acceptable. Hence, the null hypothesis H_0: $\rho_0 = 0.7$ and the alternative H_1: $\rho_1 = 0.85$. For practical reasons no child could be seen more than $k = 4$ times and approximately 30 subjects were available. Thus the design options were restricted to a choice of $k = 2$, 3 or 4.

For two-sided significance of 5% and 80% power from equation (10.27), we find that when $k = 2$, $m_{\text{Subjects}} = 42.4$ and so $N_{\text{Observations}} = k\ m_{\text{Subjects}} \approx 86$, while for $k = 3$, $m_{\text{Subjects}} = 29.3$ and $N_{\text{Observations}} = k\ m_{\text{Subjects}} \approx 90$ and when $k = 4$, $m_{\text{Subjects}} = 25.0$ and $N_{\text{Observations}} = k\ m_{\text{Subjects}} = 100$.

In the design with the minimum number of observations, $N_{\text{Observations}} = 86$, and so 43 children would each be seen twice. The restriction in numbers of children possible to about 30 eliminates the possibility of this design. The next best option is if each child is seen three times, implying $N_{\text{Observations}} = 90$, to achieve the required power. Ultimately, the investigators decided to opt for $k = 4$ observations per child. This requires more observations in total, but involves fewer children.

A useful method for planning studies of inter-rater reliability has been described by Bonett (2002). Thus, rather than specify a minimum acceptable value for ρ, as in equation (10.27), one might plan for a $100(1-\alpha)\%$ CI of width W_ρ. Then with k raters on m_{Subjects} subjects an approximate sample size is:

$$m_{\text{Subjects}} = 1 + \frac{8z_{1-\alpha/2}^2 (1 - \rho_{\text{Plan}})^2 [1 + (k-1)\rho_{\text{Plan}}]^2}{k(k-1)W_\rho^2}. \tag{10.28}$$

When there are only $k = 2$ raters and the anticipated intra-class correlation is $\rho_{\text{Plan}} > 0.7$, then the sample size required is increased from m_{Subjects} to $(m_{\text{Subjects}} + 5\rho_{\text{Plan}})$.

This formula is more robust to differing values of ρ than that given by Walter, Eliasziw and Donner (1998). For example, under a null hypothesis of $\rho_0 = 0.7$, with $\alpha = \beta = 0.05$ and $k = 3$, from equation (10.27) for $\rho_1 = 0.725$, 0.75 and 0.80, we require

3376, 786 and 167 subjects respectively. In comparison, the corresponding sample sizes required to estimate ρ with a 95% CI of $W_\rho = 0.2$ are 60, 52 and 37. This large reduction is caused by changing the value of ρ_1 which results in changing the effect size C_0 of equation (10.26), which has a big influence on the sample size.

Example *– sample size – confidence interval for the intra-class correlation*

Suppose we wished to estimate ρ in the study of Walter, Eliasziw and Donner (1998) and we wished to estimate it to within ± 0.1, or a 95% CI width of $W_\rho = 0.2$. If we assume that $\rho = 0.85$ and that we had $k = 4$ raters then equation (10.28) suggests $m = 19.2$, that is 20 children are required. Thus, if the same four therapists rate a sample of 20 children, and if r, the estimate of ρ, is close to 0.85, then we would expect the width of CI for ρ to be close to 0.2.

Design features

Careful selection of material to be reviewed

Define criteria for basis of review

Selection of observer(s)

Blind assessment of repeat reviews

Random order of material to be reviewed

Careful design of second – before-and-after – review

Crossover design – for two-observer review

11 Prognostic Factor Studies

Summary

The object of this chapter is to summarise some key aspects of the design of prognostic factor studies. These studies are usually based on regression models that help determine which of the (usually many) candidate variables, often in combination, are truly prognostic for outcome. We point out that choice of a model depends on subjective judgement, ranging from the choice of the variables to consider to the precise statistical methods used in the variable selection process. Consequently, emphasis is placed on the need to first develop a model with an index group of patients which is then validated in an entirely separate group of patients. We use a survival time endpoint to illustrate the methodology, although the same issues relate to other types of endpoint variables.

11.1 INTRODUCTION

An integral part of clinical management is concern with respect to the ultimate outcome for the patient with a specific disease or condition. In many situations, and without treatment, patients may rapidly and fully recover with no residual manifestation of the initial condition remaining. In this situation it would be natural to monitor the course of disease from onset to resolution, to measure the corresponding time interval and perhaps relate this time to features of the patient succumbing to the disease in the first place and the severity of the disease so contracted. Any features established, which appear prognostic for outcome, may then be used to counsel future patients on the anticipated time course of the disease for them. In addition these prognostic variables may provide clues to underlying aetiology of the disease and which may indicate means of eradication or prevention.

However, it is not often possible to monitor the natural history of a disease in this way. It is more likely that the responsible clinical team will institute some intervention, however benign, which may alter the natural course to some extent. Nevertheless, even in the context of patients recruited to randomised controlled trials, it may also be that prognostic factors (besides treatment itself, which it is hoped will influence outcome) will contribute to outcome. For example, it is well known that those patients with Ewing's sarcoma presenting with metastatic disease have a poorer prognosis than those who do not. Despite this, the same treatment may be appropriate for both metastatic and non-metastatic groups. So if one treatment under investigation in a clinical trial

Design of Studies for Medical Research. D. Machin and M. J. Campbell
© 2005 John Wiley & Sons Ltd. ISBN 0 470 84495 7

turns out to be better than the standard, the relative prognostic effect of the presence of metastatic disease may or may not be modified.

It is common to find, although it is by no means always the case, that several variables contribute to the ultimate prognosis. For example, if in Ewing's sarcoma a pelvic site is involved this too is is an adverse prognostic feature for subsequent survival. Thus note has to be taken of the four metastases by site combinations in judging prognosis for these patients.

Factors prognostic for outcome are often determined by using multiple regression techniques relating, for example, the time to resolution of the condition to the potential explanatory variables. Thus for Ewing's sarcoma the regression model for the ultimate survival time will include information on both the presence or absence of metastic disease and pelvic involvement at diagnosis. Once established, this regression model can help to quantify the risk, with respect to the endpoint of concern, associated with these factors.

Often there may be many potential features of the patient, such as age, gender and weight, and features of the disease present, such as its severity, which may or may not influence outcome. Thus those variables that are strongly prognostic are to be identified and those clearly not prognostic set aside, whilst others may need to be more fully investigated in further studies.

The techniques used to obtain a prognostic model from a number of candidate variables are essentially statistical in nature using regression models. We will not describe this process in detail as they refer more to analysis than design. However, the discussion of the design of prognostic factor studies requires some unavoidable reference to model building and so this chapter is somewhat more technical in nature than previous ones.

As for all studies, 'good' design features are an essential ingredient for prognostic studies.

11.2   CASE STUDY

To motivate the discussion in this chapter, we use the prognostic factor study concerned with patients with inoperable hepatocellular carcinoma conducted by Tan, Law, Ng and Machin (2003). The aim was to develop a prognostic index (PI), not the very best possible using sophisticated measures, but rather one of (easy) practicable utility. This study comprised two components.

In the first, several potential variables were investigated from information provided from 397 inoperable patients with hepatocellular carcinoma (HCC) who had all been diagnosed and treated at the same institution in Singapore (the index group). The variables considered included age, gender, ethnicity, significant alcohol intake, Zubrod performance score, presence of ascites, chronic hepatitis C, chronic hepatitis B, Child–Pugh Class, TNM Stage and serum AFP. From these 11 candidate variables, Zubrod score, presence of ascites and AFP levels were identified as prognostic. These were then used to derive a prognostic index, which allowed the HCC patients to be assigned to one of three risk (Low, Medium, High) groups.

The second component, applied the prognostic index so derived to 234 new HCC patients (the validation group) recruited to a multinational randomised clinical trial

Table 11.1 Characteristics of patients with inoperable hepatocellular carcinoma of the index and validation groups (after Tan, Law, Ng and Machin, 2003. Simple Clinical prognostic model for hepatocellular carcinoma in developing countries and its validation. *Journal of Clinical Oncology*, **21**, 2294–2298 [11]

Variable		Index group n	Index group $\%$	Validation group n	Validation group $\%$
Zubrod score	0	32	8	69	21
(ZPS)	1	119	30	157	48
	2	118	30	59	18
	3	42	11	37	11
	4	8	2	—	—
	Unknown	78	20	2	1
Presence	Yes	167	42	129	40
of	No	227	57	194	60
ascites	Unknown	3	1	1	—
AFP (µg/L)	$\leqslant 49$	80	20	41	13
	50–499	55	14	21	6
	500–4999	86	22	171	53
	5000–49 999	93	23	21	6
	$\geqslant 50\,000$	84	21	17	5
Ethnic	Chinese	352	89	156	48
group	Malay	31	8	34	11
	Others	14	4	—	—
	Myanmar	—	—	103	32
	Thai	—		14	4
	Others	—	—	17	5
Gender	Male	333	84	270	83
	Female	64	16	54	17
Age (years)	$\leqslant 39$	21	5		
	40–49	37	9		
	50–59	92	23		
	60–69	120	30		
	70–79	93	23		
	$\geqslant 80$	34	9		
Significant	Yes	68	17		
alcohol	No	277	70		
intake	Unknown	52	13		
Chronic	Yes	325	82		
hepatitis	No	21	5		
B	Unknown	53	13		
Chronic	Yes	27	7		
hepatitis	No	318	80		
C	Unknown	52	13		
Child–Pugh	A	137	35		
Class	B	184	46		
	C	76	19		
UICC TNM	I/II	64	16		
Stage	III	41	10		
	IVa	214	54		
	IVb	78	20		

reported by Chow, Tai, Tan *et al.* (2002). The purpose was to see if the PI so derived was indeed prognostic for the disease.

The basic characteristics of the index group with respect to all the candidate variables and those eventually identified as prognostic are given in Table 11.1. The corresponding numbers of patients of the validation group are also included. It should be noted that fewer variables were recorded in the validation group as it is generally good practice to keep these to key variables so as to minimise the work for the clinical teams entering patients into a trial.

The process of developing a 'simple' model in this context balances practical with statistical considerations. Practical issues include using categories for serum AFP, classifying any unknown characteristics into the worst group, and rounding the regression coefficients to obtain the relative weights attached to each variable.

11.3   CANDIDATE VARIABLES

STUDY ENDPOINT

We assume that a prognostic factor study is in design and, just as for any other study, the key endpoint has to be established. For example, in many circumstances this will be the time either to the resolution of the disease (cure) or, as would be the case in prognostic studies in patients with advanced cancer, the survival time of the patient. In this latter case, the survival time might be calculated from the date of diagnosis to the date of death. The outcome for a group of such patients with survival times is summarised using the Kaplan–Meier estimate of the corresponding survival curve. One such example has been given in Figure 9.3 which shows the survival curves of patients with hepatocellular carcinoma treated with three doses of tamoxifen as reported by Chow, Tai, Tan *et al.* (2002).

Although we will use an illustrative example involving survival time, and hence the Cox proportional hazards model is appropriate, for other outcome measures differing models would be required. Thus for binary outcomes this would be expressed via logistic regression and for continuous outcomes multiple (least squares) regression. All of which are available in standard statistical computer packages.

The univariate Cox proportional hazards regression model of a single potential prognostic variable, x is

$$h = \exp(\beta x), \tag{11.1}$$

where h represents the risk and β is the corresponding regression coefficient to be estimated from the survival times of the patients, each with associated value for x. In the simplest case, x is a binary variable, for example, taking the value 0 for males and 1 for females. In this case if b, the estimate of β of equation (11.1), turns out to be zero, then $h = \exp(0) = 1$. This implies that, whatever the value of x, $h = 1$ and the risk for males and females is the same. Thus gender is not prognostic for outcome. On the other hand, if $b = 2$ say, then if $x = 0$, $h_{\text{Male}} = 1$ but when $x = 1$, $h_{\text{Female}} = \exp(2)$, implying a greater risk for the females. In general, the associated hazard ratio is $HR = h_{\text{Female}}/h_{\text{Male}} = \exp(\beta \times 1)/\exp(\beta \times 0) = \exp(\beta)$. Since log $HR = \beta$, the regression coefficient itself is often termed the log hazard ratio.

For v potential prognostic variables, $x_1, x_2, x_3, \ldots, x_v$ the Cox model becomes/takes the multivariable form

$$h = \exp(\beta_1 x_1 + \beta_2 x_2 + \beta_3 x_3 + \ldots + \beta_v x_v), \tag{11.2}$$

where $\beta_1, \beta_2, \beta_3, \ldots, \beta_v$ are the corresponding regression coefficients to be estimated in the modelling process.

The basic structure of a prognostic factor study is to record, for each of the N patients recruited, their basic characteristics at the time of diagnosis of their disease and their ultimate survival, t. As we noted in Chapter 3, for survival time studies these times may be censored for some subjects in which case $T+$ is recorded. In very simple terms, once the regression model is fitted to these data, those $\xi (\leqslant v)$ variables for which a null hypothesis that the corresponding regression coefficient β_i is zero is rejected, are retained in the model and are termed prognostic. The remaining $v - \xi$ variables that are 'not statistically different' from zero are removed from the model and are considered as not prognostic for outcome.

IDENTIFYING THE SUBJECTS

Before establishing which individual patients are to be included in the prognostic factor investigation the basic patient population of interest has to be defined. So, just as one would do for any clinical study, clear eligibility criteria have to be established. Such eligibility requirements will usually include the particular diagnoses of interest as well as precise details of how these diagnoses are established. Further, it may be necessary to restrict the patients so selected to those that will receive a particular form of therapy. In some situations, this restriction may be made to ensure a relatively homogeneous set of patients so that the potential prognostic indicators are not obscured by varying degrees of efficacy of the (possibly) uncontrolled choice of therapies that may have been given to such patients.

Clearly if the patients used for a prognostic study are those recruited to a randomised trial, then differences between patients (due to treatment received) can be accommodated in the prognostic modelling process in a systematic way. The choice of subjects may also (and should) be influenced by the quality of data that can be collected for the purposes of the study. Once again if these data come from a randomised trial then one may be reassured more easily that the data are well documented than for a study that involves extracting data from patient case notes which are designed principally for other purposes. Without good quality data, the conclusions drawn from studies of prognosis must be regarded as uncertain.

USE OF THE INDEX

One should also give some thought as to how the prognostic factors once established are to be used. If the purpose is purely scientific, then the variables considered can be very esoteric in nature (perhaps determined by very complex assays). On the other hand, if the index is to be used to guide advice that will be given to patients in the clinic then the variables for use are best established easily with minimal sophisticated (laboratory-type) measures involved.

CHOOSING THE VARIABLES

Apart from the endpoint measure itself, it is also important to determine which variables are to be the candidate variables for the prognostic factor investigation.

Help with the choice of variables to study (or not) should be obtained by reviewing the literature for variables that have been investigated in previous studies. It is clear that those that have been shown to have major prognostic influence should also be included in the planned study. We will call these 'Level–In' variables. A decision then has to be made as to which of the other variables so examined may be still unproven, 'Level–Query', and those that have already been found conclusively not to be useful, 'Level–Out'.

Of course, the purpose of the current study may be to investigate entirely new variables, 'Level–New'. For this latter category it will be advisable to consider aspects of the Bradford-Hill criteria of Figure 1.1 with respect to ultimate causality. At this stage one also has to determine whether the objective of investigating 'Level–New' variables is to replace the 'Level–In' variables or rather to ask if their added inclusion 'enhances' the ability to distinguish more clearly prognostic groups. The approach to modelling is different in these two situations.

Considerable thought at the planning stage needs to be focused on the selection of the variables and the associated Levels. There is a tendency to assign very few to 'Level–Out' for fear of 'missing something important'.

Case study – *choice of candidate variables* – *inoperable hepatocellular carcinoma*

It is well known that AFP is indeed predictive in this disease and so it was regarded as a 'Level–In' variable for the modelling. The remaining variables were all 'Level–Query' as, although most had been investigated before and some not found to be very predictive, they had usually been considered together with variables that were strongly predictive but which were not candidate variables for this study.

Example – *choice of candidate variables* – *node-positive breast cancer*

Although not using our categorisation, Sauerbrei, Royston, Bojar *et al.* (1999) imply for non-metastatic breast cancer that nodal status is the only Level–In variable associated with prognosis. In contrast Level–Query is attached to tumour size, tumour grade, histological type, oestrogen (ER) and progesterone receptor (PR), menopausal status and age despite many investigations of their respective roles. They also point out that more than 100 Level–New factors have been proposed at various times.

SCREENING THE VARIABLES

However, before going to the stage of fitting the chosen model of the form (11.2), it is often desirable to do some (often informal) preliminary screening of the variables. One such screen, for those candidate variables that are continuous in nature, is to calculate the correlation matrix of all the corresponding pairwise correlation coefficients. Should this matrix contain some large correlation coefficients then this may indicate that only one of the corresponding pair of variables contributing to any high value needs to be included in the modelling process.

The choice of which to take forward to the modelling can be made in several ways depending on circumstance. These may include the easiest or cheapest of the two measures to obtain from the patients or the variable most often used by previous studies. A common option is to begin by first modelling these variables individually by use of the univariate model equation (11.1). Suppose the variables concerned are x_1 and x_2, then the models to fit are $h_1 = \exp(\beta_1 x_1)$ and $h_2 = \exp(\beta_2 x_2)$. It is then determined which of the estimated regression coefficients (b_1 or b_2) is the 'most statistically significant' and the associated x then may be the variable that is chosen. Before the final choice, a check is made using the two-variable version of equation (11.2), that is $h_{1,2} = \exp(\beta_1 x_1 + \beta_2 x_2)$, to see that if both variables are included whether worthwhile extra information is obtained over the single variable chosen.

TRANSFORMATIONS

In the modelling process, it is often easier if a variable has a linear influence on the outcome of concern. If a variable, say x, is continuous then the direct use of equation (11.1) implies that the effect on the risk of death is log-linear, that is, the log HR increases or decreases linearly as the value of the factor increases. This may or may not be the case. This may be checked by fitting the model $h_{Quadratic} = \exp(\beta_1 x + \beta_2 x^2)$ which has algebraically a quadratic form and is estimated by $h_{Quadratic} = \exp(b_1 x + b_2 x^2)$. If a formal test of the null hypothesis, $\beta_2 = 0$, is not rejected then x is assumed to act linearly, since this implies $\beta_2 x^2 = 0$ whatever the value of x. Otherwise a more detailed examination of the relationship implied by changing values of x will need to be instituted.

If linearity is not the case, then creation of categories to reflect the shape of the relationship is recommended in preference to attempting to describe the precise detail of the non-linear relationship. Although in certain circumstances a transformation of the basic variable may achieve the desired linearity. Common transformations of the basic variable, x, are $\log x$ and $\sqrt{x}$. Complex transformations are best avoided.

Example – investigating linearity – colorectal cancer

Chung, Eu, Machin *et al.* (1998) investigated whether young age was an adverse prognostic factor for survival in patients with colorectal cancer. In general colorectal death rates increase with age (as is the case for many cancers) and so if young age ($\leqslant 39$ years) is indeed indicative of a worse prognosis, then the age-specific death rates would be U-shaped when plotted against decade. This was indeed the case, with those aged 40–59 of lowest risk whilst those of the ≤ 39 age-group were at a similar risk to those 60–79 or some 30 years older.

As a consequence, for age an unordered categorical variable was created of the age decades for the modelling process – this despite the fact that the underlying variable was continuous and hence the successive categories had a natural order. Had ordered categories been used in the modelling process, then this is equivalent to coding them as 0, 1, 2, etc. that is then treated as numerical data. If the model is then fitted with this variable, then it takes a linear form which, in this situation, is not appropriate. Using the unordered categories allows the shape of the underlying relationship to be examined without imposing an algebraic form such as the quadratic referred to previously.

One difficulty with categorising continuous variables is the fact that, once created, there is an implicit assumption that there is a step change in risk at a boundary between adjacent categories. This is unlikely to be the case. Sometimes boundaries are convenient choices, for example, decade groups for age. In other circumstances, the choice may be made by investigating a range of options and then choosing that which 'magnifies' the difference beween adjacent categories. Such devices can lead to an over-optimistic view of the prognostic variable in question. If a dichotomy is to be chosen, then one method is to take the cut at the median value but there is no guarantee that the risk will divide along these lines. Since the purpose of categorising the variable is to better investigate the 'shape' of the associated risk, a minimum number of three categories is required for this, and a maximum of five would seem reasonable (although if data are plentiful more could be taken).

Case study *– transformation of data – inoperable hepatocellular carcinoma*

The only laboratory-based variable included was AFP as it is widely used even in less developed clinical settings in other respects. This was categorised into the five groups, effectively on a logarithmic scale, as shown in Table 11.1.

MISSING VALUES

It is important that the proportion of data items that are missing or unknown in the data set is minimal. Experience suggests that as the number of variables requested of the clinical teams increases the proportion of 'missing' data also increases. Missing data cause considerable 'biases' to arise in the modelling process and should be avoided if at all possible. Although there are no formal rules attached to an acceptable level of missing data, if more than 20% are missing for a particular variable, then serious consideration should be given to excluding it from the modelling process. If the missing data comprise less than 5%, then the bias introduced may be regarded as minimal. These are only pragmatic suggestions, however, and may have to be varied with circumstance. No useful model can result if a vital piece of information cannot be easily collected.

For those variables for which data are missing, it is useful to create a category of their own. If treated like this in the modelling process, then, if the data are missing at random, this category should behave in a central manner since it will comprise a (random) mixture of the other category levels. Were it to correspond to (say) the highest risk category, then this may indicate that 'missing' is a sign of poor prognosis. Perhaps it is then 'missing' as the patient was too ill for the measure to be recorded. For example, when a patient is an emergency admission, time for less routine assessments may not be available and so they may go unrecorded. In which case the absence of these values may be indicative of a worse outcome and hence the fact of them 'missing' is prognostic for outcome.

Case study – *missing data* – *inoperable hepatocellular carcinoma*

In Table 11.1 the Zubrod score has a large proportion (19.6%) of missing values. In screening the variable, an unordered categorical variable was first created with four levels (0, 1, 2, Missing) and used in a univariate model of Zubrod score. The size of the corresponding category '2' and 'Missing' regression coefficients were similar. As a consequence, these two categories were merged for the multivariable modelling.

This device is no substitute for the 'real' data values, however, and serious concern must be raised about a variable for which there is a large proportion of missing data.

NUMBER OF VARIABLES

In equation (11.2) the number of variables, v, that can be included is clearly without end, but for every variable added there is at least one further regression coefficient to be estimated. It is easy to imagine that there can be more candidate variables than patients. So a simple rule is to never allow into the model more variables than subjects. If there are more variables than subjects, then the screening process to determine Level–In, Level–Query, and Level–Out must ensure the number is reduced accordingly. It has to be realised that if a g-group categorical variable is included, then this adds $g-1$ regression coefficients to the model. Thus it is really the number of regression coefficients, k ($\geqslant v$), to be estimated that should, at the very least, be less then N. In fact, for survival-type studies, it is the number of events observed, O, that is critical rather than N itself. Thus a very large study with few events may have the same limit to k as a small study with a proportionately larger number of events. We return to this topic when discussing an appropriate study size.

MEASUREMENT

Although we have talked in general terms about the candidate variables, as we have indicated in Chapter 2, reliable measurement of these is clearly critical to prognostic factor studies also. Thus, for example, Simon and Altman (1994) stress that any laboratory assays should be performed blinded to clinical data and outcome, and that intra- and inter-laboratory reproducibility of assays should be documented.

FITTING THE MODEL

Univariate

As there are usually several, sometimes many, variables as potential candidates for inclusion even after screening, the next step is often to reduce these numbers by options by fitting a univariate model for each in turn, then only to take forward those of the candidate variables (all of which must be either Level–In or Level–Query) for which the corresponding null hypothesis of $\beta=0$ had been rejected. The remaining variables are then studied in a multivariable regression model.

Case study – univariate models – inoperable hepatocellular carcinoma

Individual (univariate) Cox regression analysis of all the clinical parameters indicated in Table 11.1 and serum AFP level showed that the major variables influencing survival are Zubrod performance score, presence of ascites and AFP. Thus, the univariate analysis screen had reduced the k from 30 to eight regression coefficients to be estimated: two for Zubrod score, two for ascites and three for log AFP. The corresponding regression coefficients are given in Table 11.2(a). Little prognostic information was provided by age, gender, ethnicity or significant alcohol history.

Multivariable

Although individually the candidate variables in the univariate stage of the modelling are all statistically significant, when included together in a multivariable model this need no longer be the case. The next stage of the modelling process is then to select those which still appear to influence outcome and discard those which do not. There are many alternative methods for doing this, ranging from adding one variable at a time to the best univariate model to removing one variable at a time from a multivariable model that first includes all the candidate variables.

Case study – multivariable model – inoperable hepatocellular carcinoma

Candidate variables for the multivariable prognostic index were only those (shown in Table 11.2(a)) that had been found to be statistically significant (*p*-value < 0.05) in a univariate Cox model using binary, tertiary or four-group unordered categories.

Selective Cox regression using a step-down procedure was used to determine the best combination of these variables for prognosis. However, before this was undertaken, those patients with unknown Zubrod score or ascites were first recategorised into the nearest risk group. The multivariable selection process considered the three variables simultaneously but retained all of them in the resulting model given in Table 11.2(b). Thus all the variables were found to remain predictive of survival even when considered together.

A comparison of the regression coefficients with the corresponding ones of Table 11.2(a) shows little change. This suggests that the three basic variables act independently of each other.

In some instances, the regression coefficients of the multivariable model are rounded to numerically convenient values. Thus, for example, those for AFP approximated to 0, 0.3, 0.6 and 0.9 and so the corresponding categorical variable (requiring three regression coefficients) was replaced by a discrete numerical variable with values 0, 1, 2 and 3 (requiring one regression cofficient). Also the patients with Zubrod score unknown were merged with the $\geqslant 2$ group and then, because the regression coefficients approximated to 0, 0.5 and 1, the corresponding categorical variable (requiring two regression coefficients) was replaced by a discrete numerical variable with values 0, 1 and 2 (requiring one regression cofficient), and finally those with ascites unknown were merged with the ascites present group.

A multivariable analysis (but no longer selective) for these three modified variables is summarised in Table 11.2(c).

Selection

Although there may be several 'individually' predictive variables identified at the screening stage, once all these are in the same regression model some may no longer appear prognostic. Essentially this is because the same (or similar) information may be held in one or more of the other variables.

Prognostic Index

For each of the patients in the index or training set, a score can be derived by substituting the corresponding values of the variables associated with each into the regression equation of Table 11.2(c). The resulting scores, S, can then either be plotted in a frequency distribution or ranked in numerical order. From either of these the distribution of values can then be partitioned into (say) three or more groups and the corresponding Kaplan–Meier survival curves plotted for the patients of these groups.

Table 11.2 Univariate and multivariable Cox proportional hazards regression models of Zubrod score, ascites and serum AFP level for the index cases (from Tan, Law, Ng and Machin, 2003. Simple clinical prognostic model for hepatocellular carcinoma in developing countries and its validation. *Journal of Clinical Oncology*, **21**, 2294–2298 [11]

Variable	Category	n	Coefficient	Hazard ratio	95% CI
(a) Univariate					
Zubrod score	0	32	0	1	
(ZPS)	1	119	0.542	1.72	1.16 to 2.54
	$\geqslant 2$	168	1.092	2.98	2.02 to 4.41
	Unknown	78	0.811	2.25	1.48 to 3.41
Ascites	Absent	227	0	1	
	Present	167	0.668	1.95	1.59 to 2.40
	Unknown	3	1.869	6.48	2.05 to 2.46
AFP (µg/L)	$\leqslant 499$	134	0	1	
	500–4999	86	0.262	1.30	0.99 to 1.70
	5000–49 999	93	0.652	1.92	1.46 to 2.52
	$\geqslant 50\,000$	84	0.912	2.49	1.88 to 3.31
(b) Multivariable categorical					
Zubrod score	0	32	0	1	
(ZPS)	1	119	0.432	1.54	1.04 to 2.29
	$\geqslant 2$/Unknown	246	0.689	1.99	1.35 to 2.93
Ascites	Absent	227	0	1	
	Present/Unknown	170	0.663	1.94	1.57 to 2.40
AFP (µg/L)	$\leqslant 499$	134	0	1	
	500–4999	86	0.155	1.20	0.89 to 1.54
	5000–49 999	93	0.636	1.89	1.43 to 2.50
	$\geqslant 50\,000$/Unknown	84	0.818	2.27	1.70 to 3.03
(c) Multivariable ordered categorical					
Zubrod (P)	0, 1, 2		0.304		
Ascites (A)	0, 1		0.646		
AFP (F)	0, 1, 2, 3		0.290		

Case study *– prognostic groups – inoperable hepatocellular carcinoma*

The Cox regression of Table 11.2(c) gives a score, S, for each patient as

$$S = \log h = 0.646A + 0.304P + 0.290F,$$

where A denotes ascites, P physical performance by Zubrod performance score (ZPS) and F serum AFP level. Dividing the terms on the right-hand side of this equation by the smallest regression coefficient, namely 0.290, and rounding to the nearest integer gives a simplified survival score, SS, of

$$SS = 2A + P + F.$$

On this basis the minimum possible for $SS=0$ and the maximum is $SS=7$. Plots of the corresponding eight survival curves suggested that there are three groups (Low, Medium, High Risk) of sufficiently different prognosis. The Kaplan–Meier survival curves for these three groups are given in Figure 11.1(a). At 6 months the estimated proportions alive for Low, Medium and High Risk groups are approximately 60%, 20% and 5% respectively.

PREDICTED PROGNOSTIC INFORMATION

If the Kaplan–Meier plots of the different risk groups are sufficiently separated then this suggests that these groups may be used for prognosis. Altman and Royston (2000)

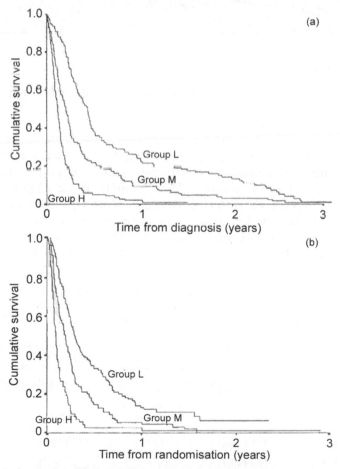

Figure 11.1 Index and validation Kaplan–Meier estimates of Low, Medium and High Risk prognostic groups for patients with inoperable hepatocellular carcinoma (from Tan, Law, Ng and Machin, 2003. Simple clinical prognostic model for hepatocellular carcinoma in developing countries and its validation. *Journal of Clinical Oncology*, **21**, 2294–2298 [11]

provide a measure of the prognostic information contained in these groups as that summarised by the predicted separation ($PSEP$)

$$PSEP = p_{High} - p_{Low}, \tag{11.3}$$

where p_{High} is the predicted probability of dying for the patients in the worst prognosis group (High Risk) at a fixed time t, and p_{Low} is the predicted probability of dying for the patients in the best prognosis group (Low Risk) at the same time point.

Case study – PSEP – inoperable hepatocellular carcinoma

The 6-month death rates for the index set of 397 patients with inoperable hepatocellular cancer are given in Table 11.3. Thus the proportions of deaths at $t=6$ months in the High and Low Risk groups are $p_{High}=0.571$ and $p_{Low}=0.947$, so $PSEP=0.947 - 0.571=0.376$.

Study Size

There is no easy way to calculate study size for prognostic modelling to cover all exigencies including the unknown number, and strength, of any truly prognostic variable of those candidates being considered.

We first consider the case of estimating a single regression coefficient in a univariate logistic regression equation including a single variable. For such a binary outcome variable, y, Hosmer and Lemeshow (2000) note that a 'relevant quantity is the frequency of the least frequent outcome'. For example, if the endpoint variable is survival status and there are 500 subjects in the study of whom 350 are alive ($y=1$) and 150 are dead ($y=0$), then the key determinate to see if the study size is adequate is $m=\min(m_1, m_0)$. Here m_1 and m_0 are the numbers in the corresponding binary groups. They suggest therefore that the most favourable situation is when $m_1=N/2$ of the

Table 11.3 Estimated 6-month death rates, $PSEP$ for index and $OSEP$ for validation groups according to survival score (SS) (from Tan, Law, Ng and Machin, 2003. Simple clinical prognostic model for hepatocellular carcinoma in developing countries and its validation. *Journal of Clinical Oncology*, **21**, 2294–2298 [11]

		Patient group			
		Index group		Validation group	
Risk group	SS	n (%)	6-month death rate (p)	n (%)	6-month death rate (p)
Low	0–2	105 (26.4)	0.571	142 (43.8)	0.666
Medium	3–4	160 (40.3)	0.787	111 (34.3)	0.855
High	5–7	132 (33.3)	0.947	71 (21.9)	0.972
		$PSEP$	0.376	$OSEP$	0.306

subjects have the event and $m_0 = N/2$ do not. In other words, the sample size N depends on the distribution of values in the endpoint variable, y.

In this situation, and based on the work of Peduzzi, Concato, Kemper *et al.* (1996), about 10 events per regression coefficient to be estimated in the prognostic factor study are necessary in order to get reasonably stable estimates of the regression coefficients. This suggests that the number of events per candidate variable (EPV) ≥ 10 (strictly events per candidate regression coefficient). Thus in total $\geq 10k$ events are required.

We can turn the problem around and ask: suppose there are N subjects, how many parameters can be estimated based on this rule of 10? The answer is no more than $m/10$. That is, the number of parameters that can be estimated is $k \leq \min(m_1, m_0)/10$. In the above example $m = \min(350, 150) = 150$ and hence the recommended maximum number of regression coefficients to be estimated is $k = (150/10) = 15$. The optimal situation is if $m = N/2$, in which case $k = N/20$.

For actual survival-time studies using Cox proportional hazards models, we suggest that k should be a maximum of $O/10$ and preferably closer to $O/20$, where O is the total number of events observed in the index group.

Case study – *number of variables – hepatocellular carcinoma*

For the Index group of Tan, Law, Ng and Machin (2003) there were $N = 397$ patients all but seven of whom had died and none were lost to follow-up. Thus the number of events is $O = 397 - 7 = 390$ and the suggested number of regression coefficients that might be estimated is between $390/10 = 39$ and $390/20 = 19$. Thus the $k = 30$ regression coefficients, from the $v = 11$ candidate variables of Table 11.1, is within the suggested range.

Example – *study size – non-small-cell lung cancer*

Piffarré, Rosell, Monzó *et al.* (1997) investigate the prognostic value on survival of replication errors (RER) on chromosomes 2p and 3p amongst 64 patients with non-small-cell lung cancer using Cox's proportional hazards model.

Amongst these patients only $O = 19$ (30%) had died, which suggests that the number of regression coefficients appropriate to estimate in a multivariable Cox model is between 19/20 and 19/10 which indicate at the most $k = 2$. In fact the authors appear to investigate, at least $v = 8$ candidate variables (involving $k \geq 10$ regression coefficients) including age, gender, histological type (squamous cell carcinoma, adenocarcinoma, large-cell carcinoma), tumour stage (I, II, IIIA), K-ras (mutated, non-mutated), p53 (mutated, non-mutated), LOH (complete loss of one or both alleles of the repeat locus) and RER (postive, negative). As a result of non-specified selection procedure they derive a prognostic model including RER and Stage. The numbers of events is clearly too few for such an investigation.

PRACTICALITIES

Once the variables to be examined in the prognostic modelling have been determined the model can be fitted and the 'important' variables identified in a number of (statistically speaking) mechanistic ways. However, there is no 'best' method and so there is some subjective choice in which to use. However, with sufficient data, strongly influential candidate variables are likely to emerge whatever the method adopted.

Some care is needed in the use of any 'mechanistic' approach. Thus a statistically significant regression coefficient for a variable may be established, perhaps in a prognostic factor study of many patients, but its actual effect on patient outcome is very small. Thus any judgement must be based on the magnitude of the regression coefficient and not just the associated p-value. Conversely in a more modest study, a variable exerting a major prognostic influence but not statistically significant, could be eliminated.

Design features – the index or training set

Determine an adequate sample size

Define eligibility carefully

Identify the variables of interest

Determine Level–In, Level–Query, Level–Out and Level–New

Ensure data are complete

Screen the Level–Query and Level–New using univariate methods

Model the Level–In variables

Add the Level–Query and Level–New

Create the PI

Estimate PSEP

11.4 VALIDATING A PROGNOSTIC FACTOR MODEL

PROCESS

As with all exploratory procedures, it is almost inevitable that a prognostic model derived from one data set will not perform as well on a second. There are many reasons for this, but an important one is because of random differences (perhaps exaggerating the effects of a particular variable on prognosis) that will be picked up by the modelling process. In contrast, where random differences happen to reduce the effects of the particular variable it will then tend to be excluded from the model chosen. In the former case, the 'exaggeration' may be revealed on later investigation whereas there is a real danger in the second case that the one omitted may go unnoticed. It is clear also from the processes we have described above that 'subjective' judgement comes into the modelling process.

1.	Are the same variables still important?
2.	Is the functional form of the prognostic model correct?
3.	Are the estimated regression coefficients compatible?
4.	How well does the new model fit the data?
5.	Is the correct ordering of the prognostic groups preserved?
6.	Are the event rates between the prognostic groups significantly different?

Figure 11.2 Items necessary for model validation (from Altman and Royston, 2000; reproduced by permission of John Wiley & Sons Ltd)

Altman and Royston (2000) state: 'These considerations argue strongly for the need to evaluate performance of a model on a new series of patients, ideally in a different location'. Thus if a research group are developing a PI, then to satisfy this requirement a validation group of patients is required. This implies that the whole exercise is a two-stage process, involving the index or training group of patients as we have described above and a second validation group of patients. Figure 11.2 details the conditions necessary for validating a PI as specified by Altman and Royston (2000).

VERIFYING A PROGNOSTIC INDEX

Published Index

If a prognostic model for a situation has been developed by others and perhaps reported in the literature, then one may reasonably wish to verify if the index so derived is applicable to another set of patients. However, before proceeding it is useful to check the exact details of how the index was produced and to be sure that the methodology is acceptable. For example, if the methodology appears flawed, then this may affect judgement with respect to the level of validation that one might expect. Of course, if 'pure' verification is required then care has to be taken in defining the eligibility in precisely the same way as for those for whom the model was constructed. On the other hand, if one is interested to see if the model is applicable to a wider range of patients, then as wide a range as considered relevant is appropriate. However, the expectations for the original model must be duly adjusted, depending on the extent of the overlap between the patient groups concerned. The criteria for judging the model must be defined in advance of the verification process.

For pure verification purposes, a measure such as *PSEP* should first be obtained for the data constructing the original model, perhaps from the relevant publication itself. Then the score for each patient in the validation group is obtained using the exact model formulation as published and, on the basis of their individual scores, they are assigned to the recommended prognostic groups. The corresponding Kaplan–Meier curves are estimated and *PSEP*, now termed the observed separation (*OSEP*), is calculated and compared to the original. Close agreement in these values would validate the model.

A common mistake, rather then to check the exact model published on the new data, is to build one's own model and see if the process of model building chooses the same variables. However, it is often quite difficult to replicate some of the more 'subjective' criteria involved in a modelling process, so differences may result as a consequence of this. Nevertheless, if this process selects the same variables, then a check is made of whether or not the corresponding regression coefficients are similar in value. This may or may not verify the prognostic value of the published index.

Developing an Index

The above process is mirrored when developing a new PI, except that one first starts with a training set and derives the PI oneself. A key feature of the design is for the research group to identify an appropriate validation group. However, an important aspect of the process is to ensure the model to be validated is derived *before* detailed knowledge of the validation group is available to the modelling team. Ideally the validation set should be obtained from patients from a different location and their data collected by a different research team.

Case study – *validation group – OSEP – inoperable hepatocellular carcinoma*

Patients from the Asia-Pacific-wide multicentre trial for treatment of inoperable HCC and recruited over the period 4 April 1997 to 8 June 2000 were used to validate the PI. These were 329 patients who were randomised in a double-blind fashion to either tamoxifen treatment or placebo. Survival information was available on all but five of these patients. All consenting patients had their baseline characteristics recorded at the time of diagnosis of HCC, following which they were randomised to the trial and routine follow-up until death.

Survival was calculated from the date of randomisation. The *SS* derived from the Index group was used to calculate, for each new patient, the corresponding value for him or her. On the basis of this score the patient was then assigned to one of the proposed Low, Medium and High Risk groups as previously defined and the survival experience summarised using the Kaplan–Meier technique. From these curves, shown in Figure 11.1 (lower panel), the proportions alive at 6 months was estimated giving $OSEP = p_{High} - p_{Low} = 0.31$. This is close to the corresponding $PSEP = 0.38$ obtained from Figure 11.1 (upper panel) demonstrating validity of the prognostic model.

In addition, the use of the validation group, obtained from a prospective multinational, multiethnic, randomised controlled clinical trial with high-quality data, provides additional reassurance. The initial model was established 3 years before the prospective validation data became available.

Study Size

It is difficult to be prescriptive about the size required of the validation group. Clearly the number of candidate variables to include is now stipulated by the PI derived from the Index group. Thus one might argue that $k_{\text{Validation}}$ is likely to be much smaller than k_{Index}, so a pragmatic way is to suggest $O_{\text{Validation}}$ is somewhere in the order of $10 \times k_{\text{Validation}}$ to $20 \times k_{\text{Validation}}$.

***Case study** – size of validation group – inoperable hepatocellular carcinoma*

The final PI derived in this study included $v=3$ variables (involving $k_{\text{Validation}}=3$ regression coefficients). Thus the above suggestion indicates that $O_{\text{Validation}}$ should be between $10 \times k_{\text{Validation}}=30$ and $20 \times k_{\text{Validation}}=60$. The data set actually used comprised 296 patients of whom 276 (93%) had died. This would appear to be more than sufficient for the validation process.

Design features – the validation set

Define eligibility cross-check with the index or training set

Cross-check with the details provided by Altman and Royston (2000)

Follow exactly the same process of scoring the individual patients as suggested by the PI

Calculate OSEP and compare with PSEP

References

A'Hern RP (2001). Sample size tables for exact single-stage phase II designs. *Statistics in Medicine*, **20**, 859–866. [8]

Altman DG, Gore SM, Gardner MJ and Pocock SJ (2000). Statistical guidelines for contributors to medical journals. In DG Altman, D Machin, TN Bryant and MJ Gardner (eds), *Statistics with Confidence* (2nd edn). British Medical Journal, London, pp. 171–190. [1, 3]

Altman DG, Machin D, Bryant TN and Gardner MJ (eds) (2000). *Statistics with Confidence* (2nd edn). British Medical Journal Books, London. [1, 3]

Altman DG and Royston P (2000). What do we mean by validating a prognostic model. *Statistics in Medicine*, **19**, 453–473. [11]

Anderson LJ, Holden S, Davis B, Prescott E, Charrier CC, Bunce NH, Firmin DN, Wonke B, Porter J, Walker JM and Pennell DJ (2001). Cardiovascular T2-star (T2*) magnetic resonance for the early diagnosis of myocardial iron overload. *European Heart Journal*, **22**, 2171–2179. [10]

Ang ES-W, Lee S-T, Gan CS-G, Chan Y-H, Cheung Y-B and Machin D (2003). Pain control in a randomized controlled trial comparing Moist Exposed Burn Ointment (MEBO) and conventional methods in patients with partial thickness burns. *Journal of Burn Care and Rehabilitation*, **24**, 289–296. [2]

Ang ES-W, Lee S-T, Gan CS-G, See PG-J, Chan Y-H, Ng L-H and Machin D (2001). Evaluating the role of alternative therapy in burn wound management: randomized trial comparing Moist Exposed Burn Ointment with conventional methods in the management of patients with second-degree burns. *Medscape General Medicine* (6 March 2001), **3**(2), 3. [3, 7]

Asch DA, Jedrziewski K, Christiakis NA (1997). Response rates to mail surveys published in medical journals. *Journal of Clinical Epidemiology*, **50**, 1129–1136. [6]

Asian Lichen Planus Study Group (2005). A randomised controlled trial to compare steroid with cyclosporine for the topical treatment of oral lichen planus. In press [2]

ATAC (Arimidex, Tamoxifen Alone or in Combination) Trialists' Group (2002). Anastrozole alone or in combination with tamoxifen versus tamoxifen alone for adjuvant treatment of postmenopausal women with early breast cancer: first results of the ATAC randomised trial. *Lancet*, **359**, 2131–2139. [7, 9]

Baldini E, Tibaldi C, Ardizzoni A, Salvati F, Antilli A, Portalone L, Barbera S, *et al.* (1998). Cisplatin-vindesine-mitomycin (MVP) vs cisplatin-ifosfamide-vinorelbine (PIN) vs carboplatin-vinorelbine (CaN) in patients with advanced non-small-cell lung cancer (NSCLC): a FONICAP randomized phase II study. *British Journal of Cancer*, **77**, 2367–2370. [8]

Barker DJP, Forsén T, Uutela A, Osmond C and Eriksson JG (2001). Size at birth and resilience to effects of poor living conditions in adult life: longitudinal study. *British Medical Journal*, **323**, 1273–1276. [6]

Begg C, Cho M, Eastwood S, Horton R, Moher D, Olkin I, Pitkin R, Rennie D, Schultz KF, Simel D and Stroup DF (1996). Improving the quality of reporting randomized controlled trials: the CONSORT statement. *Journal of the American Medical Association*, **276**, 637–639. [1, 7]

Bennet L and Berglund J (2002). Reinfection with Lyme borreliosis: a retrospective follow-up study in Southern Sweden. *Scandinavian Journal of Infectious Diseases*, **34**, 183–186. [5]

Design of Studies for Medical Research. D. Machin and M. J. Campbell
© 2005 John Wiley & Sons Ltd. ISBN 0 470 84495 7

Berglund J, Stjernberg L, Ornstein K, Tykesson-Joelsson K and Walter H (2002). 5-y follow up of patients with neuroborreliosis. *Scandinavian Journal of Infectious Diseases*, **34**, 421–425. [6]

Bhargava V, Lenfant B, Perret C, Pascual M-H, Sultan E and Montay G (2002). Lack of food on the bioavailibility of a new kerolide antibacterial, telithromycin. *Scandinavian Journal of Infectious Diseases*, **34**, 823–826. [7, 8]

Birkett MA and Day SJ (1994). Internal pilot studies for estimating sample size. *Statistics in Medicine*, **13**, 2455–2463. [3]

Bonett DG (2002). Sample size requirements for estimating intraclass correlations with desired precision. *Statistics in Medicine*, **21**, 1331–1335. [10]

Bossuyt PM, Reitsma JB, Brund DE, Gatsonis CA, Glasziou PP, Irwig LM, Lijmer LG, Moher D, Rennie D and de Vet HC (2003). Towards complete and accurate reporting of studies of diagnostic accuracy: the STARD initiative. Standards for Reporting of Diagnostic Accuracy. *Clinical Chemistry*, **49**, 19–20. [10]

Boynton PM (2004). Administering, analysing and reporting your questionnaire. *British Medical Journal*, **328**, 1372–1375. [6]

Brandes AA, Vastola F, Basso U, Berti F, Inna G, Rotilio A, Gardiman M, Scienza R, Monfardini S and Ermani M (2003). A prospective study of glioblastoma in the elderly. *Cancer*, **97**, 657–662. [7]

Brealey D, Brand M, Hargreaves I, Heales S, Land J, Smolenski R, Davies NA, Cooper CE and Singer M (2002). Association between mitochondrial dysfunction and outcome of septic shock. *Lancet*, **360**, 219–223. [5]

Browne RH (1995). On the use of a pilot study for sample size determination. *Statistics in Medicine*, **14**, 1933–1940. [3]

Bryant J and Day R (1995). Incorporating toxicity considerations into the design of two-stage phase II clinical trials. *Biometrics*, **51**, 1372–1383. [7, 8]

Butenas S, Cawthern KM, van't Meer C, DiLorenzo JB and Mann KG (2001). Antiplatelet agents in tissue-induced blood coagulation. *Blood*, **97**, 2314–2322. [5]

Calne R, Moffatt SD, Friend PJ, Jamieson NV, Bradley JA, Hale G, Firth J, Bradley K, Smith KGC and Walsdmann H (1999). Campath IH allows low-dose cyclosporine monotherapy in 32 cadaveric renal allocraft recipients. *Transplantation*, **68**, 1–10. [5]

Campbell G, Pickles T and D'yachkova Y (2003). A randomised trial of cranberry versus apple juice in the management of urinary symptoms during external beam radiation therapy for prostate cancer. *Clinical Oncology*, **15**, 322–328. [4]

Campbell MJ (2000). Cluster randomized trials in general (family) practice research. *Statistical Methods in Medical Research*, **9**, 81–94. [9]

Campbell MJ and Gardner MJ (2000). Medians and their differences. In DG Altman, D Machin, TN Bryant and MJ Gardner (eds), *Statistics with Confidence* (2nd edn). *British Medical Journal*, London. [10]

Campbell MJ and Waters WE (1990). Does anonymity increase response rate in postal questionnaire surveys about sensitive subjects? A randomised trial. *Journal of Epidemiology and Community Health*, **44**, 75–76. [6]

Campbell MK, Elbourne DR, Altman DG for the CONSORT Group (2004). The CONSORT statement: extension to cluster randomised trials. *British Medical Journal*, **328**, 702–708. [7]

Cantor AB (1996). Sample size calculations for Cohen's kappa. *Psychological Methods*, **2**, 150–153. [10]

Case LD and Morgan TM (2003). Design of Phase II cancer trials evaluating survival probabilities. *BMC Medical Research Methodology*, **3**, 6. [8]

Chow PK-H, Tai B-C, Tan C-K, Machin D, Johnson PJ, Khin M-W and Soo K-C (2002). No role for high-dose tamoxifen in the treatment of inoperable hepatocellular carcinoma: an Asia-Pacific double-blind randomised controlled trial. *Hepatology*, **36**, 1221–1226. [1, 4, 7, 9, 11]

Chung YFA, Eu K-W, Machin D, Ho JMS, Nyam DCNK, Leong AFPK and Seow-Choen F (1998). Young age is not a poor prognostic marker in colorectal cancer. *British Journal of Surgery*, **85**, 1255–1259. [11]

Cicchetti DV (2001). The precision of reliability and validity estimates re-visited: distinguishing between clinical and statistical significance of sample size requirements. *Journal of Clinical and Experimental Neuropsychology*, **23**, 695–700. [10]

Clancy L, Goodman P, Sinclair H and Dockerty DW (2002). Effect of air-pollution control on death rates in Dublin, Ireland: an intervention study. *Lancet*, **360**, 1210–1214. [5]

Cohen J (1988). *Statistical Power Analysis for the Behavioral Sciences* (2nd edn). Lawrence Erlbaum, Mahwah, NJ. [3, 5]

Collins JF (2001). Protocols. In CK Redmond and T Colton (eds), *Biostatistics in Clinical Trials*. Wiley, Chichester, pp. 373–377. [1]

Connor J, Norton R, Ameratunga S, Robinson E, Civil I, Dunn R, Bailey J and Jackson R (2002). Driver sleepiness and risk of serious injury to car occupants: population based case-control study. *British Medical Journal*, **324**, 1125–1128. [6]

CPMP Working Party on Efficacy of Medicinal Products (1995). Biostatistical methodology in clinical trials in applications for marketing authorizations for medicinal products. *Statistics in Medicine*, **14**, 1659–1682. [2, 3]

Crum NF, Utz GC and Wallace MR (2002). Stenotrophomonas maltophilia endocarditis. *Scandinavian Journal of Infectious Diseases*, **34**, 925–927. [5]

Csendes A, Burdiles P, Korn O, Braghetto I, Huertas C and Rojas J (2002). Late results of a randomized clinical trial comparing total fundoplication *versus* calibration of the cardia with posterior gastropexy. *British Journal of Surgery*, **87**, 289–297. [4]

Cuschieri A, Weeden S, Fielding J, Bancewicz J, Craven J, Joypaul V, Sydes M and Fayers P (1999). Patient survival after D1 and D2 resections for gastric cancer: long-term results of the MRC randomized surgical trial. *British Journal of Cancer*, **79**, 1522–1530. [3]

Day L, Fildes B, Gordon I, Fitzharris M, Flamer H and Lord S (2002). Randomised factorial trial of falls prevention among older people living in their own homes. *British Medical Journal*, **325**, 128–131. [9]

Day SJ and Graham DF (1991). Sample size estimation for comparing two or more groups. *Statistics in Medicine*, **10**, 33–43. [5, 9]

Devereux JG, Foster PJ, Baasanhu J, Uranchimeg D, Lee P-K, Erdenbeleig T, Machin D, Johnson GJ and Alsbirk PH (2000). Anterior chamber depth measurement as a screening tool for primary angle-closure glaucoma in an East Asian population. *Archives of Ophthalmology*, **118**, 257–263. [6, 10]

de Vet HC, van der Weijden T, Muris JW, Heyrman J, Buntinx F and Knottnerus JA (2001). Systematic reviews of diagnostic research. Considerations about assessment and incorporation of methodological quality. *European Journal of Epidemiology*, **17**, 301–306. [10]

Dickersin K and Rennie D (2003). Registering clinical trials. *Journal of the American Medical Association*, **290**, 516–523. [7]

Diletti E, Hauschke D and Steinijans VW (1991). Sample size determination for bioequivalence assessment by means of confidence intervals. *International Journal Clinical Pharmacology, Therapy and Toxicology*, **29**, 1–8. [3]

Dillman DA (2004). *Mail and Internet Surveys. The Tailored Design Method* (2nd edn). Wiley, New York. [6]

Dodd P, Day SJ, Goldhill DR, MacLeod DM, Withington PS and Yate PM (1989). Glycopyrronium requirements for antagonism of the muscarinic side effects of edrophonium. *British Journal Anaesthesia*, **62**, 77–81. [5]

Donner A and Eliasziw M (1992). A goodness-of-fit approach to inference procedures for the kappa statistics: confidence interval construction, significance testing and sample size estimation. *Statistics in Medicine*, **11**, 1511–1519. [10]

Donner A and Klar N (2000). Pitfalls of and controversies in cluster randomisation trials. *American Journal of Public Health*, **94**, 416–422. [9]

Donner A, Piaggio G, Villar J, Pinol A, Al-Mazrou Y, Ba'aqeel H, Bakketeig L, Belizán, JM, Berendes H, Carroli G, Farnot U and Lumbiganon P (1998). Methodological considerations in the design of the WHO antenatal care randomised controlled trial. *Paediatric and Perinatal Epidemiology*, **12**, Suppl. 2, 59–74. [7]

Draper B, Brodaty H, Low L-F, Richards V, Paton H and Lie D (2002). Self-destructive behaviors in nursing home residents. *Journal American Geriatric Society*, **50**, 354–358. [5]

Drasdo N, Chiti Z, Owens DR and North RV (2002). Effect of darkness on inner retinal hypoxia in diabetes. *Lancet*, **359**, 2251–2253. [3]

Drummond M and McGuire A (2002). *Economic Evaluation in Health Care: Merging Theory with Practice*. Oxford University Press, Oxford. [7]

Edwards P, Roberts I, Clarke M, Di Guiseppi C, Pratap S, Wentz R and Kwan I (2002). Increasing response rates to postal questionnaires; systematic review. *British Medical Journal*, **324**, 1183. [6]

Elashoff JD (2000). *nQuery Advisor Version 4 User's Guide*. Los Angeles. [3]

EMEA (2002). Note for Guidance on Good Clinical Practice (CPMP/ICH/135/95). European Agency for the Evaluation of Medicinal Products, London. http://www.emea.eu.int. [1, 4]

Estey EH and Thall P (2003). New designs for phase 2 clinical trials. *Blood*, **102**, 442–448. [8]

Estlin EJ, Pinkerton CR, Lewis IJ, Lashford L, McDowell H, Morland B, Kohler J, Newell DR, Boddy AV, Taylor GA, Price L, Ablett S, Hobson R, Pitsiladis M, Brampton M, Cledeninn N, Johnston A and Pearson AD (2001). A phase I study of nolatrexed dihydochloride in children with advanced cancer. A United Kingdom Children's Cancer Study Group Investigation. *British Journal of Cancer*, **84**, 11–18. [8]

Fairclough DL (2002). *Design and Analysis of Quality of Life Studies in Clinical Trials*. CRC Press, Boca Raton, FL. [7]

Farrington CP (1995). Relative incidence estimation from case series for vaccine safety evaluation. *Biometrics*, **51**, 228–235. [6]

Farrington CP (2004). Re 'Risk analysis of aseptic meningitis after measles-mumps-rubella vaccination in Korean children by using a case-crossover design' (letter). *American Journal of Epidemiology*, **159**, 717–718. [6]

Fayers PM and Machin D (1995). Sample size: how many patients are necessary? *British Journal of Cancer*, **72**, 1–9. [3]

Fayers PM and Machin D (2000). *Quality of Life: Assessment, Analysis and Interpretation*. Wiley, Chichester. [7]

FDA (Food and Drug Administration) (1988). *Guidelines for the Format and Content of the Clinical and Statistics Section of New Drug Applications*. US Department of Health and Human Services, Public Health Service, Food and Drug Administration. [3]

Fender GR, Prentice A, Gorst T, Nixon RM, Duffy SW, Day NE and Smith SK (1999). Randomised controlled trial of educational package on management of menorrhagia in primary care: the Anglia menorrhagia education study: *British Medical Journal*, **318**, 1246–1250. [9]

Fleiss JL (1986). *The Design and Analysis of Clinical Experiments*. Wiley, New York. [9]

Fleming TR (1982). One-sample multiple testing procedure for Phase II clinical trials. *Biometrics*, **38**, 143–151. [8]

Flinn IW, Goodman SN, Post L, Jamison J, Miller CB, Gore S, Diehl L, Willis C, Ambinder RF and Byrd JC (2000). A dose-finding study of liposomal daunorubicin with CVP (COP-X) in advanced NHL. *Annals of Oncology*, **11**, 691–695. [8]

Foo K-F, Tan E-H, Leong S-S, Wee JTS, Tan T, Fong K-W, Koh L, Tai B-C, Lian L-G and Machin D (2002). Gemcitabine in metastatic nasopharyngeal carcinoma of the undifferentiated type. *Annals of Oncology*, **13**, 150–156. [7, 8]

Foster PJ, Oen FTS, Machin D, Ng T-P, Devreux JG, Johnson GJ, Khaw PT and Seah SKL (2000). The prevalence of glaucoma in Chinese residents of Singapore: a cross-sectional population survey of the Tanjong Pagar District. *Archives Ophthalmology*, **118**, 1105–1111. [3, 6]

Freedman LS, Parmar MKB and Baker RG (1993). The design of observer agreement studies with binary assessments. *Statistics in Medicine*, **12**, 165–179. [10]

Gardner MJ, Machin D, Campbell MJ and Altman DG (2000). Statistical checklists. In DG Altman, D Machin, TN Bryant and MJ Gardner (eds), *Statistics with Confidence* (2nd edn). *British Medical Journal*, London, pp. 191–201. [1, 3]

Gattellari M and Ward JE (2001). Will donations to their learned college increase surgeon's participation rate in surveys? A randomized trial. *Journal of Clinical Epidemiology*, **54**, 645–649. [6]

Gehan EA (1961). The determination of the number of patients required in a preliminary and follow-up trial of a new chemotherapeutic agent. *Journal of Chronic Diseases*, **13**, 346–353. [8]

Gilliland FD, Li Y-F, Saxon A and Diaz-Sanchez D (2004). Effect of glutathione-*S*-transferase M1 and P1 genotypes on xenobiotic enhancement of allergic responses: randomised, placebo-controlled crossover study. *Lancet*, **363**, 119–125. [5]

Gilman EA, Cheng KK, Winter HR and Scragg R (1995). Trends in rates and seasonal distribution of sudden infant deaths in England and Wales, 1988–92. *British Medical Journal*, **310**, 631–632. [1]

González-Martín A, Crespo C, García-López JL, Pedraza M, Garrido P, Lastra E and Moyano A (2002). Ifosfamide and vinorelbine in advanced platinum-resistant ovarian cancer: excessive toxicity with a potentially active regimen. *Gynecologic Oncology*, **84**, 368–373. [8]

Goodman SN, Zahurak ML and Piantadosi S (1995). Some practical improvements in the continual reassessment method for phase I studies. *Statistics in Medicine*, **14**, 1149–1161. [8]

Harpenau LA, Plemons JM and Rees TD (1995). Effectiveness of low dose cyclosporine in the management of patients with oral erosive lichen planus. *Oral Surgery Oral Medicine Oral Pathology Oral Radiological Endod*, **80**, 161–167. [2]

Harris EK and Boyd JC (1995). *Statistical Bases of Reference Values in Laboratory Medicine*. Marcel Dekker, New York. [10]

Hill AB (1965). The environment and disease: association or causation. *Proceedings of the Royal Society of Medicine*, **58**, 295–300. [1]

Hong B, Ji YH, Hong JH, Nam KY and Ahn Ty (2002). A double-blind crossover study evaluating the efficacy of Korean red ginseng in patients with erectile dysfunction: a preliminary report. *Journal of Urology*, **168**, 2070–2073. [9]

Hosmer DW and Lemeshow S (2000). *Applied Logistic Regression* (2nd edn). Wiley, New York. [11]

Hovind P, Tarnow L, Rossing P, Jensen BR, Graae M, Torp I, Binder C and Parving HH (2004). Predictors for the development of microalbuminuria and macroalbuminuria in patients with type 1 diabetes: inception cohort study. *British Medical Journal*, **328**, 1105 (8 May), doi:10.1136/bmj.38070.450891.FE. [6]

Huibers MJ, Bleijenberg G, Beurkens AJ, Kant IJ, Knottnerus JA, van der Windt DA, Bazelmans E and van Schayck CP (2004). An alternative trial design to overcome validity and recruitment problems in primary care research. *Family Practice*, **21**, 213–218. [7]

ICH E9 Expert Working Group (1999). Statistical principles for clinical trials: ICH harmonised tripartite guideline. *Statistics in Medicine*, **18**, 1907–1942. [4, 7]

Itoh K, Ohtsu T, Fukuda H, Sasaki Y, Ogura M, Morishima Y, Chou T, Aikawa K, Uike N, Mizorogi F, Ohno T, Ikeda S, Sai T, Taniwaki M, Kawano F, Niimi M, Hotta T, Shimoyama M and Tobinai K (2002). Randomized phase II study of biweekly CHOP and dose-escalated CHOP with prophylactic use of lenograstim (glycosylated G-CSF) in aggressive non-Hodgkin's lymphoma: Japan Clinical Oncology Group Study 9505. *Annals of Oncology*, **13**, 1347–1355. [8]

Jensen PT, Groenwold M, Klee MC, Thranov I, Petersen MAa and Machin D (2003). Longitudinal study of sexual function and vaginal changes after radiotherapy for cervical cancer. *International Journal of Radiation Oncology Biology & Physics*, **56**, 937–949. [5, 6]

Jensen PT, Klee MC, Thranov I and Groenvold M (2004). Validation of a questionnaire for self-assessment of sexual function and vaginal changes after gynaecological cancer. *Psycho-Oncology*, **13**, 577–592. [2]

Jones B, Jarvis P, Lewis JA and Ebbutt AF (1996). Trials to assess equivalence: the importance of rigorous methods. *British Medical Journal*, **313**, 36–39. [3, 7, 9]

Julious SA (2004). Sample sizes for clinical trials with normal data. *Statistics in Medicine*, **23**, 1921–1986. [3, 8]

Julious SA and Debarnot CAM (2000). Why are pharmacokinetic data summarized by arithmetic means? *Journal of Biopharmaceutical Statistics*, **10**, 55–71. [8]

Kalantar JS and Talley NJ (1999). The effects of lottery incentive and length of questionnaire on health survey response rates: a randomized study. *Journal of Clinical Epidemiology*, **52**, 1117–1122. [6]

King EA, Baldwin DS, Sinclair JMA, Baker NG, Campbell MJ and Thompson C (2001). The Wessex Recent In-patient Suicide Study, I: Case-control study of 234 recently discharged psychiatric patient suicides. *British Journal of Psychiatry*, **178**, 531–536. [6]

Kinmonth AL, Woodcock A, Griffin S, Spiegal N and Campbell MJ (1998). Randomised controlled trial of patient centred care of diabetes in general practice: impact on current wellbeing and future disease risk. *British Medical Journal*, **317**, 1202–1208. [7]

Klee M, Groenvold M and Machin D (1997). Quality of life of Danish women: population-based norms of the EORTC QLQ-C30. *Quality of Life Research*, **6**, 27–34. [4]

Korn EL, Midthune D, Chen TT, Rubinstein LV, Christian MC and Simon RM (1994). A comparison of two Phase I trial designs. *Statistics in Medicine*, **13**, 1799–1806. [8]

Lassere M and Johnson K (2002). The power of the protocol. *Lancet*, **360**, 1620–1622. [1]

Lau WY, Leung TWT, Ho SKW, Chan M, Machin D, Lau J, Chan ATC, Yeo W, Mok TSK, Yu SCH, Leung NWY and Johnson PJ (1999). Adjuvant intra-arterial iodine-131-labelled lipiodol for resectable hepatocellular carcinoma: a prospective randomised trial. *Lancet*, **353**, 797–801. [7]

Lehnert M, Mross K, Schueller J, Thuerlimann B, Kroeger N and Kupper H (1998). Phase II trial of dexverapamil and epirubicin in patients with non-responsive metastatic breast cancer. *British Journal of Cancer*, **77**, 1155–1163. [8]

Lewis JA and Machin D (1993). Intention to treat: who should use ITT. *British Journal of Cancer*, **68**, 647–650. [7]

Li D, Dhawale P, Rubin PJ, Haacke EM and Gropler RJ (1996). Myocardial signal response to dipyridamole and dobutamine: demonstration of the BOLD effect using a double-echo gradient-echo sequence. *Magnetic Resonance in Medicine*, **36**, 16–20. [10]

Linnet K (1987). Two-stage transformation systems for normalization of reference distributions evaluated. *Clinical Chemistry*, **33**, 381–386. [10]

Lobo DN, Bostock KA, Neal KR, Perkins AC, Rowlands BJ and Allison SP (2002). Effect of salt and water balance on recovery of gastrointestinal function after elective colonic resection: a randomised controlled trial. *Lancet*, **359**, 1812–1818. [3, 4]

Lyons RA, Djahanbakhch O, Saridogan E, Naftalin AA, Mahmood T, Weekes A and Chenoy R (2002). Peritoneal fluid, endometriosis, and ciliary beat frequency in the human fallopian tube. *Lancet*, **360**, 1221–1222. [4, 5]

Machin D, Campbell MJ, Fayers PM and Pinol A (1997). *Statistical Tables for the Design of Clinical Studies* (2nd edn). Blackwell Scientific Publications, Oxford. [3]

Machin D, Cheung Y-B and Parmar MKB (2005). *Survival Analysis: A Practical Approach* (2nd edn) Wiley, Chichester. [11]

Machin D, Stenning SP, Parmar MKB, Fayers PM, Girling DJ, Stephens RJ, Stewart LA and Whaley JB (1997). Thirty years of Medical Research Council randomized trials in solid tumours. *Clinical Oncology*, **9**, 20–28. [7]

Maclure M and Mittleman MA (2000). Should we use a case-crossover design? *Annual Review of Public Health*, **21**, 193–221. [6]

Mant T and Allen E (2001). Early phase studies, pharmacokinetics and adverse drug interactions. In I Di Giovanna and G Hayes, *Principles of Clinical Research*. Wrightson Biomedical Publishing, Petersfield, pp. 117–160. [8]

Marchese VG, Chiarello LA and Lange BJ (2003). Strength and functional mobility in children with acute lymphoblastic leukemia. *Medical Pediatric Oncology*, **40**, 230–232. [5]

Matteuci E and Giampietro O (2000). Transmembrane electron transfer in diabetic nephropathy. *Diabetes Care*, **23**, 994–999. [5]

McCarthy HD, Ellis SM and Cole TJ (2003). Central overweight and obesity in British youth aged 11–16 years: cross sectional surveys of waist circumference. *British Medical Journal*, **326**, 624. [5]

McMurray JJ, Östergren J, Swedberg K, Granger CB, Held P, Michelson EL, Olofsson B, Yusuf S, Pfeffer MA (2003). Effects of candesartan in patients with chronic heart failure and reduced left-ventricular systolic function taking angiotensin-converting-enzyme inhibitors: the CHARM-Added trial. *Lancet*, **362**, 767–771. [9]

Medical Research Council (2002). *Design of Complex Intervention Trials*. Medical Research Council, London. [9]

Medical Research Council Lung Cancer Working Party (1996). Randomized trial of palliative two-fraction versus more intensive 13-fraction radiotherapy for patients with inoperable non-small cell lung cancer and good performance status. *Clinical Oncology*, **8**, 167–175. [4]

Moher D, Schultz KF, Altman DG, for the CONSORT Group (2001). The CONSORT statement: revised recommendations for improving the quality of reports of parallel-group randomised trials. *Lancet*, **357**, 1191–1194. [1, 4, 7]

Muler JH, McGinn CJ, Normolle D, Lawrence T, Brown D, Hejna G and Zalupski MM (2004). Phase I trial using time-to-event continual reassessment strategy for dose escalation of cisplatin combined with gemcitabine and radiation therapy in pancreatic cancer. *Journal of Clinical Oncology*, **22**, 238–243. [7]

Myles PS, Troedel S, Boquest M and Reeves M (1999). The pain visual analog scale: is it linear or non-linear? *Anaesthesia and Analgesia*, **89**, 1517–1520. [2]

National Cancer Institute (2003). *Common Terminology Criteria for Adverse Events* (v3.0 CTCAE). National Cancer Institute, Bethesda. http:/ctep.cancer.gov/reporting/ctc.html. [8]

Newcombe RG and Altman DG (2000). Proportions and their differences. In DG Altman, D Machin, TN Bryant and MJ Gardner (eds). *Statistics with Confidence* (2nd edn). British Medical Journal, London, 45–56. [3, 8]

Neymark N, Kiebert W, Torfs K, Davies L, Fayers P, Hillner B, Gelber R, Guyatt G, Kind D, Machin D, Nord E, Osoba D, Revicki D, Schulman K and Simpson K (1998). Methodological and statistical issues of quality of life (QoL) and economic evaluation in cancer clinical trials: report of a workshop. *European Journal of Cancer*, **34**, 1317–1333. [7]

Nicholl J and Campbell MJ (2002). Epidemiological research. *Lancet*, **360**, 258–259. [4]

Obuchowski NA and McClish DN (1997). Sample size determination for diagnostic accuracy studies involving binormal ROC curve indices. *Statistics in Medicine*, **16**, 1529–1542. [10]

Öncül O, Özsoy MF, Gul HC, Koçak N, Cavuslu S and Pasha A (2002). Cutaneous anthrax in Turkey: a review of 32 cases. *Scandinavian Journal of Infectious Diseases*, **34**, 413–416. [5]

O'Quigley J (2001). Dose-finding designs using continual reassessment method. In J Crowley (ed.), *Handbook of Statistics in Clinical Oncology*. Marcel Dekker, New York, pp. 35–72. [8]

O'Quigley J, Pepe M and Fisher L (1990). Continual reassessment method: a practical design for Phase I clinical trials in cancer. *Biometrics*, **46**, 33–38. [8]

Park T, Ki M and Yi S-G (2004). Statistical analysis of MMR vaccine adverse effects on aseptic meningitis using the case cross-over design. *Statistics in Medicine*, **23**, 1871–1884. [6]

Peduzzi P, Concato J, Kemper E, Holford TR and Feinstein AR (1996). A simulation study of the number of events per variable in logistic regression analysis. *Journal of Clinical Epidemiology*, **49**, 1372–1379. [11]

Piaggio G and Pinol APY (2001). Use of the equivalence approach in reproductive health trials. *Statistics in Medicine*, **20**, 3571–3587. [7]

Piantadosi S (1997). *Clinical Trials: A Methodologic Perspective*. Wiley, New York. [9]

Piffarré A, Rosell R, Monzó M, De Anta JM, Moreno I, Sánchez JJ, Ariza A, Mate JL, Martínez E and Sánchez M (1997). Prognostic value of replication errors on chromosomes 2p and 3p in non-small-cell lung cancer. *British Journal of Cancer*, **75**, 184–189. [11]

Pocock SJ and White I (1999) Trials stopped early: too good to be true? *Lancet*, **353**, 943–944. [7]

Prentice RL (1995). Design issues in cohort studies. *Statistical Methods in Medical Research*, **4**, 272–292. [6]

Reeder SB, Faranesh AZ, Boxerman JL and McVeigh ER (1998). In vivo measurement of T2* and field inhomogeneity maps in the human heart. *Magnetic Resonance in Medicine*, **39**, 988–998. [10]

Regidor E, Barrio G, de la Feunte L, Domingo A and Alonso J (1999). Association between educational level and health related quality of life in Spanish adults. *Journal of Epidemiology and Community Health*, **53**, 75–82. [9]

Sackett DL, Richardson WS, Rosenberg W and Haynes RB (1997). *Evidence-based Medicine: How to Practice and Teach EBM*. Churchill Livingstone, New York. [1]

Sauerbrei W, Royston P, Bojar H, Schmoor C and Schumacher M (1999). Modelling the effects of standard prognostic factors in node-negative breast cancer. *British Journal of Cancer*, **79**, 1752–1760. [11]

Scott NW, McPherson GC, Ramsay CR and Campbell MK (2002). The method of minimization for allocation to clinical trials. *Controlled Clinical Trials*, **23**, 662–674. [4]

Senn SJ (2002). *Cross-over Trials in Clinical Research*. Wiley, Chichester. [9]

Shaw MJ, Beebe TJ, Jensen HL and Adlis SA (2001). The use of monetary incentives in a community survey: impact on response rates, data quality and cost. *Health Services Research*, **35**, 1339–1346. [6]

Shepherd FA, Burkes R, Cormier Y, Crump M, Feld R, Strack T and Schulz M (1996). Phase I dose-escalation trial of gemcitabine and cisplatin for advanced non-small-cell lung cancer: usefulness of mathematic modeling to determine maximum-tolerable dose. *Journal of Clinical Oncology*, **14**, 1656–1662. [8]

Simon R (1989). Optimal two-stage designs for Phase II clinical trials. *Controlled Clinical Trials*, **10**, 1–10. [8]

Simon R (2000). Therapeutic equivalence trials. In J Crowley (ed.), *Handbook of Statistics in Clinical Oncology*. Marcel Dekker, New York, pp. 173–187. [9]

Simon R and Altman DG (1994). Statistical aspects of prognostic factor studies in oncology. *British Journal of Cancer*, **69**, 979–985. [11]

Simon R, Wittes RE and Ellenberg SS (1985). Randomized Phase II clinical trials. *Cancer Treatment Reports*, **69**, 1375–1381. [8]

Slap GP, Lot L, Huang B, Daniyam CA, Zink TM and Succop PA (2003). Sexual behaviour of adolescents in Nigeria: cross sectional survey of secondary school students. *British Medical Journal*, **326**, 15–16. [6]

Smith M, Bernstein M, Bleyer WA, Borsi JD, Ho P, Lewis IJ, Pearson A, Pein F, Pratt C, Reaman G, Riccardi R, Seibel N, Trueworthy R, Ungerleider R, Vassal G and Vietti T (1998). Conduct of Phase I trials in children with cancer. *Journal of Clinical Oncology*, 16, 966 978. [8]

Smith TL, Lee JJ, Kantarjian HM, Legha SS and Raber MN (1996). Design and results of Phase I cancer clinical trials: three-year experience at M.D. Anderson Cancer Center. *Journal of Clinical Oncology*, **14**, 287–295. [8]

Spiegelhalter DJ, Freedman LS and Parmar MKB (1994). Bayesian approaches to randomized trials (with discussion). *Journal of the Royal Statistical Society*, **A**, **157**, 357–416. [3]

Sprangers MA, Cull A and Groenvold M (1998). *EORTC Quality of Life Study Group: Guidelines for Developing Questionnaire Modules*. EORTC, Brussels. [2]

Spronk PE, Ince C, Gardien MJ, Mathura KR, Oudemans-van Straaten H and Zandstra DF (2002). Nitroglycerin in septic shock after intravascular volume resuscitation. *Lancet*, **260**, 1395–1396. [5]

Stomberg MW, Wickerström K, Joelsson H, Sjöström B and Haljamäe H (2003). Postoperative pain management on surgical wards – do strategies result in long term effects on staff member attitudes and clinical outcome? *Pain Management Nursing*, **4**, 1–12. [9]

Storer B (2001). Choosing a Phase I design. In J Crowley (ed.), *Handbook of Statistics in Clinical Oncology*. Marcel Dekker, New York, pp. 73–91. [8]

Tan C-K, Law N-M, Ng N-S and Machin D (2003). Simple clinical prognostic model for hepatocellular carcinoma in developing countries and its validation. *Journal of Clinical Oncology*, **21**, 2294–2298. [11]

Tan S-B, Dear KBG, Bruzzi P and Machin D (2003). Strategy for randomised clinical trials in rare cancers. *British Medical Journal*, **327**, 47–49. [3]

Tan S-B and Machin D (2002). Bayesian two-stage designs for Phase II clinical trials. *Statistics in Medicine*, **21**, 1991–2012. [8]

Tan S-B, Machin D, Tai B-C, Foo K-F and Tan E-H (2002). A Bayesian re-assessment of two Phase II trials of gemcitabine in metastatic nasopharyngeal cancer. *British Journal of Cancer*, **86**, 843–850. [8]

Tang C-L, Eu K-W, Tai B-C, Soh JGS, Machin D and Seow-Choen F (2001). Randomized clinical trial of the effect of open *versus* laparoscopically assisted colectomy on systemic immunity in patients with colorectal cancer. *British Journal of Surgery*, **88**, 801–807. [2, 9]

Temple R (2000). Current definitions of phases of investigation and the role of the FDA in the conduct of clinical trials. *American Heart Journal*, **139**, S133–S135. [3]

The Family Heart Study Group (1994). The British Family Heart Study: its design and methods, and prevalence of cardiovascular risk factors. *British Journal of General Practice*, **44**, 62–67. [9]

Therasse P, Arbuck SG, Eisenhauer EA, Wanders J, Kaplan RS, Rubinstein L, Verweij J, Van Glabbeke M, van Oosterom T, Christian MC and Gwyther SG (2000). New guidelines to evaluate the response to treatment in solid tumours. *Journal of the National Cancer Institute*, **92**, 205–216. [2]

Thompson C, Kinmonth AL, Stevens L, Peveler RC, Stevens A, Ostler KJ, Pickering RM, Baker NG, Henson A, Preece J, Cooper D and Campbell MJ (2000). Effects of a clinical-practice guideline and practice-based education on detection and outcome of depression in primary care: Hampshire Depression Project randomised controlled trial. *Lancet*, **355**, 185–191. [9]

Thompson SG, Pyke SDM and Hardy RJ (1997). The design and analysis of paired cluster randomized trials: an application of meta-analysis techniques. *Statistics in Medicine*, **16**, 2063–2079. [9]

Thumboo J, Fong KY, Machin D, Chan SP, Soh CH, Leong KH, Feng PH, Thio ST and Boey ML (2002). Does being bilingual in English and Chinese influence Quality-of-Life scales? *Medical Care*, **40**, 105–122. [6]

Torrance GW, Feeny D and Furlong W (2001). Visual analog scales: do they have a role in the measurement of preferences for health states? *Medical Decision Making*, **21**, 329–334. [2]

Ukoumunne OC, Gulliford MC, Chinn S, Sterne JAC and Burney PG (1999). Methods for evaluating area-wide and organisation-based interventions in health and health care: a systematic review. *Health Technology Assessment*, **3**(5), iii–92. [9]

Van der Zee J, van Rhoon GC, Wike-Hooley JL, Faithfull NS and Reinhold HS (1983). Whole-body hyperthermia in cancer therapy: a report of a Phase I-II study. *European Journal of Cancer and Clinical Oncology*, **19**, 1189–1200. [8]

Van Rijswijk REN, Vermorken JB, Reed N, Favalli G, Mendiola C, Zanaboni F, Mangili G, Vergote I, Guastalla JP, ten Bokkel Huinink WW, Lacave AJ, Bonnefoi H, Tumulo S, Rietbroek R, Teodorovic I, Coens C and Pecorelli S (2003). Cisplatin, doxorubicin and ifosfamide in carcinosarcoma of the female genital tract. A phase II study of the European Organization for Research and Treatment of Cancer Gynaecological Cancer Group (EORTC 55923). *European Journal of Cancer*, **39**, 481–487. [7]

Verhoef H, West CE, Nzyuko SM, de Vogel S, van der Valk R, Wang MA, Kuijsten A, Veenemans J and Kok FJ (2002). Intermittent administration of iron and sulfadoxine-pyrimethamine to control anaemia in Kenyan children: a randomised controlled trial. *Lancet*, **360**, 908–914. [5, 7]

Vernier JJ, Brown BW and Thall PF (1999). *Continual Reassessment Method (CRM) for Dose-finding in Phase I Clinical Trials*. CRM-Version 1.0, MD Anderson Cancer Centre, Houston, TX. [8]

Wacker CM, Bock M, Hartlep AW, Bauer WR, van Kaick G, Pfleger S, Ertl G and Schad LR (1999). BOLD-MRI in 10 patients with coronary artery disease: evidence for imaging of capillary recruitment in myocardium supplied by the stenotic artery. *MAGMA*, **8**, 48–54. [10]

Wallentin L, Wilcox RG, Weaver WD, Emanuelsson H, Goodvin A, Nyström P and Bylock A (2003). Oral ximelagatran for secondary prophylaxis after myocardial infarction: the ESTEEM randomised controlled trial. *Lancet*, **362**, 789–797. [9]

Walls C, Lewis A, Bullman J, Boswell D, Summers SJ, Dow A and Sidhu J (2004). Pharmacokinetic profile of a new form of sumatriptan tablets in healthy volunteers. *Current Medical Research and Opinion*, **20**, 803–809. [7]

Walter SD, Eliasziw M and Donner A (1998). Sample size and optimal designs for reliability studies. *Statistics in Medicine*, **17**, 101–110. [10]

Ware JE, Snow KK, Kosinski M and Gandek B (1993). *SF-36 Health Survey Manual and Interpretation Guide*. New England Medical Centre, Boston, MA. [2, 6]

Weir NH, Fiaschi K and Machin D (1998). The distribution and latency of the auditory P300 in schizophrenia and depression. *Schizophrenia Research*, **31**, 151–158. [3, 5]

Wickramaratne PJ (1995). Sample size determination in epidemiologic studies. *Statistical Methods in Medical Research*, **4**, 311–337. [3]

Wittes J and Brittain E (1990). The role of internal pilot studies in increasing the efficiency of clinical trials. *Statistics in Medicine*, **9**, 65–72. [3]

Wooding WM (1994). *Planning Pharmaceutical Clinical Trials*. Wiley, New York. [8]

Young T, de Haes JCJM, Curran D, Fayers PM and Bradberg Y (1999). *Guidelines for Assessing Quality of Life in EORTC Trials*. EORTC, Brussels. [2]

Zelen M (1992). Randomised consent trials. *Lancet*, **340**, 375. [7]

Tables

Table T1 Percentage points of the Normal distribution

Two-sided	One-sided	z
0.001	0.0005	3.2905
0.005	0.0025	2.8070
0.010	0.0050	2.5758
0.020	0.0100	2.3263
0.025	0.0125	2.2414
0.050	0.0250	1.9600
0.100	0.0500	1.6449
0.200	0.1000	1.2816
0.300	0.1500	1.0364
0.400	0.2000	0.8416
0.500	0.2500	0.6745
0.600	0.3000	0.5244
0.700	0.3500	0.3853
0.800	0.4000	0.2533

(Column header group: α)

Design of Studies for Medical Research. D. Machin and M. J. Campbell
© 2005 John Wiley & Sons Ltd. ISBN 0 470 84495 7

Table T2 Sample sizes to estimate a proportion π for a given 95% confidence interval of width ω

π_{Plan}	ω_{Plan}			
	0.05	0.10	0.15	0.20
0.01	108	43	25	17
0.02	152	52	29	19
0.03	201	61	33	21
0.04	252	72	37	23
0.05	304	83	41	25
0.06	356	95	46	28
0.07	407	107	50	30
0.08	458	118	55	32
0.09	508	130	60	35
0.10	557	141	64	37
0.11	604	153	69	40
0.12	651	164	74	42
0.13	696	175	78	44
0.14	741	186	83	47
0.15	784	196	87	49
0.16	826	206	92	51
0.17	867	216	96	54
0.18	907	226	100	56
0.19	945	236	104	58
0.20	982	245	108	60
0.25	1150	286	126	70
0.30	1288	320	141	78
0.35	1395	347	152	84
0.40	1472	366	161	89
0.45	1518	377	166	92
0.50	1533	381	167	93

Table T3 Random numbers. Each digit, 0 to 9, is equally likely to appear and cannot be predicted from any combination of other digits

75792	78245	83270	59987	75253	42729	98917	83137	67588	93846
80169	88847	36686	36601	91654	44249	52586	25702	09575	18939
94071	63090	23901	93268	53316	87773	89260	04804	99479	83909
67970	29162	60224	61042	98324	30425	37677	90382	96230	84565
91577	43019	67511	28527	61750	55267	07847	50165	26793	80918
84334	54827	51955	47256	21387	28456	77296	41283	01482	44494
03778	05031	90146	59031	96758	57420	23581	38824	49592	18593
58563	84810	22446	80149	99676	83102	35381	94030	59560	32145
29068	74625	90665	52747	09364	57491	59049	19767	83081	78441
90047	44763	44**534**	**55425**	**67**170	67937	88962	49992	53583	37864
54870	35009	84524	32309	88815	86792	89097	66600	26195	88326
23327	78957	50987	77876	63960	53986	46771	80998	95229	59606
03876	89100	66895	89468	96684	95491	32222	58708	34408	66930
14846	86619	04238	36182	05294	43791	88149	22637	56775	52091
94731	63786	88290	60990	98407	43437	74233	25880	96898	52186
96046	51589	84509	98162	39162	59469	60563	74917	02413	17967
95188	25011	29947	48896	83408	79684	11353	13636	46380	69003
67416	00626	49781	77833	47073	59147	50469	10807	58985	98881
50002	97121	26652	23667	13819	54138	54173	69234	28657	01031
50806	62492	67131	02610	43964	19528	68333	69484	23527	96974
43619	79413	45456	31642	78162	81686	73687	19751	24727	98742
90476	58785	15177	81377	26671	70548	41383	59773	59835	13719
43241	22852	28915	49692	75981	74215	65915	36489	10233	89897
57434	86821	63717	54640	28782	24046	84755	83021	85436	29813
15731	12986	03008	18739	07726	75512	65295	15089	81094	05260
34706	04386	02945	72555	97249	16798	05643	42343	36106	63948
16759	74867	62702	32840	08565	18403	10421	60687	68599	78034
11895	74173	72423	62838	89382	57437	85314	75320	01988	52518
87597	21289	30904	13209	04244	53651	28373	90759	70286	49678
63656	28328	25428	38671	97372	69256	49364	35398	30808	59082
72414	71686	65513	81236	26205	10013	80610	40509	50045	70530
69337	19016	50420	38803	55793	84035	93051	57693	33673	67434
64310	62819	20242	08632	83905	49477	29409	96563	86993	91207
31243	63913	66340	91169	28560	69220	14730	19752	51636	59434
39951	83556	88718	68802	06170	90451	58926	50125	28532	17189
57473	53613	76478	82668	28315	05975	96324	96135	14255	29991
50259	80588	94408	55754	79166	20490	97112	25904	20254	08781
48449	97696	14321	92549	95812	78371	77678	56618	44769	57413
50830	52921	41365	46257	66889	29420	95250	24080	08600	04189
94646	37630	50246	53925	95496	82773	41021	95435	83812	52558
49344	07037	24221	41955	47211	43418	45703	78779	77215	44594
49201	66377	64188	50398	33157	87375	55885	14174	03105	85821
57221	54927	59025	46847	35894	14639	38452	89166	72843	40954
65391	57289	67771	99160	08184	26262	46577	32603	21677	54104
01029	99783	63250	39198	51042	36834	40450	90864	49953	61032
23218	67476	45675	17299	85685	57294	30847	39985	44402	76665
35175	51935	85800	91083	97112	20865	96101	83276	84149	11443
28442	12188	99908	51660	34350	66572	43047	30217	44491	79042
89327	26880	83020	20428	87554	33251	80684	01964	04106	28243

Table T4   The 12 possible randomisations of the one basic 3×3 Latin square

	[1]				[2]				[3]				[4]	
A	B	C		A	C	B		A	B	C		A	C	B
B	C	A		B	A	C		C	A	B		C	B	A
C	A	B		C	B	A		B	C	A		B	A	C

	[5]				[6]				[7]				[8]	
B	C	A		B	A	C		B	C	A		B	A	C
C	A	B		C	B	A		A	B	C		A	C	B
A	B	C		A	C	B		C	A	B		C	B	A

	[9]				[10]				[11]				[12]	
C	A	B		C	B	A		C	A	B		C	B	A
A	B	C		A	C	B		B	C	A		B	A	C
B	C	A		B	A	C		A	B	C		A	C	B

To use these squares:

(1) Label the three options A, B and C in any order
(2) If one square is required, choose a random number between 1 and 12, say 5, then use this square for the design
(3) If two squares are required, choose a second random number (avoiding 5), say 9, then use this second square in the design
(4) If 12 squares are required, then use all the squares in random order

Table T5   The four basic 4×4 Latin squares

[1]	[2]	[3]	[4]

A	B	C	D
B	A	D	C
C	D	B	A
D	C	A	B

A	B	C	D
B	C	D	A
C	D	A	B
D	A	B	C

A	B	C	D
B	D	A	C
C	A	D	B
D	C	B	A

A	B	C	D
B	A	D	C
C	D	A	B
D	C	B	A

To use these squares:

(1) Label the four options A, B, C and D in any order
(2) Choose one of the basic squares at random, (say) [1]
(3) Randomise the four columns of the square to give (say) 1, 4, 2 and 3, to obtain a new square
(4) Randomise the four rows of the new square to give (say) 2, 3, 4 and 1, to obtain the final square for use in the design
(5) If two or more squares are required, select from those not already chosen

Table T6   The two basic 4×4 Graeco-Latin squares

1	2

$A\alpha$	$B\beta$	$C\gamma$	$D\beta$
$B\delta$	$A\gamma$	$D\beta$	$C\alpha$
$C\beta$	$D\alpha$	$A\delta$	$B\gamma$
$D\gamma$	$C\delta$	$B\alpha$	$A\beta$

$A\alpha$	$B\beta$	$C\gamma$	$D\delta$
$B\gamma$	$A\delta$	$D\alpha$	$C\beta$
$C\delta$	$D\gamma$	$A\beta$	$B\alpha$
$D\beta$	$C\alpha$	$B\delta$	$A\gamma$

To use these squares:

(1) Label the four options A, B, C and D in any order
(2) Label the four options α, β, γ and δ in any order
(3) If one square is required, choose a random number from 1 and 2, say 2, then use this square for the design
(4) Randomise the four columns of the square to give (say) 1, 4, 2 and 3, to obtain a new square
(5) Randomise the four rows of the new square to give (say) 2, 3, 4 and 1, to obtain the final square for use in the design
(6) If two squares are required, choose the other square from that just selected and repeat the randomisation of the columns and rows

Table T7 Values for the multiplier R for calculating sample sizes for repeated measures designs

							ρ						
v	w	0.0	0.1	0.2	0.3	0.4	0.5	0.6	0.65	0.7	0.75	0.8	0.9
0	1	1.00	1.00	1.00	1.00	1.00	1.00	1.00	1.00	1.00	1.00	1.00	1.00
	2	0.50	0.55	0.60	0.65	0.70	0.75	0.80	0.83	0.85	0.88	0.90	0.95
	3	0.33	0.40	0.47	0.53	0.60	0.67	0.73	0.77	0.80	0.83	0.87	0.93
	4	0.25	0.33	0.40	0.48	0.55	0.63	0.70	0.74	0.77	0.81	0.85	0.93
	5	0.20	0.28	0.36	0.44	0.52	0.60	0.68	0.72	0.76	0.80	0.84	0.90
1	1	1.00	0.99	0.96	0.91	0.84	0.75	0.64	0.58	0.51	0.44	0.36	0.19
	2	0.50	0.54	0.56	0.56	0.54	0.50	0.44	0.40	0.36	0.31	0.26	0.14
	3	0.33	0.39	0.43	0.44	0.44	0.42	0.37	0.34	0.31	0.27	0.23	0.12
	4	0.25	0.32	0.36	0.39	0.39	0.38	0.34	0.32	0.28	0.25	0.21	0.12
	5	0.20	0.27	0.32	0.35	0.36	0.35	0.32	0.30	0.27	0.24	0.20	0.11
2	1	1.00	0.98	0.93	0.86	0.77	0.67	0.55	0.49	0.42	0.36	0.29	0.15
	2	0.50	0.53	0.53	0.51	0.47	0.42	0.35	0.31	0.27	0.23	0.19	0.10
	3	0.33	0.38	0.40	0.39	0.37	0.33	0.28	0.25	0.22	0.19	0.16	0.08
	4	0.25	0.31	0.33	0.34	0.32	0.29	0.25	0.23	0.20	0.17	0.14	0.07
	5	0.20	0.26	0.29	0.30	0.29	0.27	0.23	0.21	0.18	0.16	0.13	0.07
3	1	1.00	0.98	0.91	0.83	0.73	0.63	0.51	0.45	0.39	0.32	0.26	0.13
	2	0.50	0.53	0.51	0.48	0.43	0.38	0.31	0.27	0.24	0.20	0.16	0.08
	3	0.33	0.37	0.38	0.36	0.33	0.29	0.24	0.22	0.19	0.16	0.13	0.07
	4	0.25	0.30	0.31	0.31	0.28	0.25	0.21	0.19	0.16	0.14	0.11	0.06
	5	0.20	0.25	0.27	0.27	0.25	0.22	0.19	0.17	0.15	0.13	0.10	0.05

v = number of pre-intervention observations; w = number of post-intervention observations; ρ = autocorrelation assuming compound symmetry.

Table T8 Sample sizes (rounded upwards to the nearest 10) for given coefficient of variation Ω and proportion width of the $100(1-\alpha)\%$ CI ε

α			0.05					0.01		
			Ω					Ω		
ε	0.20	0.25	0.30	0.35	0.40	0.20	0.25	0.30	0.35	0.40
0.025	990	1540	2220	3020	3940	1700	2660	3830	5210	6800
0.05	250	390	560	760	990	430	670	960	1300	1700
0.075	110	180	250	340	440	190	300	430	580	760
0.100	70	100	140	190	250	110	170	240	330	430
0.125	40	70	90	120	160	70	110	160	210	280
0.150	30	50	70	90	110	50	80	110	150	190
0.200	20	30	40	50	70	30	50	60	90	110

Table T9 Student's t-distribution. The value tabulated is t_α, such that if X is distributed as Student's t-distribution with f degrees of freedom, then α is the probability that $X \leqslant -t_\alpha$ or $X \geqslant t_\alpha$

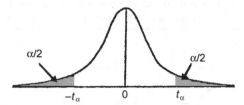

| | α | | | | | | | |
df	0.20	0.10	0.05	0.04	0.03	0.02	0.01	0.001
1	3.078	6.314	12.706	15.895	21.205	31.821	63.657	636.6
2	1.886	2.920	4.303	4.849	5.643	6.965	9.925	31.60
3	1.634	2.353	3.182	3.482	3.896	4.541	5.842	12.92
4	1.530	2.132	2.776	2.999	3.298	3.747	4.604	8.610
5	1.474	2.015	2.571	2.757	3.003	3.365	4.032	6.869
6	1.439	1.943	2.447	2.612	2.829	3.143	3.707	5.959
7	1.414	1.895	2.365	2.517	2.715	2.998	3.499	5.408
8	1.397	1.860	2.306	2.449	2.634	2.896	3.355	5.041
9	1.383	1.833	2.262	2.398	2.574	2.821	3.250	4.781
10	1.372	1.812	2.228	2.359	2.528	2.764	3.169	4.587
11	1.363	1.796	2.201	2.328	2.491	2.718	3.106	4.437
12	1.356	1.782	2.179	2.303	2.461	2.681	3.055	4.318
13	1.350	1.771	2.160	2.282	2.436	2.650	3.012	4.221
14	1.345	1.761	2.145	2.264	2.415	2.624	2.977	4.140
15	1.340	1.753	2.131	2.249	2.397	2.602	2.947	4.073
16	1.337	1.746	2.120	2.235	2.382	2.583	2.921	4.015
17	1.333	1.740	2.110	2.224	2.368	2.567	2.898	3.965
18	1.330	1.734	2.101	2.214	2.356	2.552	2.878	3.922
19	1.328	1.729	2.093	2.205	2.346	2.539	2.861	3.883
20	1.325	1.725	2.086	2.196	2.336	2.528	2.845	3.850
21	1.323	1.721	2.079	2.189	2.327	2.517	2.830	3.819
22	1.321	1.717	2.074	2.183	2.320	2.508	2.818	3.790
23	1.319	1.714	2.069	2.178	2.313	2.499	2.806	3.763
24	1.318	1.711	2.064	2.172	2.307	2.492	2.797	3.744
25	1.316	1.708	2.059	2.166	2.301	2.485	2.787	3.722
26	1.315	1.706	2.056	2.162	2.396	2.479	2.779	3.706
27	1.314	1.703	2.052	2.158	2.291	2.472	2.770	3.687
28	1.313	1.701	2.048	2.154	2.286	2.467	2.763	3.673
29	1.311	1.699	2.045	2.150	2.282	2.462	2.756	3.657
30	1.310	1.697	2.042	2.147	2.278	2.457	2.750	3.646
∞	1.282	1.645	1.960	2.054	2.170	2.326	2.576	3.291

Table T10 Two-stage Phase II designs to jointly evaluate response and toxicity – if $\geqslant t_1$ or $\leqslant r_1$ responses are observed in Stage 1 the trial is closed; if at the close of Stage 2 $\geqslant t$ or $\leqslant r$ responses are observed then the regimen is not considered suitable for further development (after Bryant and Day, 1995, Table 1; reproduced by permission of Blackwell Publishers Ltd)

Design criteria									
Toxicity		Response		Stage 1			Final		
π_{T0}	π_{TNew}	π_{R0}	π_{RNew}	n_1	t_1	r_1	N	t	r
		$\alpha_T=0.15$		$\alpha_R=0.15$		$1-\beta=0.85$			
0.6	0.8	0.05	0.25	12	7	0	30	20	2
		0.1	0.3	15	9	1	30	20	4
		0.2	0.4	17	10	3	36	24	9
		0.3	0.5	19	11	5	33	22	12
		0.4	0.6	20	12	8	37	25	17
		0.6	0.8	14	8	8	33	22	22
0.75	0.95	0.05	0.25	9	7	0	28	22	2
		0.1	0.3	12	9	1	22	18	3
		0.2	0.4	12	9	2	28	23	7
		0.3	0.5	13	9	3	27	22	10
		0.4	0.6	17	13	7	30	24	14
		0.6	0.8	14	11	8	25	20	17
		$\alpha_T=0.1$		$\alpha_R=0.1$		$1-\beta=0.9$			
0.6	0.8	0.05	0.25	22	14	1	43	29	4
		0.1	0.3	21	13	2	46	31	7
		0.2	0.4	24	15	5	54	36	14
		0.3	0.5	23	14	7	57	28	21
		0.4	0.6	25	15	10	53	36	25
		0.6	0.8	20	12	12	49	33	33
0.75	0.95	0.05	0.25	11	11	0	29	24	3
		0.1	0.3	14	14	1	34	28	5
		0.2	0.4	18	18	3	37	31	10
		0.3	0.5	22	22	7	46	38	17
		0.4	0.6	22	22	9	46	38	22
		0.6	0.8	19	19	12	43	35	29

More extensive tables are available via anonymous ftp (atonal.pci.upmc.edu).

Table T11 Sample size per treatment group for a Phase II randomised selection design for different response rates and 0.9 correct selection probability (part from Simon, Wittes and Ellenberg, 1985. Randomized phase II clinical trials. *Cancer Treatment Reports*, **69**, 1375–1381. [8])

Response rates		Number of groups (g)		
π_i, $i=1$ to $g-1$	π_{New}	2	3	4
0.10	0.25	21	31	37
	0.30	13	19	23
0.15	0.30	26	38	45
	0.35	16	23	27
0.20	0.35	29	44	52
	0.40	18	26	31
0.25	0.40	32	48	58
	0.45	19	28	34
0.30	0.45	35	52	62
	0.50	20	30	36
0.35	0.50	36	54	65
	0.55	21	31	37
0.40	0.55	37	55	67
	0.60	**21**	**31**	**38**
0.45	0.60	**37**	**55**	**67**
	0.65	21	31	37
0.50	0.65	36	54	65
	0.70	20	30	36
0.55	0.70	35	52	63
	0.75	19	28	34
0.60	0.75	32	49	59
	0.80	18	26	32
0.65	0.80	29	44	53
	0.85	16	23	28
0.70	0.85	26	39	47
	0.90	13	20	24
0.75	0.90	21	32	38
	0.95	11	16	19
0.8	0.95	16	24	29

Table T12 Samples sizes to establish a 95% or 99% reference interval (RI) for a continuous variable assumed to have a Normal distribution, with varying CIs for the cut-points

	Reference interval $100(1-\alpha)\%$				
	95%		99%		
ρ	CI – cut-point $100(1-\gamma)\%$		CI – cut-point $100(1-\gamma)\%$		
	90%	95%	90%	95%	99%
0.10	211	300	122	174	300
0.11	175	248	101	144	248
0.12	147	208	85	121	208
0.13	125	178	72	103	178
0.14	108	153	62	89	153
0.15	94	133	54	77	133
0.16	83	117	48	68	117
0.17	73	104	42	60	104
0.18	65	93	38	54	93
0.19	59	83	34	48	83
0.20	53	75	31	43	75
0.21	48	68	28	40	68
0.22	44	62	25	36	62
0.23	40	57	23	33	57
0.24	37	52	21	30	52
0.25	34	48	20	28	48
0.26	31	44	18	18	44
0.27	29	41	17	24	41
0.28	27	38	16	22	38
0.29	25	36	15	21	36
0.30	23	33	14	19	33

ρ is the ratio of the width of the CI for the cut divided by the width of the CI of the RI.

Table T13 Multiplier for calculation of the standard error of the non-parametric cut-points of a reference interval (RI)

γ	η	$\eta/\sqrt{3}$
0.01	2.1132	1.22
0.05	2.6713	1.54
0.1	4.8779	2.82
0.005	6.4345	3.71
0.001	12.5789	7.26

Table T14 Total sample size required (cases and healthy controls) to estimate the 95% CI of the area beneath a ROC to have width w

		Width	TPR					
R	FPR	w	0.4	0.5	0.6	0.7	0.8	0.9
1	0.05	0.10	320	254	190	128	74	28
		0.15	142	114	84	58	32	12
		0.20	80	64	48	32	18	8
	0.10	0.10	402	348	284	212	138	64
		0.15	178	154	126	94	62	28
		0.20	100	86	70	54	34	16
	0.20	0.10	464	434	390	328	244	138
		0.15	206	194	174	146	108	62
		0.20	116	108	98	82	62	34
1.5	0.05	0.10	353	283	213	145	85	33
		0.15	158	125	95	65	38	15
		0.20	88	70	53	38	20	8
	0.10	0.10	435	380	315	238	155	73
		0.15	193	170	140	105	70	33
		0.20	110	95	78	60	40	18
	0.20	0.10	493	465	423	360	273	155
		0.15	218	208	188	160	120	70
		0.20	123	118	105	90	68	40

R is the ratio of non-diseased to diseased subjects.

Index

Note: page numbers in *italics* refer to tables, those in **bold** refer to figures.

Design of Studies for Medical Research. D. Machin and M. J. Campbell
© 2005 John Wiley & Sons Ltd. ISBN 0 470 84495 7